THE
ANESTHESIA
MACHINE

THE ANESTHESIA MACHINE

CLAYTON PETTY, M.D.
Professor of Anesthesiology
University of Utah School of Medicine
University of Utah Medical Center
Salt Lake City, Utah

CHURCHILL LIVINGSTONE
New York, Edinburgh, London, Melbourne 1987

Library of Congress Cataloging-in-Publication Data

Petty, Clayton.
   The anesthesia machine.

   Includes bibliographies and index.
   1. Anesthesiology—Apparatus and instruments.
I. Title. [DNLM: 1. Anesthesiology—instrumentation.
WO 240 P512a]
RD78.8.P48   1987   617'.96   86–21574
ISBN 0–443–08405-X

Distributed in the United Kingdom by Churchill Livingstone, Robert
Stevenson House, 1–3 Baxter's Place, Leith Walk, Edinburgh EH1 3AF,
and by associated companies, branches, and representatives throughout
the world.

Accurate indications, adverse reactions, and dosage schedules for drugs
are provided in this book, but it is possible that they may change. The
reader is urged to review the package information data of the
manufacturers of the medications mentioned.

Copy Editor: *Leslie Burgess*
Production Designer: *Gloria Brown Milner*
Production Supervisor: *Jane Grochowski*

Printed in the United States of America

First published in 1987

Second printing in 1988

To those who provide the greatest blessings in my life I owe the most. To Zoe Leone, my wife, for her continued love, encouragement, and support. To Mason, Yvonne, Kendall, Valerie, Craig, Ember, and Laura, my children, for recognizing my desire to write this book. To God the Father for good health, inspiration, and the opportunities of life.

FOREWORD

In the past, introduction of a new subject treatise in anesthesia was saluted with encomium. The times are such that it is now in keeping with reality to preface a new anesthesia text with an *apologia pro vita sua* instead. In other words, instead of the usual praise, justification for a new book in a field severely overpopulated with texts becomes mandatory.

The Anesthesia Machine by Dr. Petty provides the anesthesiologist with insights into this device—the fulcrum of the discipline—compacted into one convenient source. Certain areas are particularly welcome: condensation of various anesthesia machine hazards into one volume; manufacturing protocols; hospital gas piping systems; etc. That factual data abound cannot be denigrated, yet, implicit in this monograph is a philosophy of great importance to anesthesiology as a medical specialty. Elaboration of this belief is interesting.

Deep insight into mechanisms of high technology is not necessary for an individual to produce results and use such advances in a safe and meaningful fashion. For example, a sophisticated computer can be used with preprogrammed software without user knowledge of circuitry or of computer languages; an automobile can safely be driven by a person who is totally ignorant of the complexities of fuel injection engines or automatic transmissions; one does not need to know the electronic circuitry of a VCR-CRT system in order to enjoy a taped version of *Tosca*. Does the anesthesiologist really need to know the intricacies of the anesthesia machine and its various inputs and ancillaries to practice safe anesthesia?

This is a difficult question and any answer is speculative because no data have been accumulated. There are many phenomena in anesthesiology of which even sophisticated physicians are totally ignorant. The basic explanation of how anesthetics produce the state of anesthesia is still totally beyond our ken. This does not preclude the use of powerful drugs and the confidence that this near-death state can be reversed by knowledge of pharmacokinetics, although in truth the corresponding essential pharmacodynamics are unknown. Anesthesia machines can be employed by individuals who know little or nothing about the enclosed contents of the devices; still, insight into the components and circuitry of the machine is not only important from a purely academic viewpoint, it can save lives.

An example of this was observed years ago in the methoxyflurane era. The copper kettle or its variant was frequently used to vaporize this drug—a good marriage because of the unusually low volatility of methoxyflurane. A very popular anesthesia machine had the direction lever for oxygen shunting to the copper kettle vaporizer and the oxygen flush valve lever the same. When the lever was turned to the vaporizer the corresponding oxygen flowmeter volume was delivered into the copper kettle. Because of the low volatility of methoxyflurane this oxygen was the only oxygen delivered to the patient! If a flush was required and the lever returned to the neutral position rather than fully to the left (copper kettle "on" position), the entire oxygen flow to the patient was diverted to the room before entry into the copper kettle. Just how many users of the machine had the ostensibly trivial knowledge that the oxygen flow could be diverted to the room with changed lever position? Unfortunately, not all.

This little parable would seem sufficient justification for this text. The reader is invited to formulate his or her own opinions.

Burnell R. Brown, Jr., M.D., Ph.D.
Professor and Head
Department of Anesthesiology
The University of Arizona
College of Medicine
Tucson, Arizona

PREFACE

Anesthesia machines are vital to the practice of anesthesia. Current anesthesia machines are being developed with a number of alarm systems and attachments relatively unfamiliar to the anesthesiologist. Many of these additions are being added to try to combat the proverb "Nothing can be made foolproof because fools are so ingenious." Technical manuals that accompany the anesthesia machine are usually not conducive to study. I have attempted to provide information in a form that will be easily understood by anesthesiologists in private practice, medical students, nurse anesthetists, and residents. The concepts discussed encompass all anesthesia machines, but the North American Drager Narkomed IIA and the Ohmeda Modulus II anesthesia machines are used when specific examples are necessary.

The history chapter is included to give a feeling of how we got to where we are today. The risk management and quality assurance chapters try to bring into perspective some of the vital issues regarding anesthesia machines that are rapidly becoming a part of our practice.

From the inception of this idea by Lewis Reines, to the follow-up by Toni Tracy, Churchill Livingstone has provided me with flexibility and encouragement.

Appreciation must be given to Sam Collett of Medical Illustration for providing the artistic skills for the figures; Margo Riese, my secretary, for the many trips she took to the library; Professional Control Group, Inc., for providing the word processor program and a disc drive; K. C. Wong, M.D., for providing financial and moral support, and Kyle Enslin, M.D., and Scott Hurst, M.D., two anesthesiologists in private practice, for reading the manuscript for clarity, organization, and practical application.

A special thank you to the many friends from Ohmeda and North American Drager. Both the local and national representatives have been very cooperative in providing technical information, photos, and advice. I am grateful for the opportunity I had to visit the assembly plants of North American Drager in Telford, Pennsylvania, and the two plants of Ohmeda in Madison, Wisconsin, and El Paso, Texas. In addition to moral support, both North American Drager and Ohmeda have given financial support toward the completion of this book.

As you read this book I hope you will find it interesting and informative. Most of all, I would like you to gain a better understanding and appreciation of the valuable anesthesia machine.

Clayton Petty, M.D.

CONTENTS

History of the Development of the Anesthesia Machine

The great English scientist Sir Humphry Davy (1778-1829) was plagued with the same mundane maladies which we acquire today, that is, the headache and the toothache. Sir Davy, however, has the distinction of being the first to obtain pain relief from the inhalation of an anesthetic[1]:

In one instance, when I had head-ache from indigestion, it was immediately removed by the effects of a large dose of gas; though it afterwards returned, but with much less violence. . . .

In cutting one of the unlucky teeth called dentes sapientiae, I experienced an extensive inflammation of the gum, accompanied with great pain, which equally destroyed the power of repose, and of consistent action.

On the day when the inflammation was most troublesome, I breathed three large doses of nitrous oxide. The pain always diminished after the first four or five inspirations, the thrilling came on as usual, and uneasiness was for a few minutes, swallowed up in pleasure. As the former state of mind however returned, the state of organ returned with it; and I once imagined that the pain was more severe after the experiment than before.

The simple anesthetic apparatus used by Sir Humphry Davy was called the "mercurial air-holder and breathing machine" (see Fig. 1-1). The apparatus was similar to the stationery respiratory spirometer of today. Nitrous oxide was first made by the process described by Joseph Priestley[2, 3] in 1772. Nitrous air (nitric oxide) was exposed to a paste made from iron filings and brimstone (sulfur) over water to produce nitrous oxide (dephlogisticated nitrous air), which was then collected in a spirometer. Valves in the spirometer allowed one to breathe undiluted, purified nitrous oxide.

The public demonstration of general anesthesia by William Thomas Greene Morton on October 14, 1846 in Boston heralded a new epoch in medicine. The *Morton inhaler* for ether was simple but had features destined to dominate the administration of anesthesia for many years. The first model of the ether inhaler was made by Wrightman, a Boston instrument maker, but it proved to be unsatisfactory. Two days before the demonstration, Dr. Augustus A. Gould suggested the incorporation of inspiratory and expiratory valves to prevent to-and-fro breathing in the flask.[4] Wrightman was able to make the final addi-

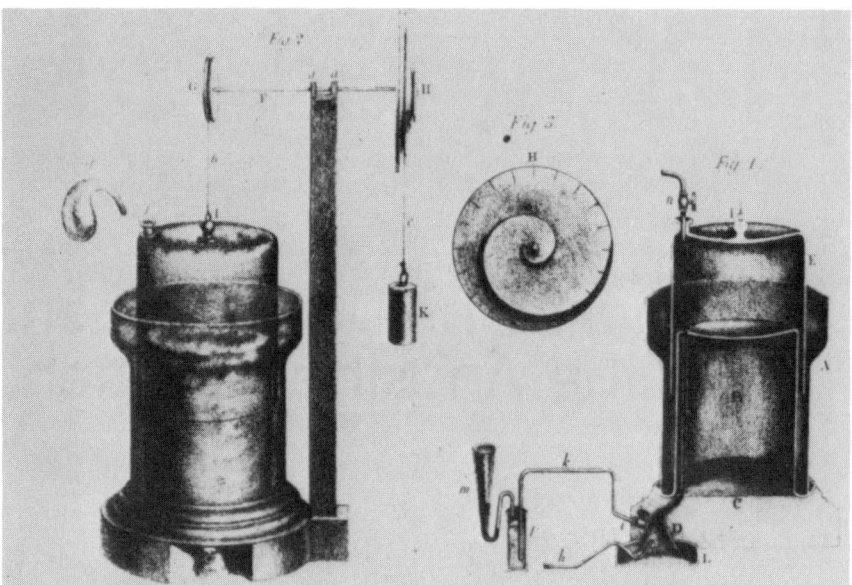

Fig. 1-1 The mercurial airholder and breathing machine (ca. 1800) used by Davy and designed by Clayfield. The bell was made of glass and had a capacity of 200 in³. Mercury replaced water as a seal for the bell. Manufactured nitrous oxide was stored in the large spirometer. Samples of gas were breathed directly from the spirometer. (Smith WDA: Under the Influence: A History of Nitrous Oxide and Oxygen Anaesthesia. ASA Wood Library–Museum of Anesthesiology, Park Ridge, IL, 1982.)

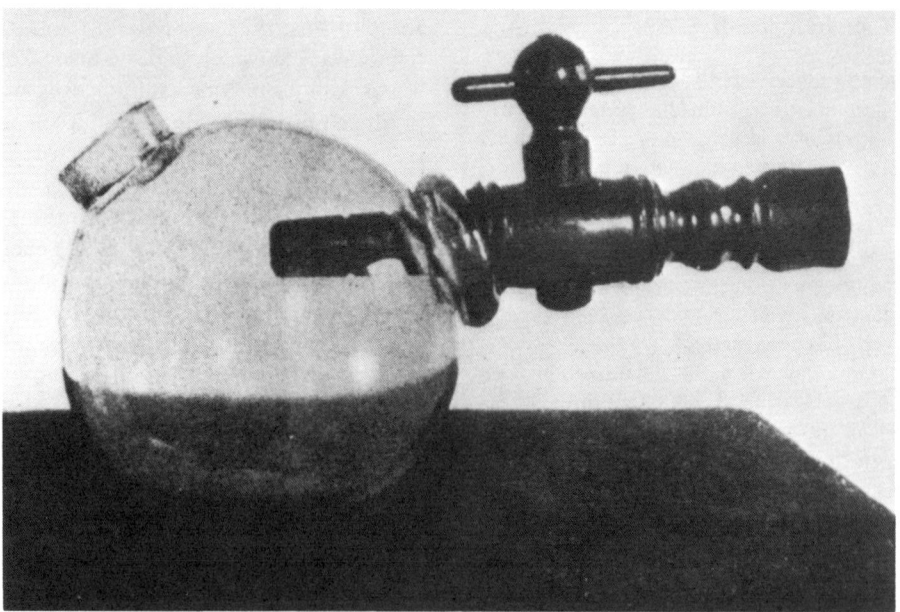

Fig. 1-2 The ether inhaler most likely used for the first public demonstration of general anesthesia, by William Morton on October 14, 1846. (Courtesy of ASA Wood Library–Museum of Anesthesiology, Park Ridge, IL.)

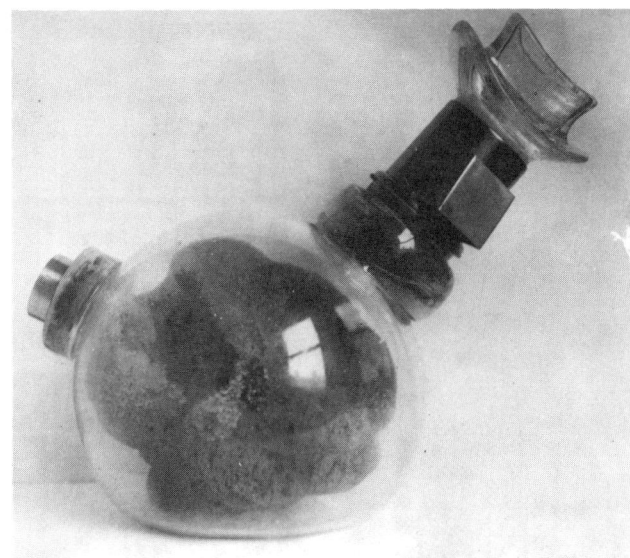

Fig. 1-3 Ether inhaler with a sponge inside the glass container. The inscription reads, "Dr TG Morton to Mason Warren, Original Ether Inhaler 1846." The wooden spigot in the first design has been replaced by a one-way nonre-breathing valve system. (Courtesy of ASA Wood Library–Museum of Anesthesiology, Park Ridge, IL.)

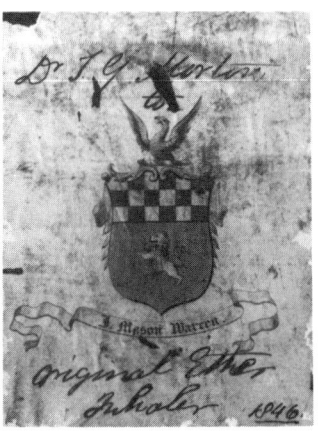

tions on the second model of the inhaler just in time for the famous demonstration. Morton later abandoned the apparatus for a sponge held over the nose and mouth.[5]

The ether inhaler was vividly described by Dr. Henry Jacob Bigelow,[4] a visiting surgeon present at the first demonstration of ether anesthesia:

> A small two-necked glass globe contains the prepared vapour with sponges to enlarge the evaporating surface. One aperture admits the air to the interior of the globe, whence, charged with vapour is drawn through the

second into the lung. The inspired air passes through the bottle, but the expiration is diverted by a valve in the mouth piece, and escaping into the apartment is thus prevented from vitiating the medicated vapour.

A model of the Morton inhaler with a wooden spigot for the control of unidirectional flow is shown in Figure 1-2. The wooden spigot model was most likely the inhaler used in the first demonstration of ether anesthesia. An improved Morton inhaler (Fig. 1-3) is described in detail in U.S. Patent 5,365, dated November 13, 1847 and issued to Augustus

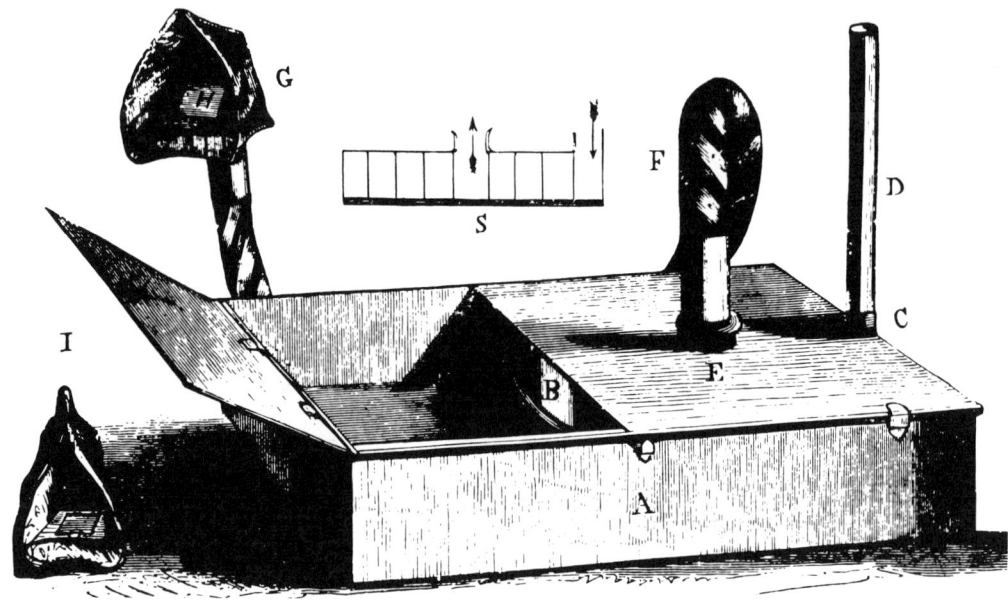

Fig. 1-4 Ether inhaler designed by Dr. John Snow in 1847. The round chamber (B) below the lid (E) contains a spiral baffle system (see Fig. 1-5). The left half of the rectangular box is a large water reservoir. Air enters the vaporizing chamber through tube D. The breathing tube (F) connects to the face mask (G). Section S is a cross section of the baffle system (B) to illustrate the path of air in the vaporizing chamber. The solid line at the bottom of S represents liquid ether. (Snow J: On the Inhalation of the Vapour of Ether. John Churchill, London, 1847.)

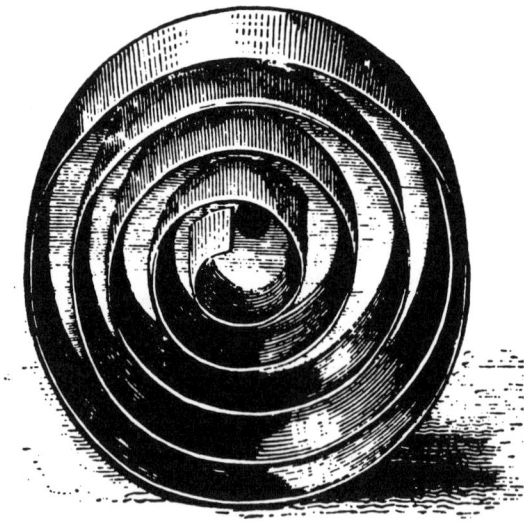

Fig. 1-5 A bottom view of the baffle system for Snow's ether inhaler. Each baffle reached within 1.6 mm of bottom (see side view schematic in Fig. 1-4). Efficiency of vaporization was better here than for the Morton inhaler because of a longer air–ether exposure time and an expanded air–ether vapor surface area. (Snow J: On the Inhalation of the Vapour of Ether. John Churchill, London, 1847.)

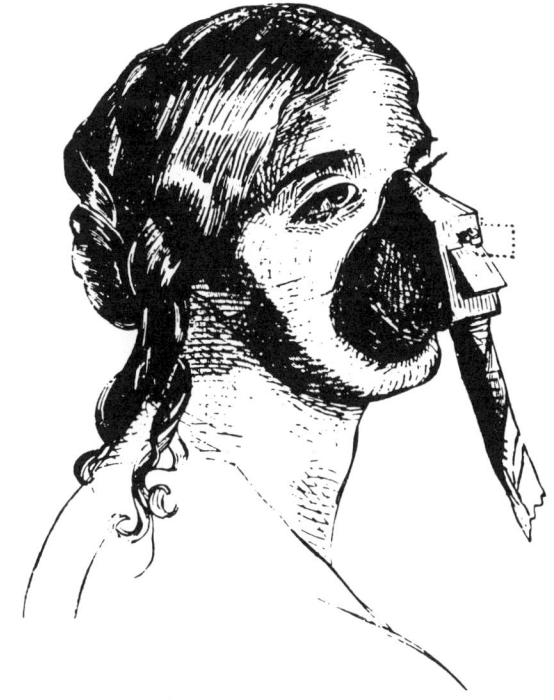

Fig. 1-6 A nonrebreathing face mask designed by Snow. Note that the expiratory valve can be turned aside to admit room air. (Snow J: On the Inhalation of the Vapour of Ether. John Churchill, London, 1847.)

A. Gould and W. T. G. Morton.[6] Ether was placed in the flask bottom and on the sponge. A leather expiration valve was located on a brass cylinder connecting the glass globe with the mouthpiece. A leather inspiration valve hung near the mouthpiece ensured unidirectional air flow through the flask. Air was thus "drawn over" the ether liquid. Only 3 minutes of ether inhalation was required for the first surgical operation under general anesthesia. Ether's high vapor pressure and potent analgesic effect were most likely responsible for the successful demonstration.

Morton's drawover ether vaporizer had a defective design. Ether vaporization caused rapid cooling and poor control of concentration. The vaporizer design was improved by Dr. John Snow[7] of England in 1847. Figure 1-4 illustrates the vaporizer. A round chamber is filled with a large reservoir of water. The left-hand portion of the vaporizer, filled with water, provides a heat sump. As ether cools during vaporization, heat is drawn through the metal adjacent to the water to maintain the ether liquid at a stable temperature. An internal baffle system (Fig. 1-5) in the vaporizer increases the air–ether surface area and allows a longer exposure time for air at the liquid surface. Vaporization efficiency was markedly improved, thus making anesthesia induction smoother and faster. However, the vaporizer apparatus still used air as the carrier gas.

A successful *nonrebreathing mask* (Fig. 1-6) with valves was designed by Snow[7] from an original idea of Sibson's. The central part of the mask was made of brass, tinned iron, or plated copper. Thin, pliable sheet-lead allowed the mask to be adapted to the patient's facial features. All metal parts touching the face were lined with oil-silk. The valves were made of vulcanized India rubber.[7]

A remarkably safe method for administering chloroform was introduced by Clover.[8] Clover made such outstanding contributions to the early scientific understanding of anesthesia that he has been described "as a creator, an inventor—with a quality of mechani-

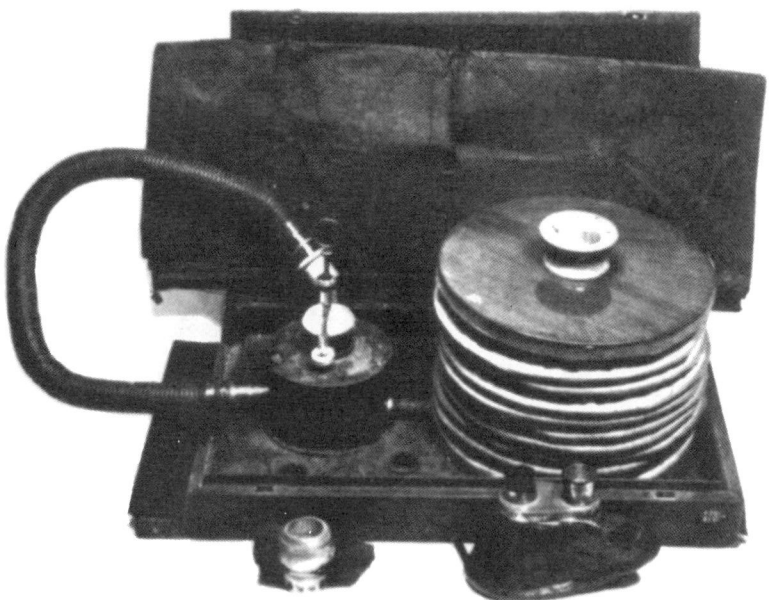

Fig. 1-7 The entire chloroform apparatus of Clover. Vaporizer, face mask, concertina bag, and 7.2-L reservoir bag are contained in a compact box. (Macintosh R, Mushin WW, Epstein HG: Physics for the Anaesthetist. 3rd Ed. Blackwell, Oxford, 1963.)

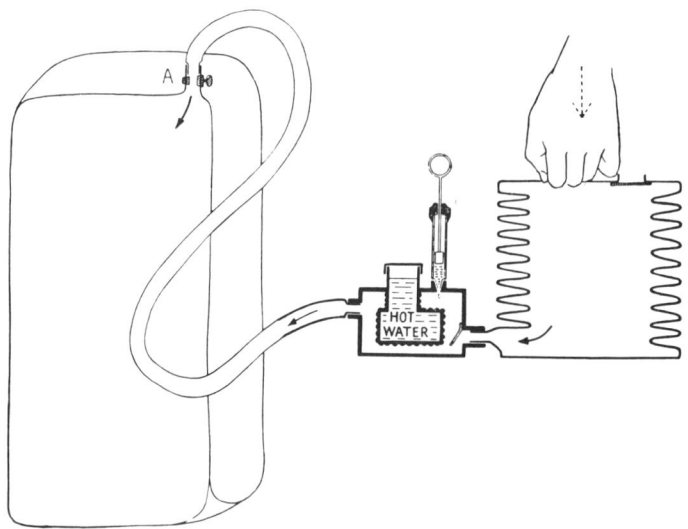

Fig. 1-8 Vaporization of chloroform with the Clover apparatus: A concertina bag is first filled with room air and then forced through the vaporizing chamber by applying downward pressure on the bag. Chloroform is injected onto the hot water plate during fillings of the 7.2-L reservoir bag. When 1 ml of liquid chloroform has been vaporized in 7.2-L of air, the final concentration of chloroform in the reservoir bag is 4 percent. (Macintosh R, Mushin WW, Epstein HG: Physics for the Anaesthetist. 3rd Ed. Blackwell, Oxford, 1963.)

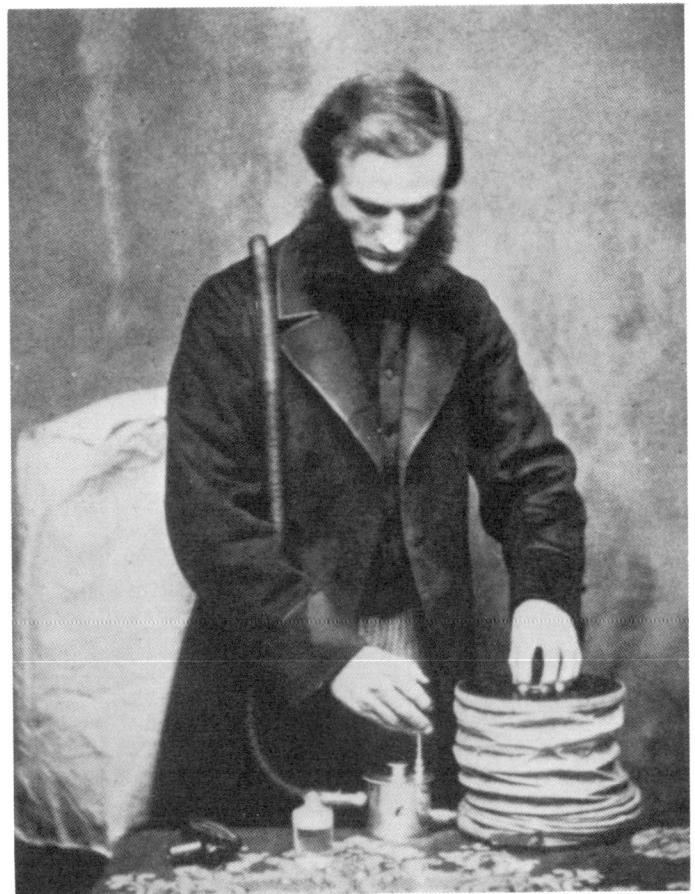

Fig. 1-9 Clover fills the reservoir bag prior to administering chloroform anesthesia. (Macintosh R, Mushin WW, Epstein HG: Physics for the Anaesthetist. 3rd Ed. Blackwell, Oxford, 1963.)

Fig. 1-10 A face mask devised by Clover in 1862. Features include a spring-loaded expiratory valve, an inflatable rim, and an adjustable port on the connecting tube that allows the addition of room air to the breathing mixture. (Macintosh R, Mushin WW, Epstein HG: Physics for the Anaesthetist. 3rd Ed. Blackwell, Oxford, 1963.)

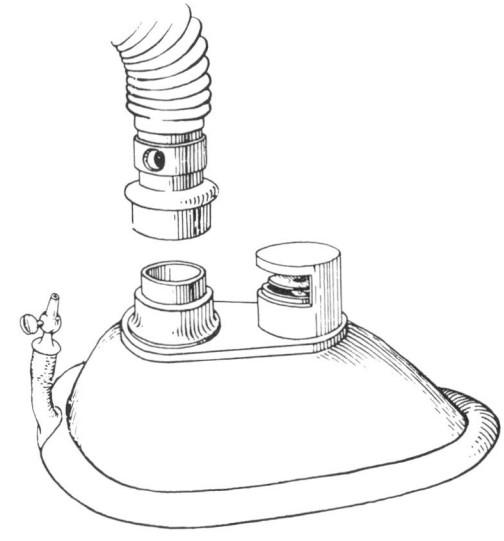

cal invention which deserves to be called genius."[9] The chloroform apparatus in Figures 1-7 to 1-10 accurately vaporized liquid chloroform to a concentration of 4 percent. Maximum chloroform vaporization was obtained by dropping liquid chloroform onto a wick in close contact with a metal surface interfaced with hot water. A total of 1 ml of liquid chloroform gave a mixture of 7.2 L of 4 percent chloroform in air.[8] Much of the guesswork associated with imprecise drawover vaporizers was eliminated by administration of a known concentration of chloroform to the patient. Disadvantages included a single, fixed anesthetic concentration and the need to change holding bags during anesthesia.

Oxygen and nitrous oxide were mixed by Andrews[10] around 1868. He quoted, "It is my impression that the best proportion of oxygen will be found to be one-fifth by volume." Oxygen added to the anesthetic mixture was not immediately accepted as an advance in anesthesia, as evidenced by this pessimistic statement of one of the earliest suppliers of *compressed oxygen,* S. S. White Dental Manufacturing Company, in 1888: "The use of oxygen is new, and its value as a remedial agent unsettled; there is even a possibility that its employment is a mere fad which when it has run its brief day of popularity will vanish into the limbo of buried hopes."[11]

Nitrous oxide was liquefied to achieve greater purity by an American dentist in Paris in 1868.[12] Liquid nitrous oxide was introduced commercially in the United States by the Johnston Brothers' Dental Depot in 1872 in a "strong iron flask about four inches wide and twelve inches long." Each flask contained about 454 L of gas.[12]

Compressed oxygen, liquid nitrous oxide, and mixtures of the two gases led to further advances in anesthetic techniques. High pressures in nitrous oxide (750 psig) and oxygen (2,000 psig) tanks required *reducing valves* to decrease pressure to approximately 45 to 55 psig in the anesthesia machine pipeline. Early reducing valves had a spring which controlled a brass diaphragm in a side drum. Figure 1-

11 is a reducing valve made between 1899 and 1910 that incorporates a safety valve, a steel pin to assist flow control, and tightly packed wool to facilitate fine flow control adjustments. Flanges on the valve body controlled temperature changes, which reduced freezing. Control of spring tension was accomplished by a carrying pin and toggle mechanism which caused movement of a brass diaphragm. Pressure changes were reflected by a graded reduction from the compressed gas cylinder to the delivery outlet in direct relationship to changes in diaphragm pressure.[11]

The first machines in which a sequence of ether and/or nitrous oxide anesthetic was attempted are illustrated in Figure 1-12. These two anesthesia machines were used by Clover[13] in 1876 to administer over 2,300 safe anesthetics. Anesthesia consisted of ether or nitrous oxide or a mixture of the two in air.

Distinction for developing the "first . . . apparatus at all applicable to general surgical use" has been given to Dr. Frederick Hewitt of England.[14] Two semielastic bags were filled from hand valves attached to high-pressure tanks of oxygen and nitrous oxide. A second graduated valve from each semielastic bag regulated the proportions of gas administered to the patient. The device was cumbersome and stimulated Cotton and Boothby[14] to develop the nitrous oxide–oxygen–ether "perfected apparatus" in 1912 (Fig. 1-13). This anesthesia machine incorporated separate automatic reducing valves for liquefied nitrous oxide and compressed oxygen. Pressures were reduced to a common line pressure of 20 psig. Another feature was the incorporation of the *first reliable flowmeters.* Each gas bubbled separately through a water container prior to mixing in a glass chamber. These "bubble-bottle" or wet flowmeters allowed the anesthesiologist to estimate the rate of individual gas flows. The flow rate from the common glass mixing chamber was controlled by a hand-adjusted valve. Mixed gas flow was controlled and could bypass the ether container or, after entering the ether container, be bubbled through or pass over the surface of the liquid ether.[14]

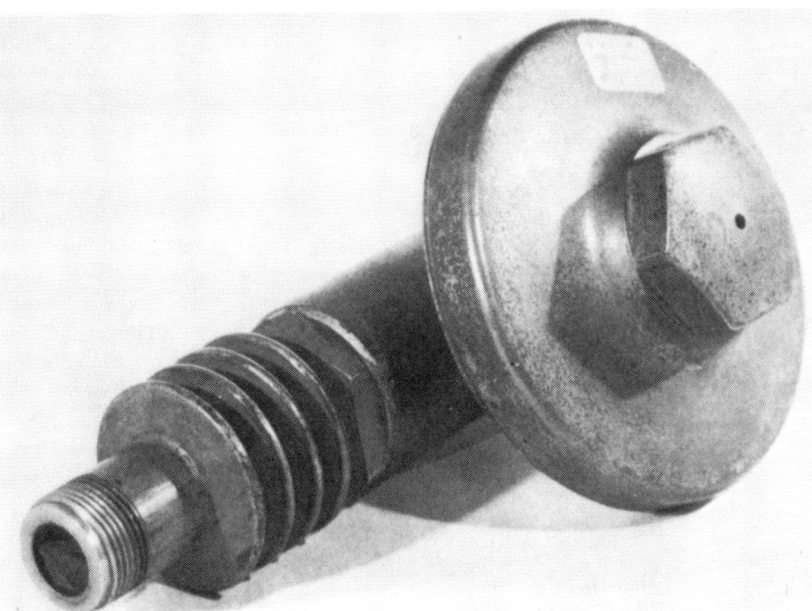

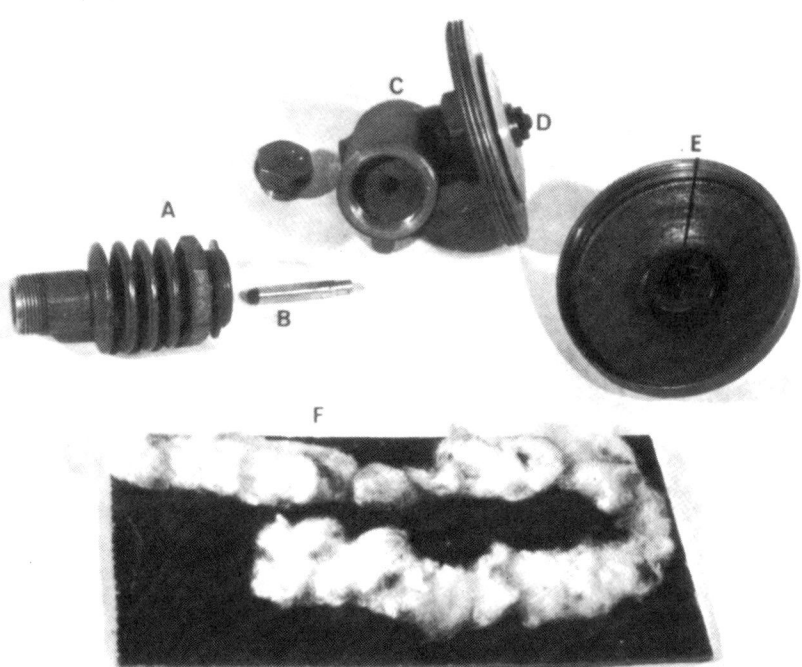

Fig. 1-11 An early reducing valve. The parts of the assembled reducing valve are seen in the bottom half: (A) flanges to prevent freezing, (B) steel pin to help control the flow rate, (C,D) housing for the brass diaphragm, (E) spring to counteract the force of the diaphragm, (F) wool for packing tube A, which improves flow rate control. A safety valve for the release of excess pressure is found on the left end of the housing for the brass diaphragm. (Thomas KB: The Development of Anaesthetic Apparatus. Blackwell, Oxford, 1980.)

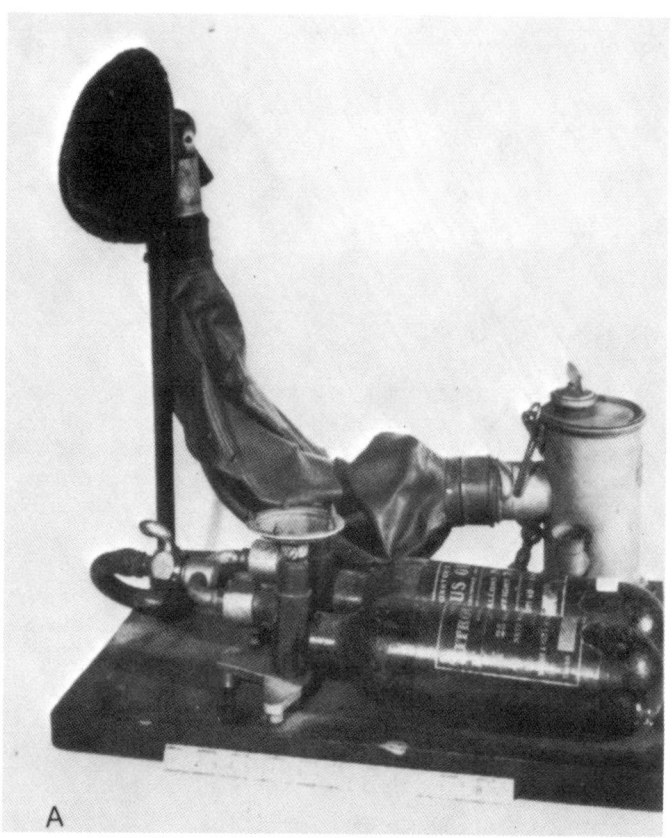

Fig. 1-12 Two apparatuses (ca. 1876) used by Clover to administer nitrous oxide and ether either singly or combined. No supplemental oxygen was used. (A) Nitrous oxide from two cylinders could be diverted into the ether chamber. Room air content was controlled by the top tap. (Thomas KB: The Development of Anaesthetic Apparatus. Blackwell, Oxford, 1980.) (B) Nitrous oxide from a cylinder (K) was passed through a gas rarefier (R) and into the reservoir bag (G). The tube inside the rubber bag (G) allowed a mixture of either air and ether or nitrous oxide, air, and ether to be delivered. (Smith WDA: Under the Influence: A History of Nitrous Oxide and Oxygen Anaesthesia. ASA Wood Library–Museum of Anesthesiology, Park Ridge, IL, 1982.)

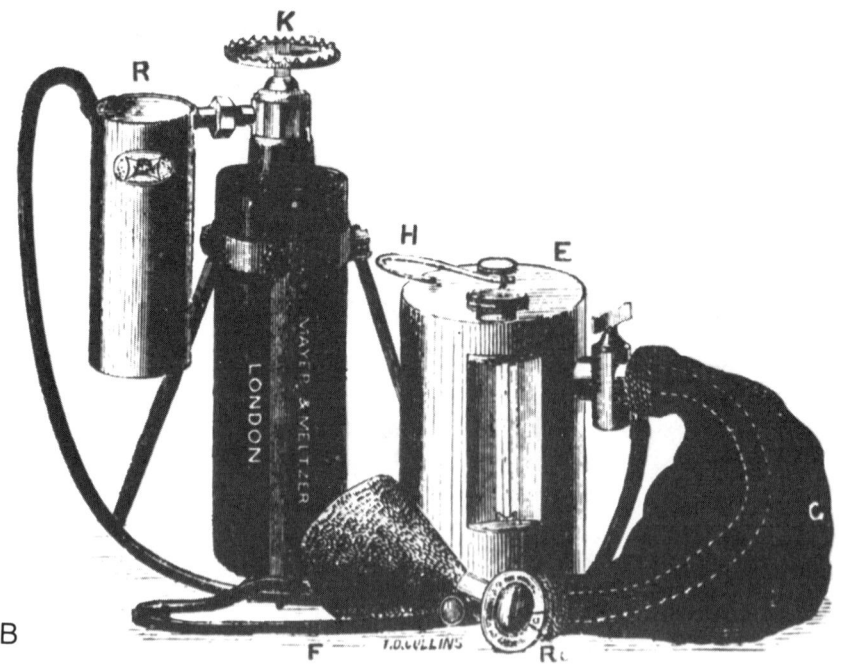

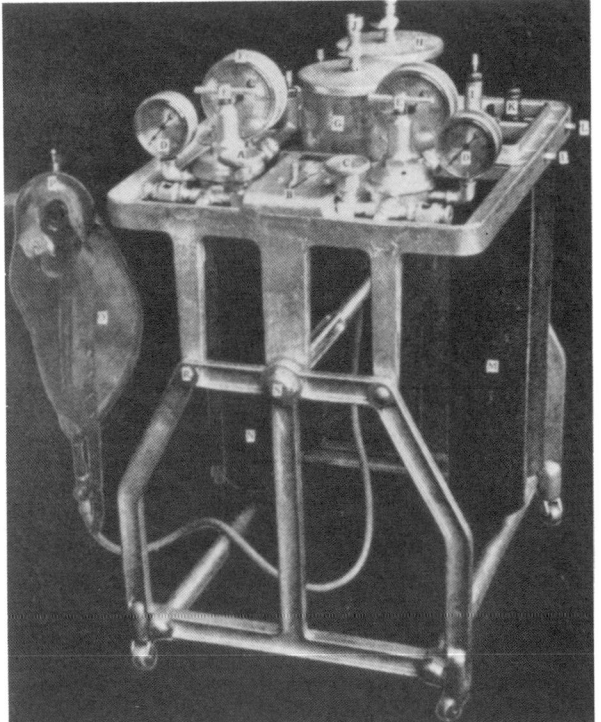

Fig. 1-13 Nitrous oxide–oxygen–ether anesthesia apparatus (ca. 1912). Unique features include (1) the reduction of high-pressure tank pressures to an anesthesia machine pipeline pressure of 20 psig, (2) the first flowmeters (bubble-through), and (3) pass-by or pass-over bubble-through ether vaporization. (From Faulconer A, Jr, Keys TE: Foundations of Anesthesiology, 1965. Courtesy of Charles C Thomas, Publisher, Springfield, IL.)

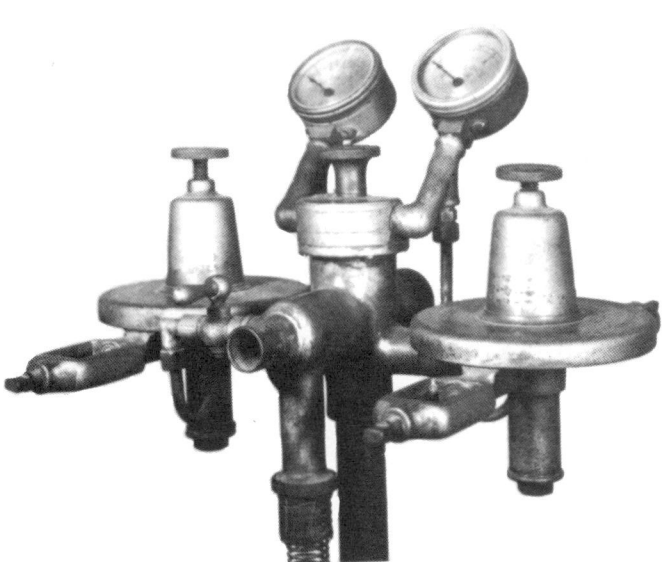

Fig. 1-14 Heidbrink nitrous oxide–oxygen anesthesia machine featuring four cylinder yokes and two flat reducing valves. The mixing chamber control knob can divide gas delivery into forty equal parts, representing a maximum of 20 gals. of nitrous oxide per minute. (Thomas KB: The Development of Anaesthetic Apparatus. Blackwell, Oxford, 1980.)

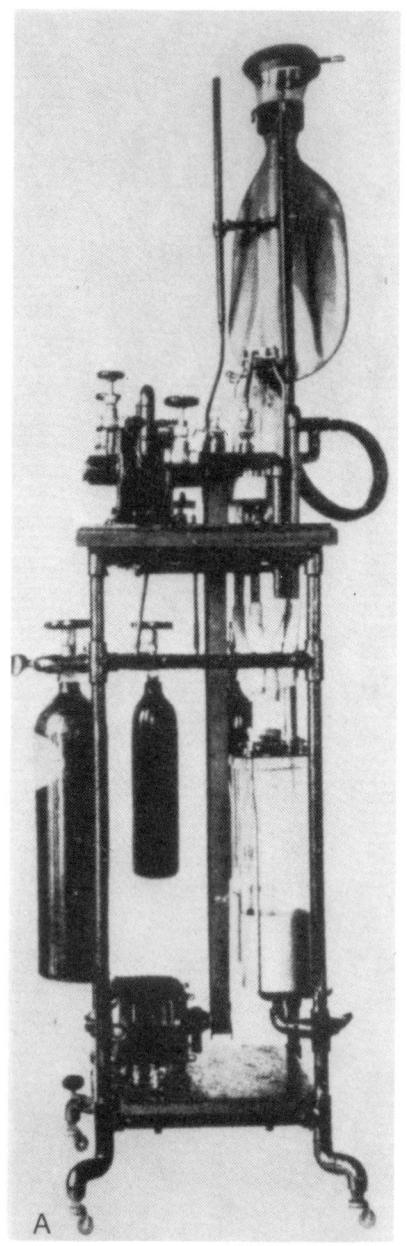

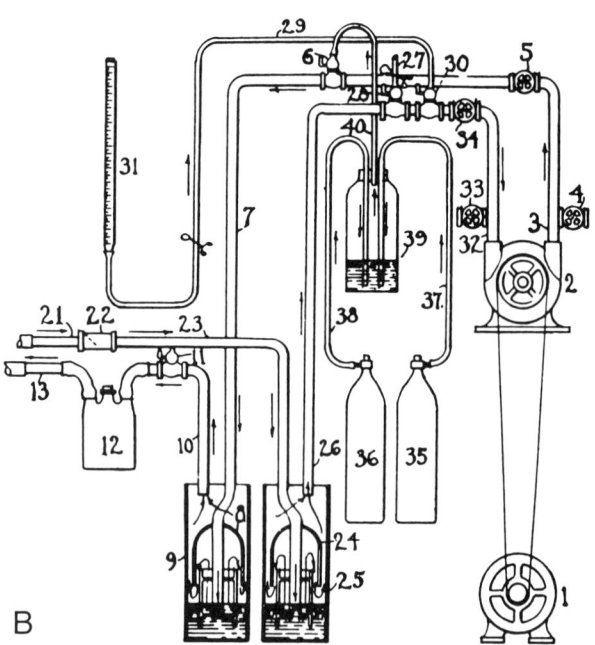

One of the *first commercial gas anesthesia machines* was designed by Jay A. Heidbrink[15, 16] in 1906. The anesthesia machine was a modification of an earlier design by Teter.[11] New design features included (1) equalization of nitrous oxide and oxygen pressures delivered to the mixing chambers by the placement of two bags of equal size between bread toasters hinged at the back and weighted on top, (2) the reservoir bag being positioned in front for easy observation, and (3) placement of an electric light bulb in the mixing chamber to warm the gases and prevent freezing of the nitrous oxide cylinder valve.[17] Heidbrink[15] further modified the anesthesia machine and marketed the "Model A" an-

Fig. 1-15 Jackson anesthesia machine (ca. 1915). (A) Right-hand side of the machine with the reservoir bag and face mask. (B) Schematic of the anesthesia machine. Interesting features include (1, 2) an electric motor and an air pump to provide circulation in the system, (9) a glass jar filled with a strong aqueous solution of sodium hydroxide and calcium hydrate to absorb carbon dioxide, (12) oil of bitter orange peel put in the container to perfume the anesthetic mixture, (25) a wash jar containing sulfuric acid to extract water, (30) an air cock for the injection of ether or chloroform, and (35, 36) cylinders for oxygen and nitrous oxide. (From Faulconer A, Jr, Keys TE: Foundations of Anesthesiology, 1965. Courtesy of Charles C Thomas, Publisher, Springfield, IL.)

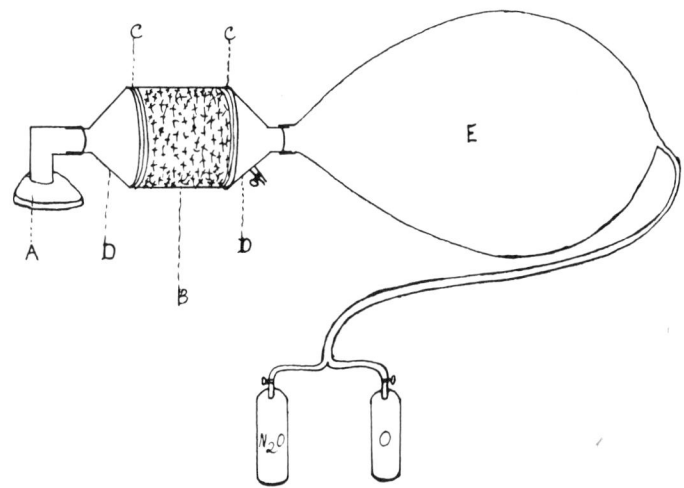

Fig. 1-16 Carbon dioxide filtration in the to-and-fro anesthetic apparatus designed by Ralph Waters (ca. 1924): (A) face mask, (B–D) cylinder containing granular sodium and calcium hydrate, and (E) reservoir bag. (From Faulconer A, Jr, Keys TE: Foundations of Anesthesiology, 1965. Courtesy of Charles C Thomas, Publisher, Springfield, IL.)

esthesia machine (see Fig. 1-14) in 1913 at a cost of $1.00 a pound, or $32.00 a machine! An automatic reducing valve was incorporated as well as a newly designed dial valve which proportioned the amount of nitrous oxide and oxygen in the gas mixture. The oxygen gauge was calibrated in "oxygen percent" and allowed oxygen to be immediately available through a stopcock (the first oxygen flush?). A bubble-through ether vaporizer completed the machine.[17] In the 1920s Heidbrink collaborated with John Lundy to fabricate the Lundy Rochester machine specifically designed for surgical anesthesia.[16] The anesthesia machine held tanks of nitrous oxide, oxygen, ethylene, and carbon dioxide.[18]

An anesthesia machine with two *carbon dioxide absorption cannisters* was designed by Franz Kuhn of Kassel, Germany, and manufactured by Drager Werk in 1906. The cannister design was taken from the respiratory apparatus developed by Schwann[19] in 1876 for mine rescue work.

A *circle system* was built into the anesthesia machine introduced in 1915 by Jackson.[20] The machine was complex (see Fig. 1-15) and must have been a maintenance nightmare. Carbon dioxide was absorbed by bubbling expired gases through 3 to 4 in. of "strong aqueous solution of sodium hydrate and calcium hydrate." Another reservoir was filled with water

when humidity was required in the breathing mixture, but it was usually used to hold a small amount of "oil of bitter orange peel . . . to perfume the air breathed by the patient." Excess water vapor was absorbed by a solution of sulfuric acid. A small air pump was required to maintain circulation within the circuit. Oxygen, nitrous oxide, ether, and carbon dioxide were "injected into the system" as required.

Granules for the absorption of carbon dioxide were introduced by Waters[21] in 1924. Granular sodium and calcium hydrate of "sufficient diameter to allow unobstructed respiration" were placed in a container between the face mask and the reservoir bag as illustrated in Figure 1-16. This "to and fro" method required minimal anesthesia equipment, saved expensive nitrous oxide (total cost for nitrous oxide, oxygen, and filter replacements per hour was 25 to 50 cents in 1924), and was convenient for many surgical cases. Some anesthesiologists found the proximity of the cannister in the field of operation to be unsatisfactory.

The *first closed-circle anesthesia apparatus* to absorb carbon dioxide by dry granules was described[22] in 1930. Figure 1-17 depicts the cannister and breathing tubes of the circle system. An 8×10 mesh was recommended with a soda lime mixture of 50 percent calcium oxide and 50 percent sodium hydroxide.

A "bobbin meter" was introduced by the Coxeter Company[8] of Great Britain to replace the popular "bubble-bottle" or wet flowmeter. The wet flowmeter worked on the principle of matching the bubble rates of nitrous oxide and oxygen. Rates of bubbling could be set

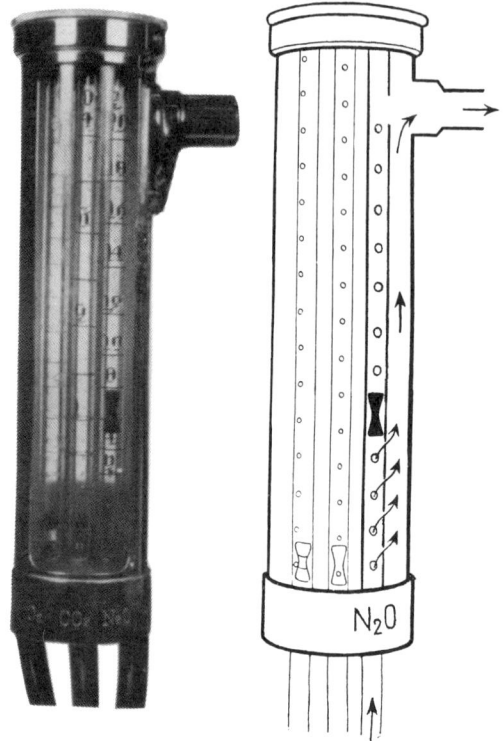

Fig. 1-18 Coxeter dry gas meter (ca. 1930). The gas flows up a vertical tube, lifting a bobbin. As the bobbin passes a vertical hole, gas escapes into the common outlet. Dirt, bobbin friction, and large steps between orifices limited the accuracy of the apparatus. (Macintosh R, Mushin WW, Epstein HG: Physics for the Anaesthetist. 3rd Ed. Blackwell, Oxford, 1963.)

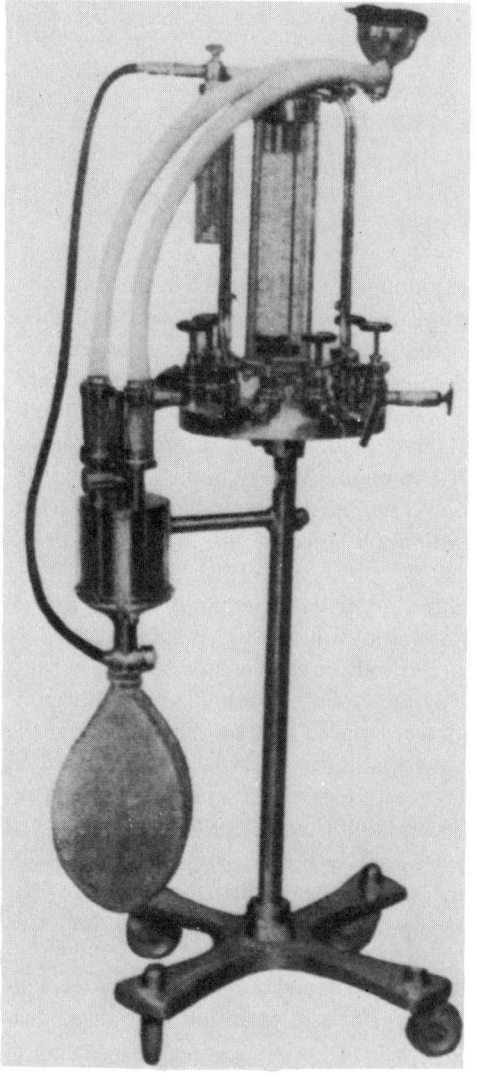

Fig. 1–17 Closed-circle anesthesia machine (ca. 1930). The cannister was filled with a soda lime mixture of 50 percent calcium oxide and 50 percent sodium hydroxide. (From Faulconer A, Jr, Keys TE: Foundations of Anesthesiology, 1965. Courtesy of Charles C Thomas, Publisher, Springfield, IL.)

but the volumes and percent concentrations of gases in the mixture were unknown. With the new bobbin meters, or dry flowmeters, gas raised a small bobbin in a tube with sidewall perforations. A high rate of flow pushed the bobbin higher in the tube and a proportional amount of gas escaped via exposure to larger numbers of perforations (see Fig. 1-18). Dry flowmeters solved many of the inherent problems of wet flowmeters but were soon found to have a few problems of their own. The bobbin could drag on the sides of the tube, an orifice could become obstructed with dirt, access for cleaning was difficult, and the orifices were not close enough together for fine adjustments of gas flow. Coxeter dry flowmeters

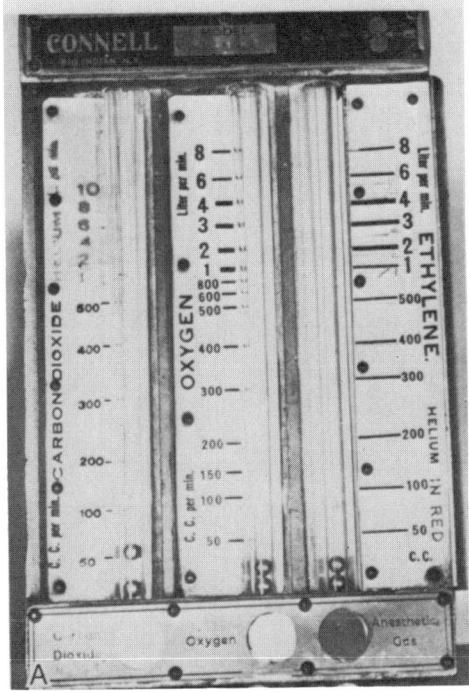

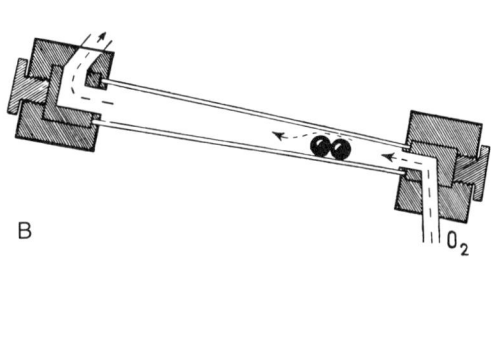

Fig. 1-19 Connell ball-bearing flowmeter. The flow tubes are tapered on an inclined plane and contain two ball bearings. (A) The 1937 Connell apparatus with carbon dioxide, oxygen, ethylene, and helium. (Thomas KB: The Development of Anaesthetic Apparatus. Blackwell, Oxford, 1980.) (B) Schematic side view of the inclined plane. Gas flow rates were read between the two balls. (Macintosh R, Mushin WW, Epstein HG: Physics for the Anaesthetist. 3rd Ed. Blackwell, Oxford, 1963.)

were adapted into the head unit of the Model 1933 Boyle Machine, destined to become recognized as the forerunner of modern anesthetic equipment.[8]

Accuracy in flowmeters was improved by combining a tapered tube and two steel balls on an inclined plane[11] in 1930. The idea for the inclined plane gas flowmeter probably originated from Ewing's description[23] in 1924 of a similar flowmeter designed for liquids. Figure 1-19 shows two steel balls being pushed up an inclined plane by a gas. Each flowmeter was calibrated for a specific gas. Two balls were required to ensure steady movement, since one steel ball by itself was found to oscillate with gas flow. The makers claimed, "the ball flow meter as now constructed is the most sensitive, accurate and compact dry flow-meter as yet devised."[11] Taper inside the 6-in.-

long glass tube was intentionally nonuniform to allow precise control at low and high flow rates. The lower 3 in. of the meter was claimed to have an accuracy of 10 ml/min.[11]

The *rotameter* was designed by Küppers[24] in Aachen, Germany, in 1908 and manufactured by Deutsche Rotawerke. The physical working principles of the rotameter are best described by Küppers.[25]

The gas streams up, through a vertical tube in which the bore gradually increases, lifting a "rotor," a rotating bobbin to varying levels depending on the velocity of the gas. Part of the gas streams through small oblique grooves in the cylindrical part of the circumference of the rotor, causes it to spin, keeps it vertical and prevents it from adhering to the wall. . . . The calibration is done empirically and individually for each glass tube.

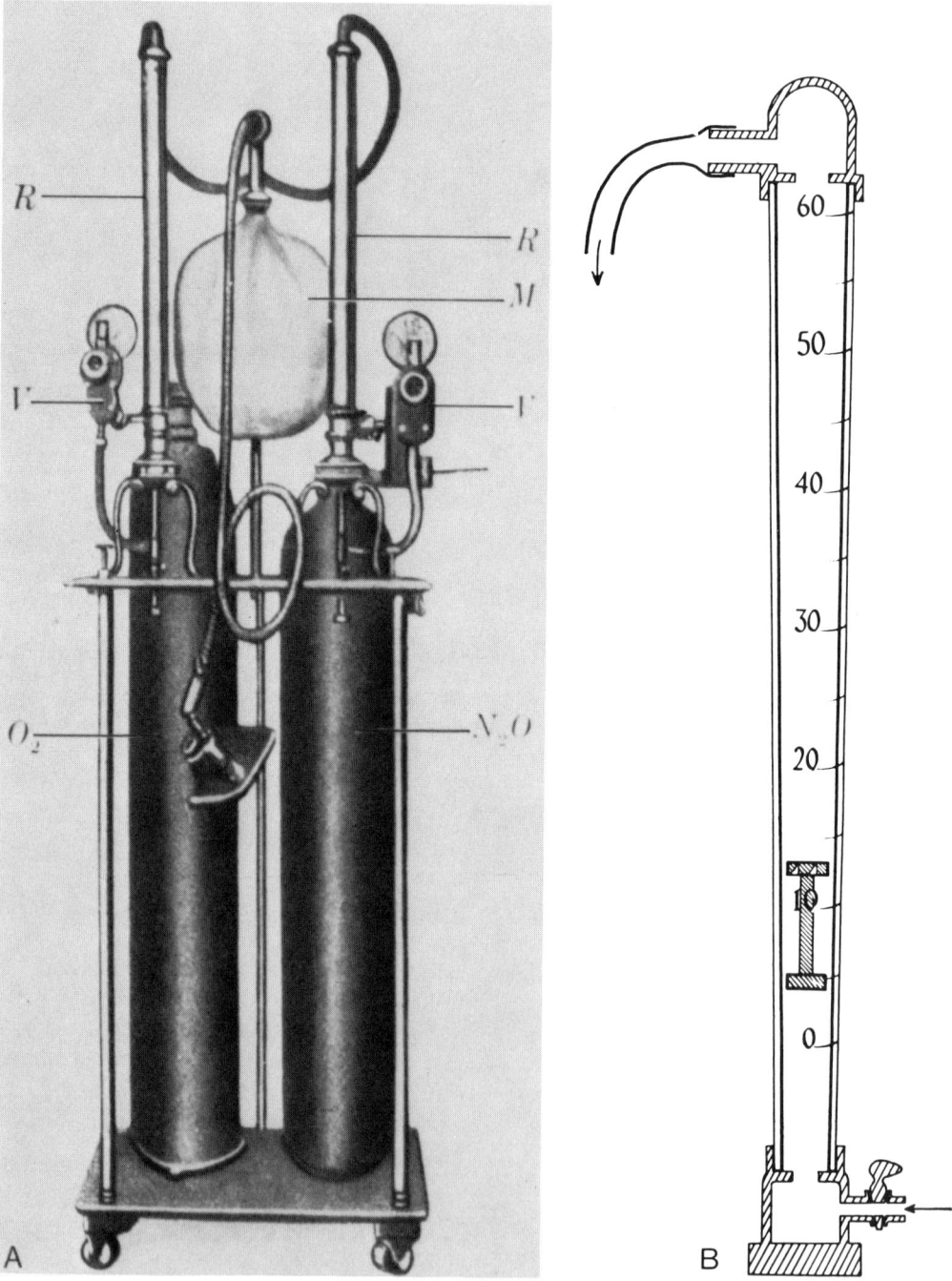

Fig. 1-20 (A) Maxmilian Neu's anesthetic machine with rotameters (1910). Oxygen and nitrous oxide were mixed in the bag (M) prior to being delivered to the patient. (Morch ET: Rotameters in anaesthesia. Br J Anaesth 24:196, 1952.) (B) A simplified diagram of the original rotameter designed by Karl Küppers in 1908. The principle features were a tapered tube, a rotating float, and individual gas calibration. (Macintosh R, Mushin WW, Epstein HG: Physics for the Anaesthetist. 3rd Ed. Blackwell, Oxford, 1963.)

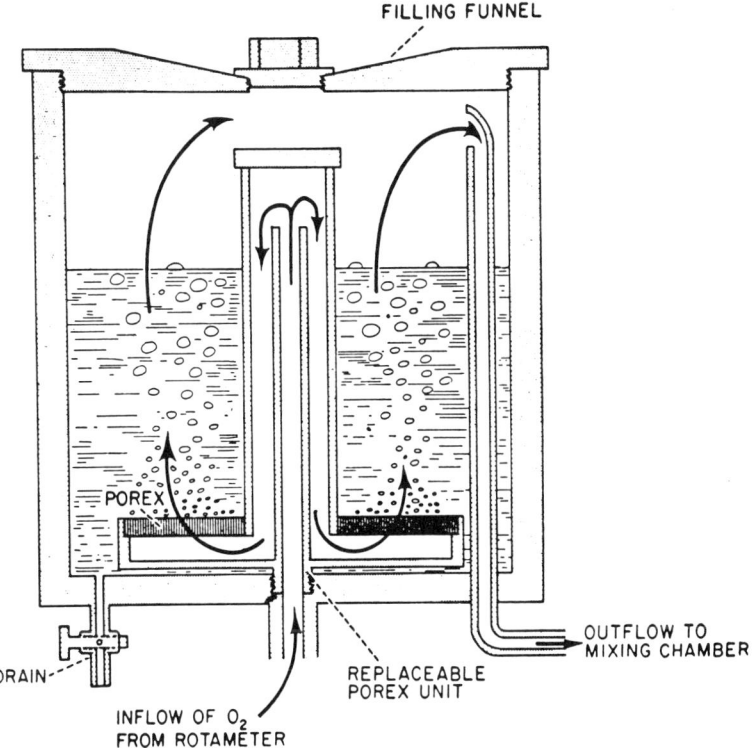

Fig. 1-21 The copper kettle bubble-through vaporizer designed by Lucien E. Morris. Hallmarks in this vaporizer design included efficiency and accurate control of concentration. (Morris LE: A new vaporizer for liquid anesthetic agents. Anesthesiology 13:587, 1952.)

Rotameters were first used in anesthesia by Dr. Maxmilian Neu of Heidelberg in 1910 (see Fig. 1-20). Unfortunately their configuration did not allow the simultaneous vaporization of ether. Widespread use of the rotameter was curtailed because its cost was twice as high as that of any other apparatus. Nitrous oxide was very expensive, which negated its widespread use and required accurate rotameters.[24] The English give credit to Richard Salt for the introduction of the rotameter "in a form suitable for anaesthetic apparatus."[26] Since 1937 the rotameter has been used to meter known quantities of gases.

A major advance in the vaporization of anesthetics was the introduction of the *copper kettle* (Fig. 1-21) by Morris.[27] Efficiency of vaporization combined with the precision con-

trol of concentration was made possible. Temperature compensation was afforded by the use of copper. Vaporization was maximized by bubbling oxygen through the liquid using an accurate flowmeter. Known quantities of anesthetic vapor were mixed with known quantities of oxygen and/or nitrous oxide.

Our anesthesia machines are the results of the developing technology taken from roots established by previous scientists. The principles are the same; only the device design has really changed (see Fig. 1-22). Portable anesthesia machines and fixed anesthesia machines are much more accurate in the delivery of anesthesia vapors owing to the application of sophisticated engineering knowledge. Nevertheless, we remain indebted to those who pioneered the vaporizer, the flowmeter, the

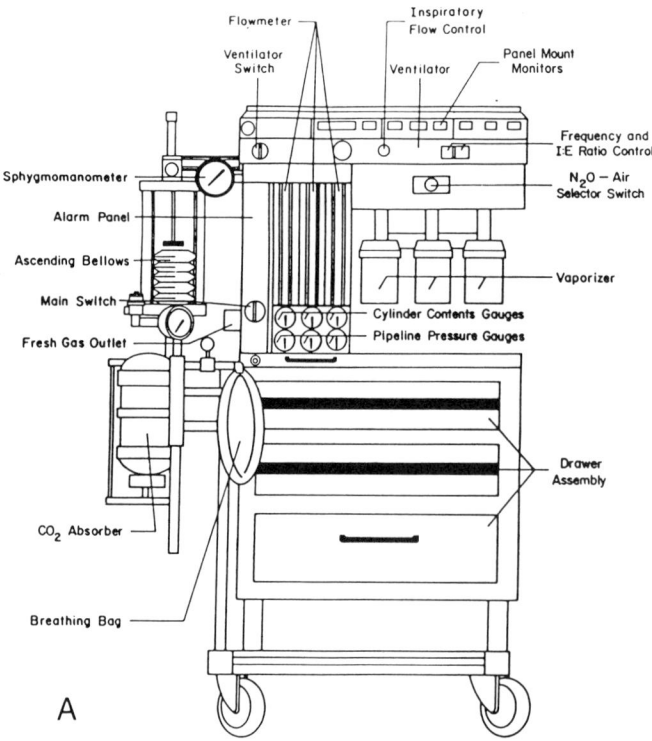

Flowmeter
Ventilator Switch
Inspiratory Flow Control
Ventilator
Panel Mount Monitors
Frequency and I·E Ratio Control
N_2O – Air Selector Switch
Sphygmomanometer
Alarm Panel
Ascending Bellows
Main Switch
Fresh Gas Outlet
Vaporizer
Cylinder Contents Gauges
Pipeline Pressure Gauges
Drawer Assembly
CO_2 Absorber
Breathing Bag

A

Fig. 1-22 Features of the Drager Narkomed IIA anesthesia machine. Front (A) and rear (B) views show the combining of many of the apparatuses developed by early pioneers in anesthesia. (Technical Service Manual. North American Drager, Telford, PA, 1985.)

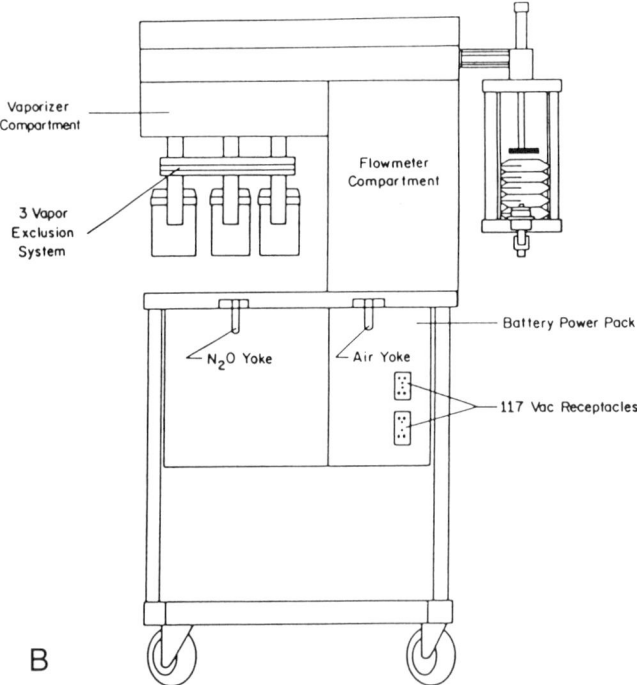

Vaporizer Compartment
3 Vapor Exclusion System
Flowmeter Compartment
Battery Power Pack
N_2O Yoke
Air Yoke
117 Vac Receptacles

B

pressure-reducing valve, and the multitude of other devices necessary for the functioning of our anesthesia machine.

REFERENCES

1. Davy H: Researches, chemical and philosophical; chiefly concerning nitrous oxide, or dephlogisticated nitrous air, and its respiration. J. Johnson, London, 1800
2. Priestley J: The discovery of nitrous oxide. Observations on different kinds of air. Philos Trans, R Soc London 62:210, 1772
3. Smith WDA: Under the Influence: a History of Nitrous Oxide and Oxygen Anaesthesia. ASA Wood Library–Museum of Anesthesiology, Park Ridge, IL, 1982
4. The Morton Inhaler. Pamphlet ca. 1968. ASA Wood Library–Museum of Anesthesiology, Park Ridge, IL.
5. Morton WTG: Letter to the editor. Lancet 2:80, 1847
6. U.S. Patent Office. Augustus A. Gould and W.T.G. Morton. Apparatus for inhaling ether. Patent 5,365, November 13, 1847
7. Snow J: On the Inhalation of the Vapour of Ether. John Churchill, London, 1847
8. Macintosh R, Mushin WW, Epstein HG: Physics for the Anaesthetist. 3rd Ed. Blackwell, Oxford, 1963
9. Marston AD: First Clover lecture. Ann R Coll Surg Engl 4:267, 1949
10. Andrews E: The oxygen mixture, a new anaesthetic combination. Chicago Med Exam 9:656, 1868
11. Thomas KB: The Development of Anaesthetic Apparatus. Blackwell, Oxford, 1980
12. Andrews E: Liquid nitrous oxide as an anaesthetic. Med Exam 13:34, 1872
13. Clover JT: On an apparatus for administering nitrous oxide gas and ether, singly or combined. Br Med J 2:74, 1876
14. Cotton FJ, Boothby WM: Nitrous oxide–oxygen–ether anaesthesia: notes on administration; a perfected apparatus. Surg Gynecol Obstet 15:281, 1912
15. Heidbrink JA: Memoirs. Newsmonth Am Dent Soc Anesth, 1, 1957
16. OHIO Chemical Manufacturing Co. (Ohmeda). In the Beginning. Internal publication. OHIO Chemical Manufacturing Co. (Ohmeda), Madison, 1967
17. Clark BJ, Heidbrink JA: A brief history. Internal publication. OHIO Chemical Manufacturing Co. (Ohmeda), Madison, 1940
18. Beck HW: Historical highlights—OHIO medical products. Internal publication. OHIO Chemical Manufacturing Co. (Ohmeda), Madison, 1981
19. Foregger R: Respiratory apparatus of Theodor Schwann. Anesthesiology 27:187, 1966
20. Jackson DE: A new method for the production of general analgesia and anaesthesia with a description of the apparatus used. J Lab Clin Med 1:1, 1915
21. Waters RM: Clinical scope and utility of carbon dioxide filtration in inhalation anesthesia. Anesth Analg 3:20, 1924
22. Sword BC: The closed circle method of administration of gas anesthesia. Anesth Analg 9:198, 1930
23. Ewing JA: A ball-and-tube flowmeter. Proc R Soc Edinburgh 65:308, 1924-25
24. Foregger R: Early use of rotameter in anaesthesia. Br J Anaesth 24:187, 1952
25. Morch ET: Rotameters in anaesthesia. Br J Anaesth 24:196, 1952
26. Flowmeters for gas or liquid. Lancet 214:718, 1941
27. Morris LE: A new vaporizer for liquid anesthetic agents. Anesthesiology 13:587, 1952

2

The Making of the Anesthesia Machine

Anesthesia machines can at times be frustrating. When faced with the purchase of an anesthesia machine, we find ourselves lost in the technical aspects of specifications and tolerances. The background of the anesthesiologist is usually clinically oriented and only a blessed few of our species can comprehend the jargon surrounding the technical intricacy of the anesthesia machine. We adjust, sometimes with difficulty, to the new devices designed for safety, the placement of the ventilator in a fixed position in the anesthesia shell, the new vaporizer designs, the lack of universal vaporizers, and many other changes which are at first unfamiliar to us.

The final blow to our patience comes when the cost of the anesthesia machine is revealed. Our question is almost always the same: Why does an anesthesia machine cost so much? The answer is somewhat dubious, depending on which viewpoint we accept. Many factors enter into the cost of the final product: (1) research and development, (2) labor, (3) materials, (4) maintenance of quality assurance, (5) product liability insurance, (6) federal regulatory bodies, and (7) reasonable profit margin. Sustaining a high standard of quality assurance can account for up to 40 to 50 percent of the overall cost of the anesthesia machine.

The physical characteristics of liquids and gases become of paramount importance in the design and manufacture of an anesthesia machine. Gas densities are especially important in flowmeter design. Temperature changes become critical in the design of vaporizers. The accurate control of gas mixtures is very important because of the marked potency of the general anesthetics. Building a well-made machine is a challenge as we reflect on the daily rigors of many different users with a multitude of anesthetic techniques.

The manufacturing plants of North American Drager and Ohmeda were toured by the author. Each company has excellent facilities which produce a high-quality anesthesia machine, that is, NarcoMed IIA (North American Drager) and Ohmeda Modulus II. Research and development activities are certainly evident in both plants. Competition in the marketplace has stimulated each manufacturer to improve the quality, design, and function of their anesthesia machine. Developments in recent years have included such items as disconnect alarms, markedly improved single-agent vaporizers, redesigned carbon dioxide absorber heads, the modulus concept of addi-

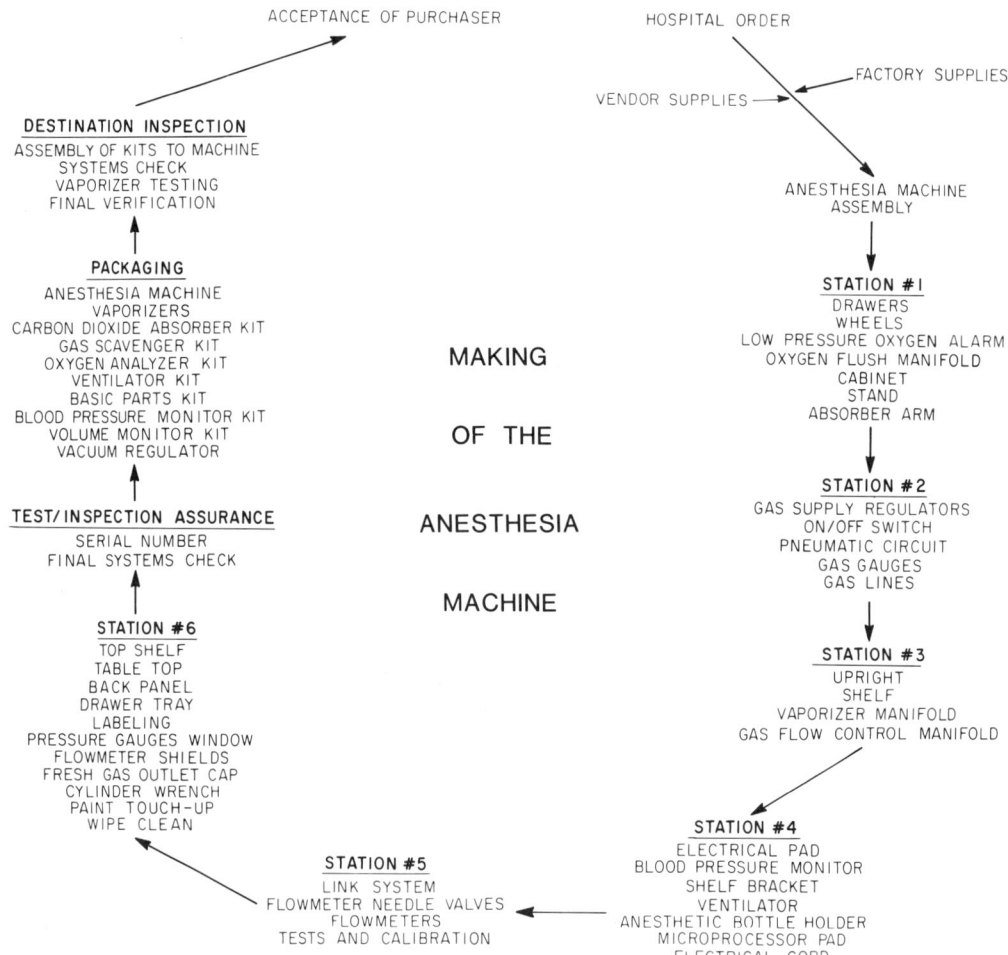

ACCEPTANCE OF PURCHASER

HOSPITAL ORDER

FACTORY SUPPLIES

VENDOR SUPPLIES

DESTINATION INSPECTION
ASSEMBLY OF KITS TO MACHINE
SYSTEMS CHECK
VAPORIZER TESTING
FINAL VERIFICATION

ANESTHESIA MACHINE
ASSEMBLY

PACKAGING
ANESTHESIA MACHINE
VAPORIZERS
CARBON DIOXIDE ABSORBER KIT
GAS SCAVENGER KIT
OXYGEN ANALYZER KIT
VENTILATOR KIT
BASIC PARTS KIT
BLOOD PRESSURE MONITOR KIT
VOLUME MONITOR KIT
VACUUM REGULATOR

MAKING

OF THE

ANESTHESIA

MACHINE

STATION #1
DRAWERS
WHEELS
LOW PRESSURE OXYGEN ALARM
OXYGEN FLUSH MANIFOLD
CABINET
STAND
ABSORBER ARM

STATION #2
GAS SUPPLY REGULATORS
ON/OFF SWITCH
PNEUMATIC CIRCUIT
GAS GAUGES
GAS LINES

TEST/INSPECTION ASSURANCE
SERIAL NUMBER
FINAL SYSTEMS CHECK

STATION #3
UPRIGHT
SHELF
VAPORIZER MANIFOLD
GAS FLOW CONTROL MANIFOLD

STATION #6
TOP SHELF
TABLE TOP
BACK PANEL
DRAWER TRAY
LABELING
PRESSURE GAUGES WINDOW
FLOWMETER SHIELDS
FRESH GAS OUTLET CAP
CYLINDER WRENCH
PAINT TOUCH-UP
WIPE CLEAN

STATION #4
ELECTRICAL PAD
BLOOD PRESSURE MONITOR
SHELF BRACKET
VENTILATOR
ANESTHETIC BOTTLE HOLDER
MICROPROCESSOR PAD
ELECTRICAL CORD

STATION #5
LINK SYSTEM
FLOWMETER NEEDLE VALVES
FLOWMETERS
TESTS AND CALIBRATION

Fig. 2-1 Summary flow chart for the making of an anesthesia machine, beginning with the *hospital order* (top right) and proceeding clockwise to the *acceptance of the purchaser* (top left).

tions to the anesthesia machine, high- and low-circuit pressure alarms, and improved ventilators.

Excessive and unjustified product liability claims could result in the existence of only one manufacturer of anesthesia machines. Lack of competition would lead to a decrease in quality and limit the research and development of improved anesthesia machines.

The assembly of an anesthesia machine is a fascinating sequence of events. The majority

of anesthesiologists will never have the opportunity to see an anesthesia machine assembled. It is appropriate to document how an anesthesia machine is made. Knowing the quality checks done and the care taken by the manufacturer to provide a superior product will help us understand the anesthesia machines we use. Each major addition is checked and rechecked for quality and function. The sequence of anesthesia machine assembly presented will be that of the Ohmeda plant in

El Paso, Texas. Elements of both American and Japanese mass production are welded into a smooth, efficient flow pattern. The Japanese concept of *kanban,* frequently translated by Americans as the "just-in-time" (JIT) inventory system, is combined with well-proven American know-how. The JIT system eliminates expensive inventories of finished goods and manufacturing parts in warehouses, stockrooms, or storage yards. This reduction of emphasis to build up inventories decreases warehousing costs, ensures faster identification of poor-quality parts, and permits the manufacturer to change to new products without being stuck with thousands of surplus components.

Assembly-line work is divided into stations for the addition and testing of specific parts. An overall view of the entire assembly process is summarized in Figure 2-1. Each section will be examined, discussed, and illustrated in detail.

Quality assurance begins prior to the addition of the first component to the anesthesia machine. Each critical item and random samples of noncritical items purchased from outside vendors are checked for quality and function in the receiving department. Items that meet the standard are shuttled to the appropriate assembly point.

Standards of quality for anesthesia components are only as good as the test apparatus used in making quality/performance checks. Each test apparatus on the assembly line has scheduled and documented tests it must undergo to ensure its proper calibration. The test apparatus to calibrate assembly-line test apparatus must meet rigid standards, some

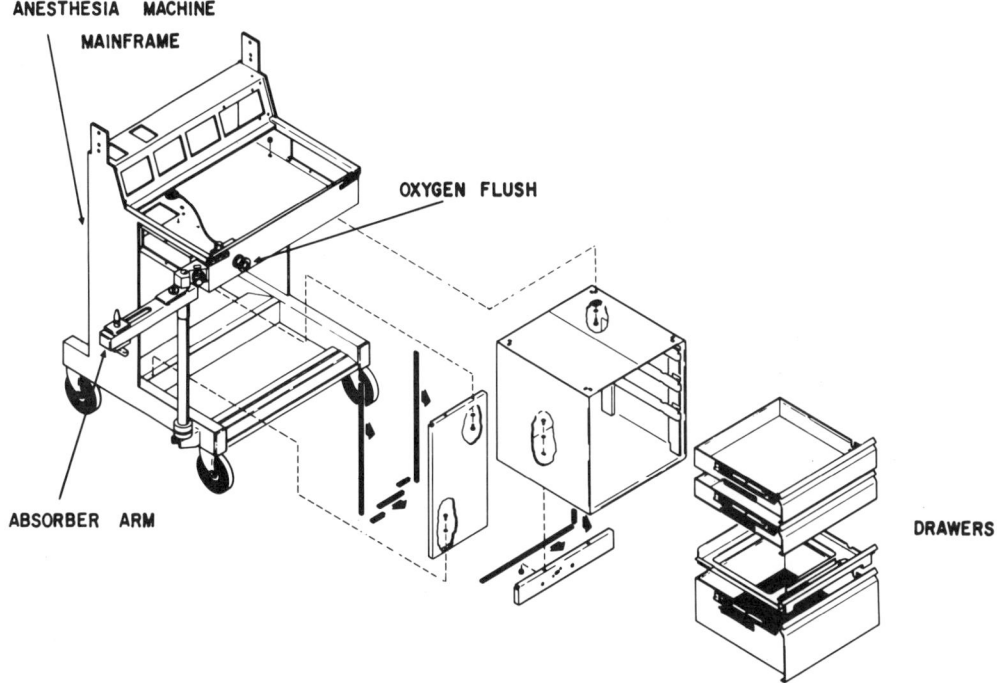

Fig. 2-2 Assembly of the cabinets and drawers to the mainframe of the anesthesia machine (station 1). (Courtesy of Ohmeda, The BOC Group, Inc.)

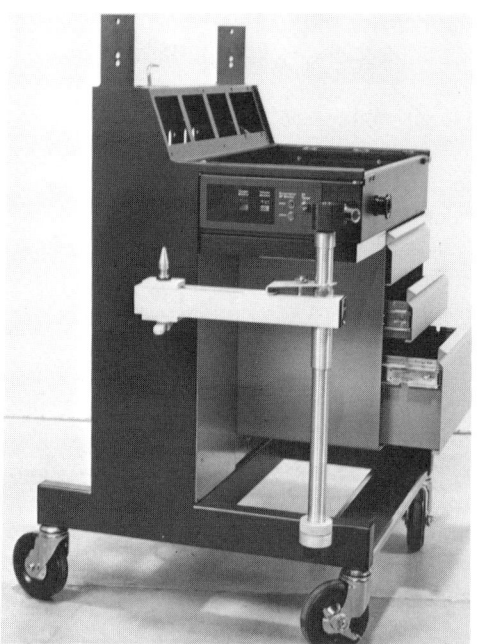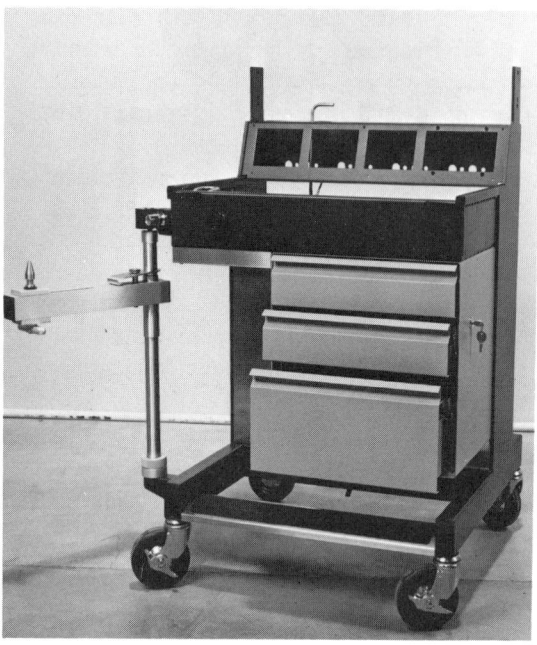

Fig. 2-3 Front and side view of the assembled stand, cabinet, and absorber arm (station 1). (Courtesy of Ohmeda, The BOC Group, Inc.)

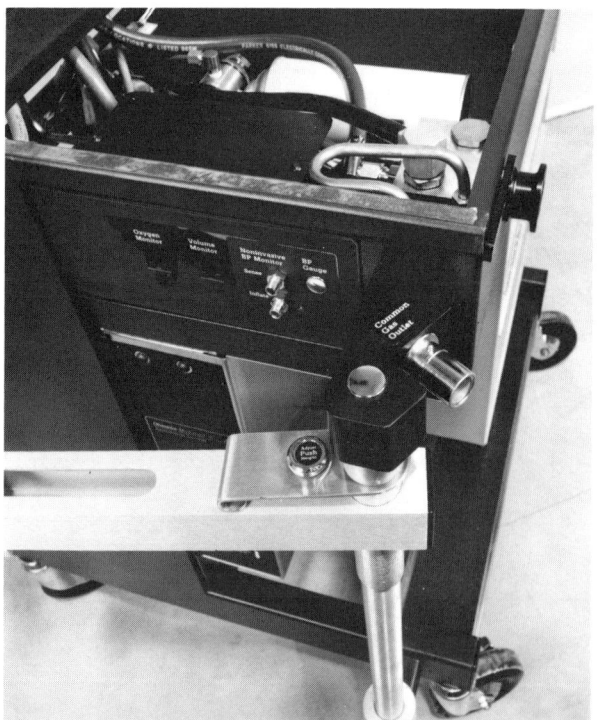

Fig. 2-4 A close-up view of the absorber arm showing the common gas outlet. Note the oxygen flush valve activator button on the front of the cabinet surrounded by a protective rim. A patient interface panel has been mounted to accept connections from the oxygen, volume, and blood pressure monitors (station 1). (Courtesy of Ohmeda, The BOC Group, Inc.)

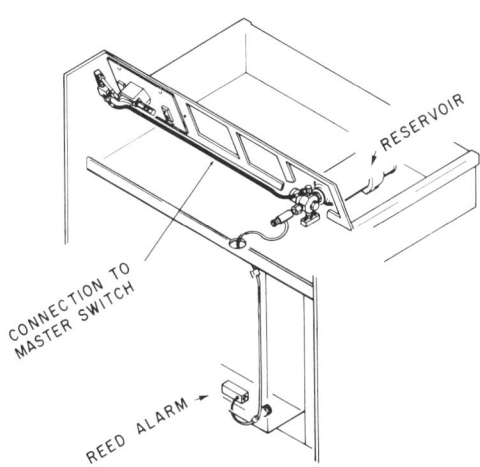

Fig. 2-5 Diagram illustrating the position of components in the oxygen supply failure alarm system. The pressure reservoir is under the table top of the anesthesia cabinet and the reed is inside the bottom portion of the rear panel (station 1). (Courtesy of Ohmeda, The BOC Group, Inc.)

of which can be linked directly to the U.S. Bureau of Standards. The Ohmeda and North American Drager factories each have a highly trained full-time staff devoted to testing and calibrating the test apparatus.

ANESTHESIA MACHINE ASSEMBLY

Station 1

The first station involves stand, cabinet, and absorber arm assembly (Figs. 2-2 to 2-4). The low-pressure oxygen alarm is tested to confirm that (1) the reed alarm sounds when the oxygen pressure is 30 psig or less and (2) the subassembly does not leak during the application of negative pressure during an observation period of 10 seconds. The low-pressure oxygen alarm (Figs. 2-5 and 2-6) and the oxygen flush manifold (Figs. 2-4 and 2-6) are then installed.

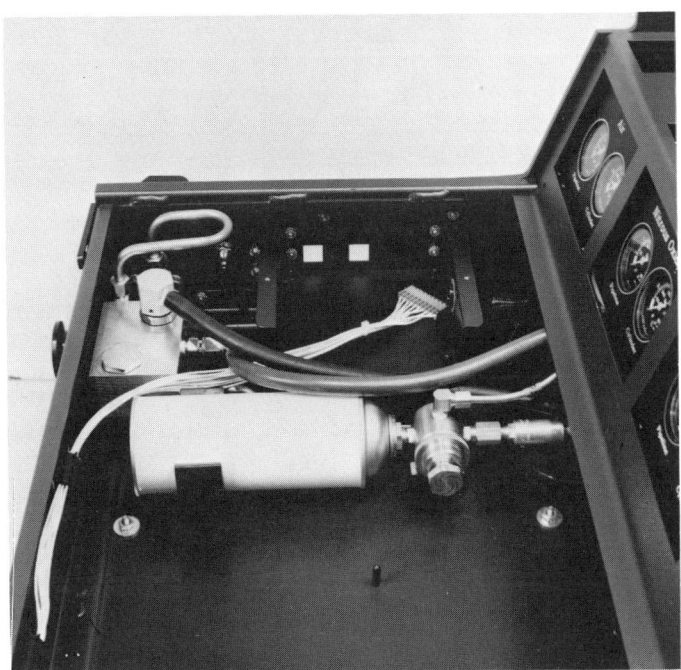

Fig. 2-6 Top view of the anesthesia machine cabinet. The oxygen reservoir, which "powers" the oxygen supply-failure alarm system, is installed. The oxygen flush valve is mounted in the top left portion of the cabinet, as viewed in this photograph (station 1). (Courtesy of Ohmeda, The BOC Group, Inc.)

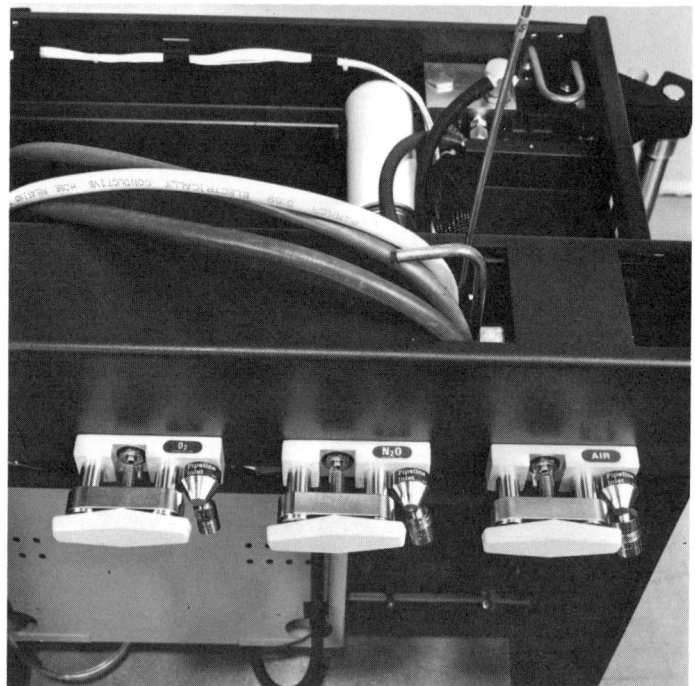

Fig. 2-7 Rear view of the anesthesia machine showing the yokes and the pipeline inlets for oxygen, nitrous oxide, and medical air (station 2). (Courtesy of Ohmeda, The BOC Group, Inc.)

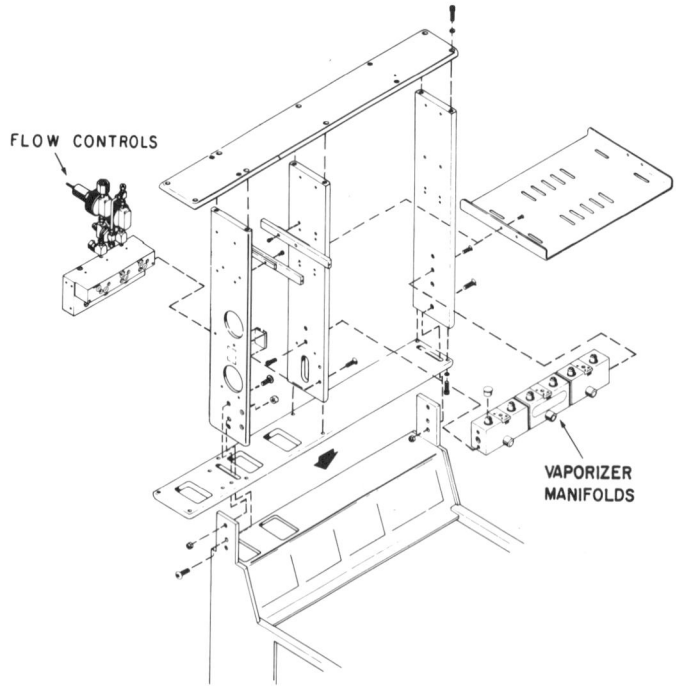

Fig. 2-8 Installation of the shelves and upper support structure of the anesthesia machine. The vaporizer manifolds and flow controls are installed in the upper support structure (station 3). (Courtesy of Ohmeda, The BOC Group, Inc.)

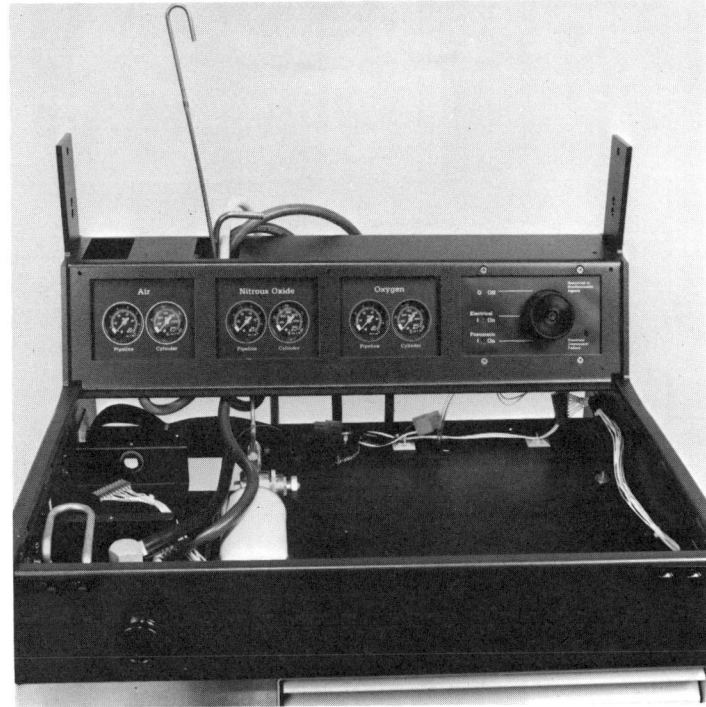

Fig. 2-9 The machine on/off switch has been installed. Gas supply modules for oxygen, nitrous oxide and purchaser-selected gas (in this case, medical air) are in place (station 3). (Courtesy of Ohmeda, The BOC Group, Inc.)

Station 2

Gas lines and yokes are added for nitrous oxide, oxygen, and one additional purchaser-selected gas (Fig. 2-7). The majority of the gas lines are made of copper to meet U.S. government standards.

Station 3

The flowmeter control manifold is installed after each specific gas regulator has been tested (Fig. 2-8). No leakage of gas is accepted across the operating seat of the regulator at a pressure of 50 ± 3 psig. The output pressure of the nitrous oxide regulator is adjusted to 26 ± 0.25 psig at 90 to 100 ml/min three successive times to confirm repeatability. The test gas flow at three ranges determines pressure stability at different flow rates. The output pressure cannot vary by more than 1.00 psig over the entire range. A final check ensures that no spontaneous cycling of the regulator occurs between 12 and 100 L/min. Testing of the oxygen regulator is essentially the same as for the nitrous oxide regulator, except the output pressure is adjusted to 14 ± 0.25 psig at 90 to 100 ml/min.

The machine on/off switch assembly, consisting of a pneumatic circuit and an electronic switching mechanism, is installed as shown in Figure 2-9. The dual-acting switch provides an on/off control to the electronic monitoring equipment and the gas circuit. Indicator lights provide visual affirmation of on/off conditions and proper gas supply pressures. Switch calibration and testing are done prior to assembly.

A safety device that ensures the presence of oxygen and prevents the flow of nitrous oxide is tested by maintaining a negative pressure created by a squeeze bulb for more than 60 seconds. Nitrous oxide flow must begin before the oxygen pressure increases to 30 psig

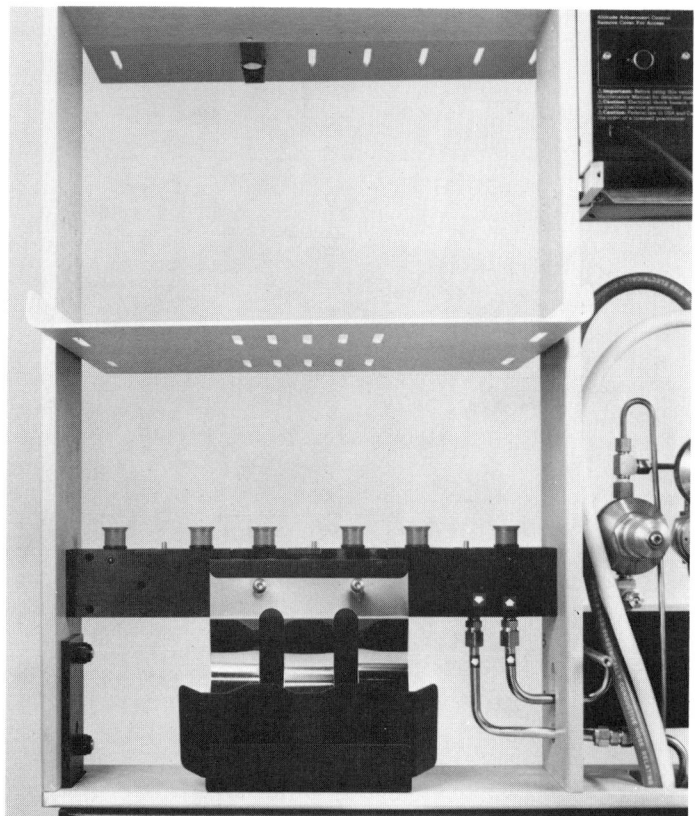

Fig. 2-10 Rear view of the anesthesia machine. On the right is the secondary oxygen regulator. The six "spool-like" forms shown are actually protective caps that cover the three vaporizer mounting positions during shipping. Monitor shelves have been added (station 3). (Courtesy of Ohmeda, The BOC Group, Inc.)

and stop before the oxygen pressure decreases to 20 psig.

Pressure regulators with gauges for oxygen, nitrous oxide, and a purchaser-selected gas (carbon dioxide, nitrogen, air, or helium) are mounted on the machine main frame (see Fig. 2-9). Low-pressure gauges for oxygen, nitrous oxide, and air are tested at 55 psig and high-pressure gauges for all gases are checked at 1,800 psig. The regulator outlet safety valve pressure is raised incrementally to 100 psig to make sure the valve does not open prior to 65 psig and is completely open at 75 psig. A continuous 1,800-psig pressure is then applied and observed for 1 hour to detect the presence of leaks. Cylinder pressure gauge readings may not drop by more than 100 psig and pipeline pressure gauge readings may not change by more than ±5 psig when confined to the machine circuit volume.

The vaporizer manifold, the upright, and the monitor shelf are attached to the main frame (see Fig. 2-10).

Station 4

A preassembled electrical pod that houses the oxygen analyzer, noninvasive blood pressure box, and the electrical controls of the ventilator is attached. The noninvasive blood pressure box or the Tyco sphygmomanometer box is placed in the designated area of the electrical pod (see Fig. 2-11). An additional shelf bracket, electrical wall cord, and an anesthetic agent bottle holder are added (Fig. 2-12). Microprocessor pods for the oxygen analyzer and volume monitor input are placed (Fig. 2-13).

A ventilator control box is mounted. The

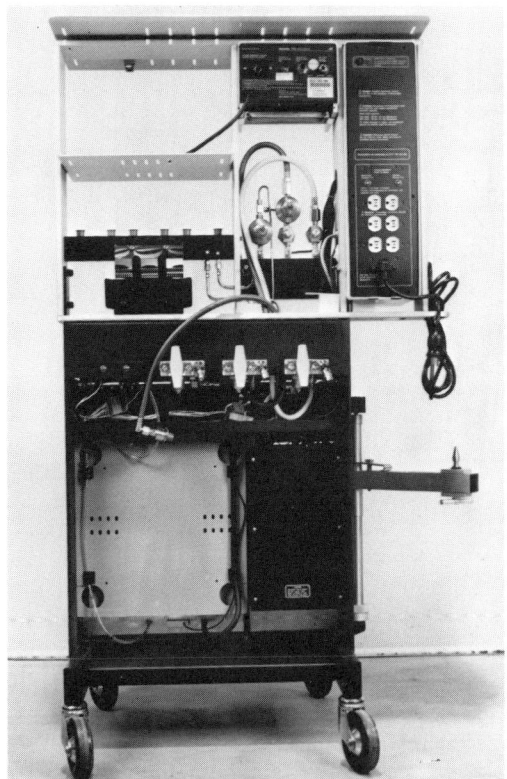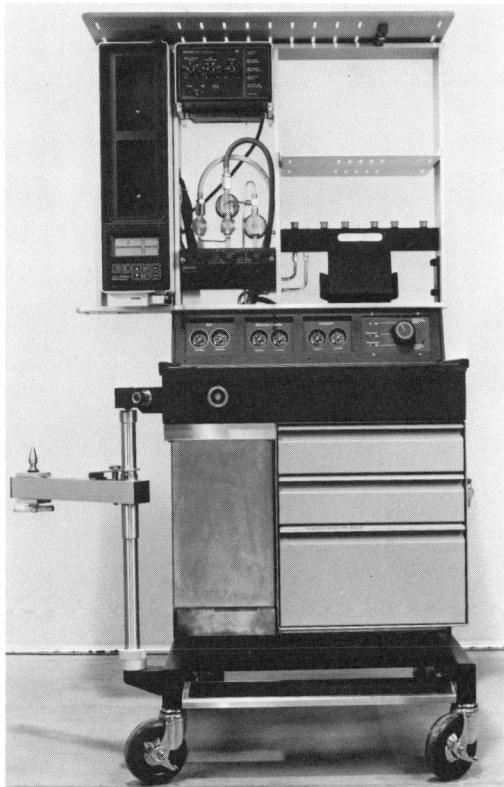

Fig. 2-11 Front and rear view of the anesthesia machine as it leaves Station 4. A ventilator control box is mounted directly above the gas regulators and to the right of the electrical pod when facing the front of the machine. The lower position in the electrical pod has been filled with an automatic noninvasive blood pressure monitor in this machine (station 4). (Courtesy of Ohmeda, The BOC Group, Inc.)

Fig. 2-12 Rear panel installation to the anesthesia machine. A storage rack for anesthetic agent bottles is attached. Cylinder supports are attached to the lower portion of the panel (station 4). (Courtesy of Ohmeda, The BOC Group, Inc.)

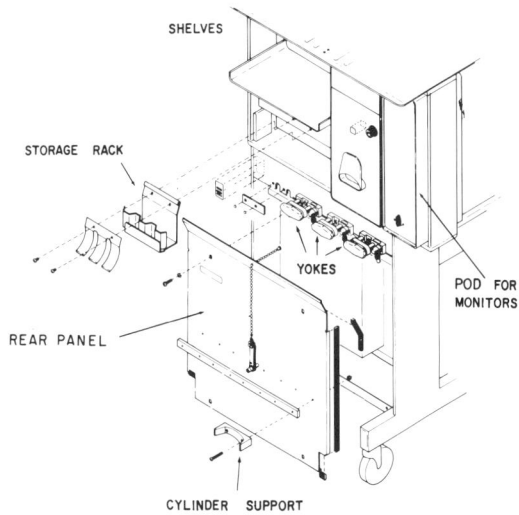

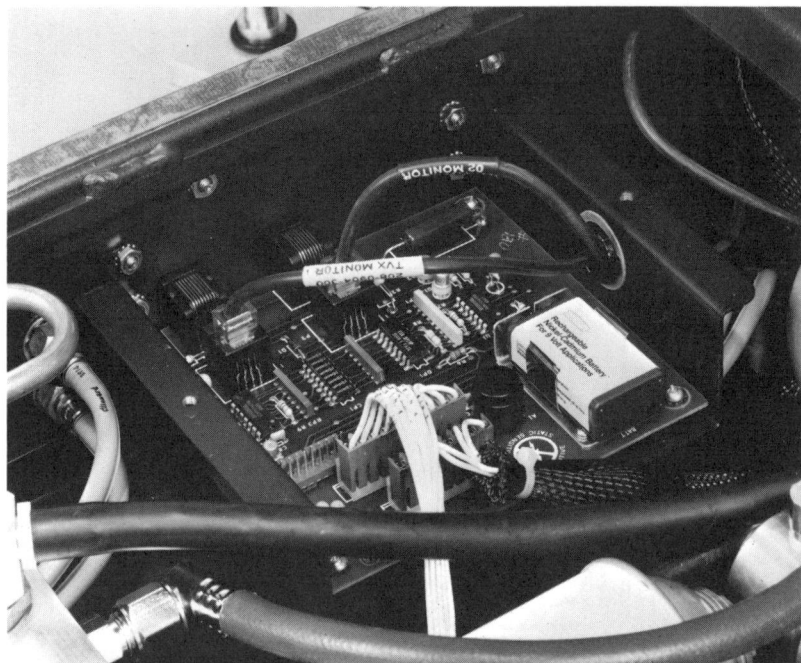

Fig. 2-13 Close-up view (underneath the table top) of the circuitry for providing alarm activation in the event of electrical power interruption. Note also the electrical interface connectors for the oxygen monitor and the volume monitor. For orientation, note the gas reservoir for the oxygen supply-failure alarm system on the bottom right (station 4). (Courtesy of Ohmeda, The BOC Group, Inc.)

ventilator was tested at another factory prior to installation. Electronic component reliability was determined by a burn-in period. A tub-shaped curve is a common characteristic of the life of electronic components (see Fig. 2-14). The highest rate of failure for electronic components occurs during the initial power up. However, once the components withstand the initial stress period, they can be expected to have a long life.

Routine electrical tests are performed on a number of additional elements: display voltage calibration, system and software clock, watchdog timer, audio oscillation, low minute volume alarm, alarm silence, high minute volume alarm, apnea alarm, minute volume accuracy, volume reverse flow alarm, microprocessor fail alarm, display, thumbwheel switch operation, mode switch, TVX transducer, undervoltage alarm, and external battery power switch.

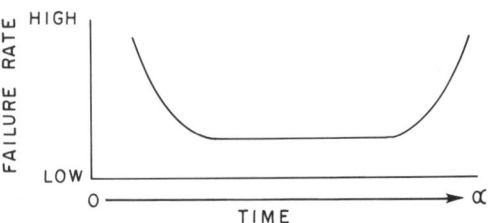

Fig. 2-14 The tub-shaped failure rate curve used for testing before shipment is characteristic of many electronic components. During the initial power-up (left-hand side of the curve) the rate of failure is greatest. Initial stressing ("burn in") can detect a large number of failures and insure an expected long life in those electronic components that survive. (Redrawn from photo, courtesy of Ohmeda, The BOC Group, Inc.)

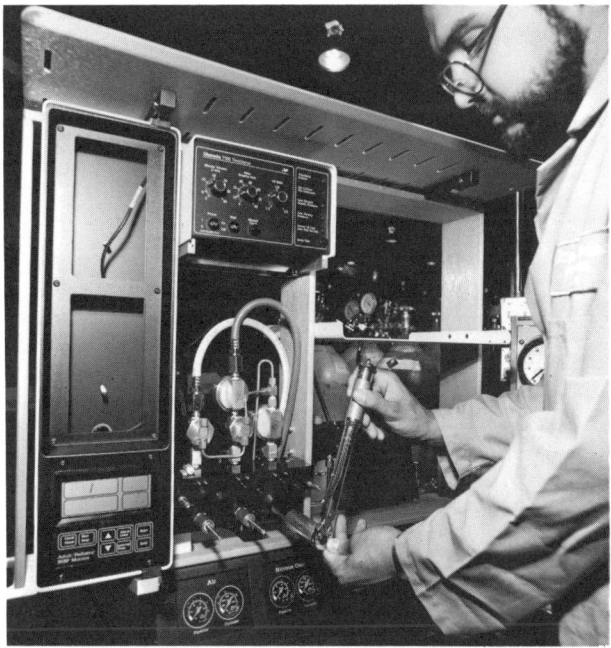

Fig. 2-15 Installation of the flow control valves (station 5). (Courtesy of Ohmeda, The BOC Group, Inc.)

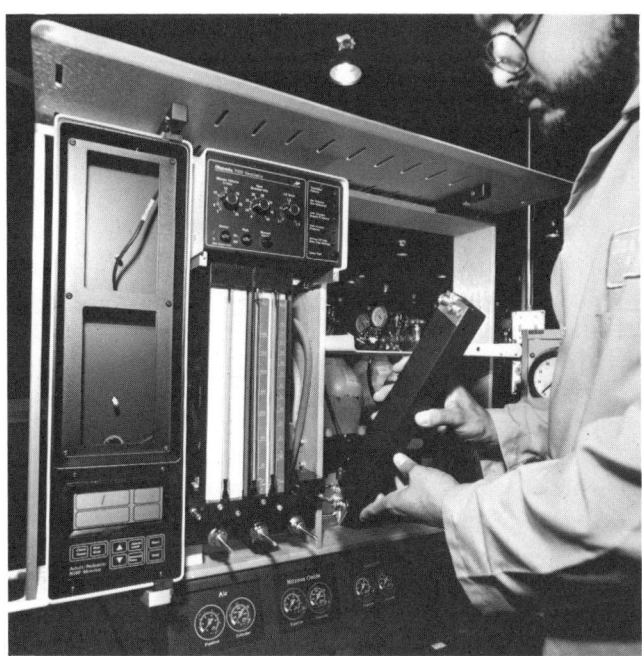

Fig. 2-16 Gas-specific pretested flowmeter modules are carefully placed in position (station 5). (Courtesy of Ohmeda, The BOC Group, Inc.)

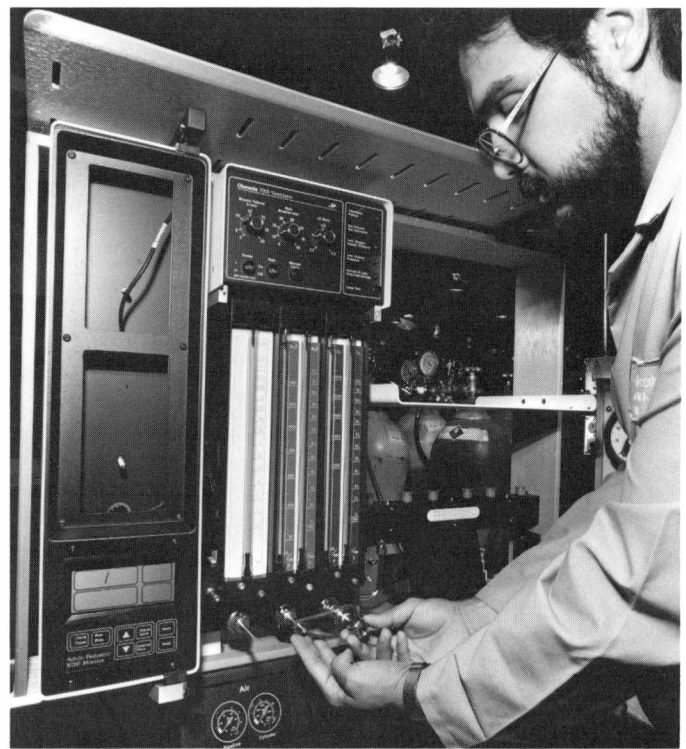

Fig. 2-17 Attachment of the Link-25 system between the nitrous oxide and oxygen flow control valves. The link system will maintain a minimum ratio of oxygen to nitrous oxide (station 5). (Courtesy of Ohmeda, The BOC Group, Inc.)

Station 5

Flowmeter needle valves are installed (Fig. 2-15) after they have been immersed in water and leak-tested at 20 psig. Previously calibrated flowmeters are then carefully installed (Fig. 2-16). Individual flowmeters have been previously calibrated to accuracies of ±2.5 percent at each individual scale mark. Each flowmeter is matched to a rotameter float and calibrated with the specific gas it will receive. Calibration is performed in a special, environmentally controlled room to maintain manufacturing constancy with changing ambient conditions. A link system (see Fig. 2-17) is attached between the nitrous oxide flowmeter needle valve and the oxygen flowmeter needle valve to maintain a minimum ratio of oxygen to nitrous oxide.

Additional electrical tests are performed on previously installed items. A dielectric test with 1,250 V for 60 to 65 seconds and a current leakage test are done to test electrical insulation properties. The alarm is checked to make sure that it sounds intermittently (3 seconds on and 12 seconds off). Back panel electrical outlets are checked for malfunction. The electrical failure/disconnect light must flash during simulated failures. The noninvasive blood pressure unit must beep within 30 seconds and the light-emitting diode (LED) hold must turn on. The ventilator unit must give the alarm by flashing the low oxygen supply pressure LED within 30 seconds. An additional test is done with the Norland Controller PMA9633.

The oxygen flush manifold is tested and calibrated. A seat leakage test, a manometer pressure test, and a check value test are then performed. A successful flow capacity test means an inlet pressure of less than 5 mmHg with a buzz or whistle at 30 ± 3 psig and a flow rate of 15 L/min. During the sealing qualities test no immediate rise in the pressure of the testing manometer at 1,000 ml/min is allowed. A leak test and a flow capacity test are done on the flush valve. The flush valve cannot have a leak greater than 0.003 L/min at 50 ± 3 psig. The oxygen flush button must activate a flow of 45 to 75 L/min.

Quality Assurance Station (Initial)

At the quality assurance station all the tests previously performed are repeated and confirmed (see Fig. 2-18).

Station 6

A noise level limit of 62 dB is checked on the oxygen loss alarm. The electrical integrity of the noninvasive blood pressure and ventilator control units is verified.

The following are then installed: tabletop, back panel, drawer tray, labels, air gauge window, flowmeter shields, cylinder wrench, and a protective cap for the fresh gas outlet. Owner's machine manuals are placed in the drawers, a paint touch-up is completed, and the machine is wiped clean. The anesthesia machine is now ready for the final quality assurance testing to be followed by packaging and shipping (Fig. 2-19).

Station 7

Before the serial and stock numbers are placed on the machine (Fig. 2-20), a final quality assurance check is done. Anesthesia machine manufacturers are required to maintain a record of each quality assurance test by machine serial number. Malfunctions which might occur during use can then be traced by component and compared to the original test results.

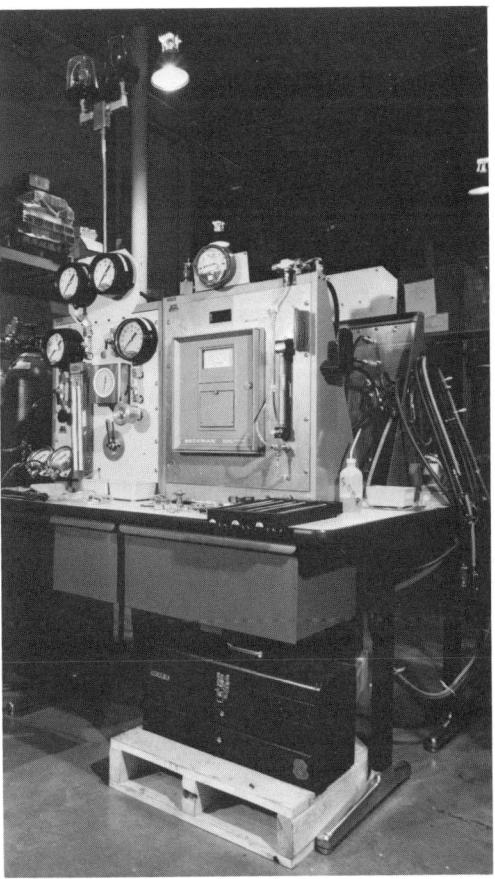

Fig. 2-18 Quality assurance testing apparatus, which is needed to test the assembled components up to Station 5. (Courtesy of Ohmeda, The BOC Group, Inc.)

The test and inspection assurance form lists criteria which each machine must meet before shipping and packing:

1. The master switch is turned to the electrical setting and the flowmeters turned on. No flow should be indicated on any flowmeter.
2. Leaks at low pressure are tested with a deflated bulb (cannot refill over 60 seconds).
3. The electrical "on" light must be on with 0 psig and the master switch on pneumatic.
4. Only oxygen should flow at 20 psig.
5. The oxygen supply pressure is activated.

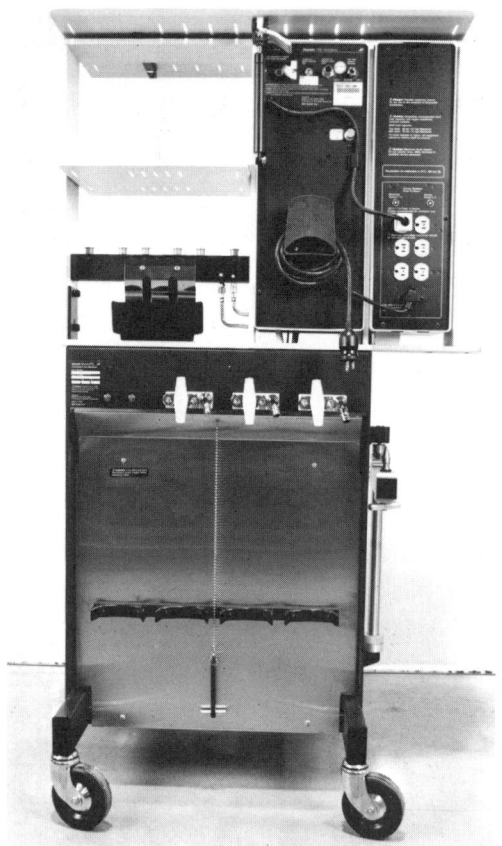 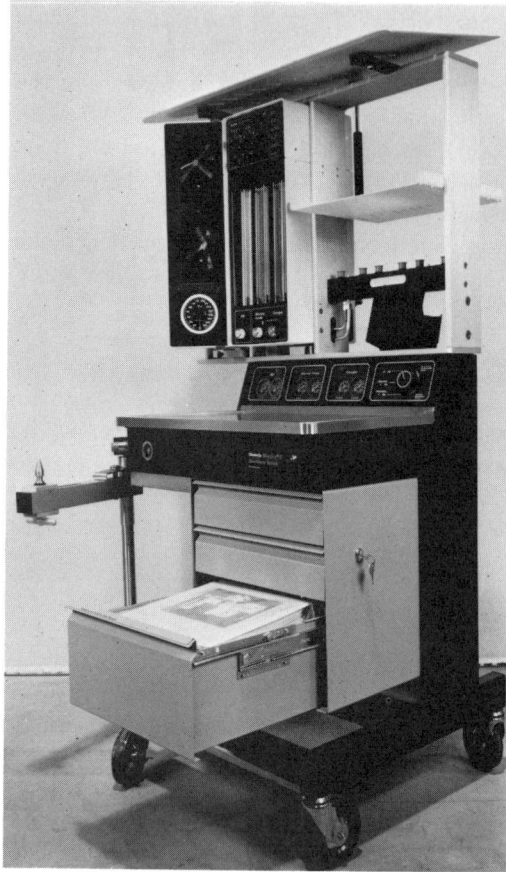

Fig. 2-19 Rear and front view of the anesthesia machine just prior to the final quality assurance testing. All the components installed at the factory are in place; additional accessories and/or monitors will be installed by service personnel at the hospital of purchase (station 6). (Courtesy of Ohmeda, The BOC Group, Inc.)

The oxygen supply failure alarm should stop between 28 and 33 psig, all gases begin to flow before 30 psig, and the light for pneumatic "on" activates between 34 and 39 psig.

6. Flow control valves must rotate smoothly, providing a uniform increase in flow, and at the stop position must flow between the maximum calibration mark and the top of the engraved scale.

7. Proportion-limiting control must provide 22 to 28.5 percent oxygen when oxygen is mixed with nitrous oxide at flows from 300 ml/min to 16 L/min.

8. Pressure should increase from 120 to 150 mmHg in the outlet relief valve.

9. A decrease in the oxygen pipeline supply pressure must turn the pneumatic "on" light out between 30 and 35 psig, the oxygen failure alarm sounds between 33 and 28 psig, and all gases except oxygen stop flowing before a pipeline pressure of 20 psig is reached.

10. The cylinder supply pressure must not fall by more than 2 psig in 120 seconds during the high-pressure leak test.

11. The electrical disconnect failure alarm must sound intermittently at 62 dB and the oxygen failure alarm should sound for more than 7 seconds at less than 62 dB.

12. The ventilator lamps should light and the nonvasive blood pressure unit switches be functional.

Packing and Shipping

The assembled anesthesia machine is bolted to a prefabricated shipping crate. Before the crate is sealed and shipped, the following pre-packaged items are added:

Specific agent vaporizers which are factory-tested by Cyprane in Leeds, England, and re-checked by Ohmeda, Madison.

The *carbon dioxide absorber*, packaged after testing. The selector valve of the absorber must not leak by more than one bubble in 30 seconds at 60 cmH_2O. At a flow rate of 100 ml/min the entire absorber system should read and hold over 30 cmH_2O in "bag and vent" mode. An incline manometer must read between 1 and 5 cmH_2O of pressure at 30 L/min when testing the adjustable pressure-limiting (APL) or pop-off valve. The maximum APL setting on the incline manometer must be between 72 and 78 cmH_2O at 3 to 30 L/min. No leak above 30 cmH_2O at 100 ml/min can occur during the APL leak test. No oscillation noise is allowed in the APL valve at a flow rate of 6 L/min when the reservoir bag is being squeezed.

An *oxygen analyzer kit*, which connects to the electrical component of the electrical pod. The chemical detector head of the oxygen analyzer is purchased from an outside vendor. Testing of the oxygen analyzer consists of verifying switch and functions and the limits for the high- and low-limit switch settings.

A *volume monitor kit*, which consists of a flow transducer cartridge clip and a flow transducer cartridge. The flow transducer cartridge clip must meet rigid output voltage, output timing, and heater continuity standards. Disposable flow transducer cartridges must (1) measure flow in 22 mm outer diameter to 22 mm inner diameter direction, (2) have a reso-

lution of 0.4 percent and an accuracy of ±0.4 percent of the reading during frequency measurements, and (3) must remain within limits at flow inputs of 6 ± 2, 30 ± 2, and 60 ± 2 L/min.

The remaining kits necessary for a complete anesthesia machine are a *vacuum regulator and a wall slide, ventilator housing, basic parts, a Tycos blood pressure monitor cuff and inflation bulb, a noninvasive blood pressure cuff and hoses, and a gas scavenger.*

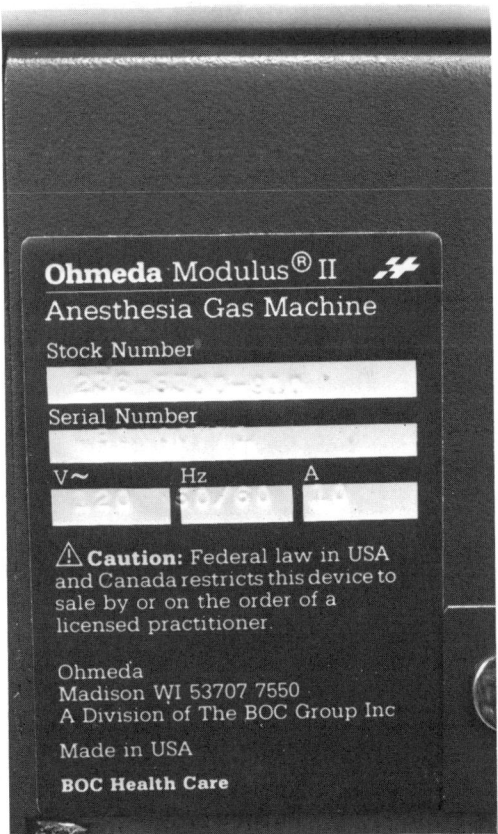

Fig. 2-20 Rating plate placed after the anesthesia machine has successfully passed the final quality assurance tests. Each machine has a serial and stock number, which are used for reference by both the operator and the manufacturer (station 7). (Courtesy of Ohmeda, The BOC Group, Inc.)

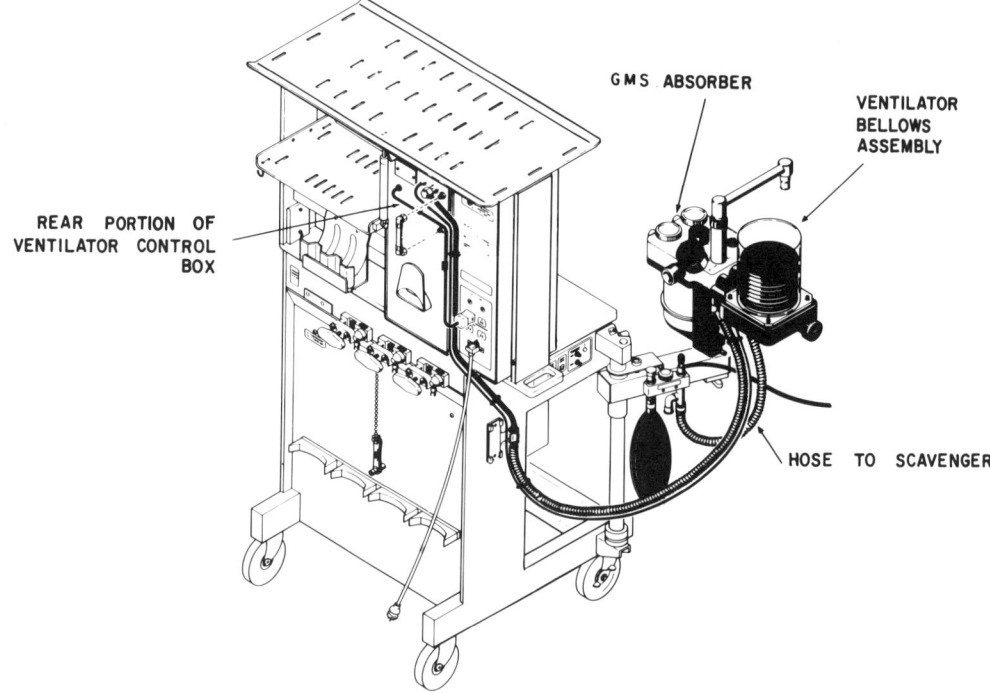

REAR PORTION OF
VENTILATOR CONTROL
BOX

GMS ABSORBER

VENTILATOR
BELLOWS
ASSEMBLY

HOSE TO SCAVENGER

Fig. 2-21 Assembly of the ventilator and the GMS absorber at the hospital. (Courtesy of Ohmeda, The BOC Group, Inc.)

ON-SITE ASSEMBLY AND CALIBRATION

Factory-trained service personnel unpack the anesthesia machine at the site and begin the final assembly (Fig. 2-21). A number of items are verified: (1) adequate pipeline supply, reserve cylinder supply, and vacuum source, (2) integrity of low-pressure gas circuitry, (3) proper functioning of electrical systems and gas flow control systems, and (4) integrity and proper functioning of gas-scavenging interface valve. Prior to turning the anesthesia machine over to the anesthesiologist, specific detailed testing is done on the absorber, vaporizers, ventilator, oxygen monitor, and volume monitor. As an example of the detail involved in testing, the following are requirements for checking the oxygen monitor.

1. Verify the battery power switch is set to the "O (off)" position.

2. Verify the proper connection of the sensor to the anesthesia machine.

3. Verify the monitor is operational when the "systems master" switch is turned to the "1 (on)" position.

4. Depress the "circuit test" switch. The display must read between 99 and 100.

5. Calibrate to 21 percent in room air. Turn the "low O_2" alarm adjustment to 22 percent. The alarm must sound. Set "low O_2" to below 21 percent and turn the "high O_2" alarm adjustment to 20 percent. The alarm must sound.

6. Calibrate to 99 percent. The display must return to 21 ± 1 percent within 3 minutes after returning to room air.

7. If the unit will not calibrate at either 21 or 99 percent, place the "probe select"

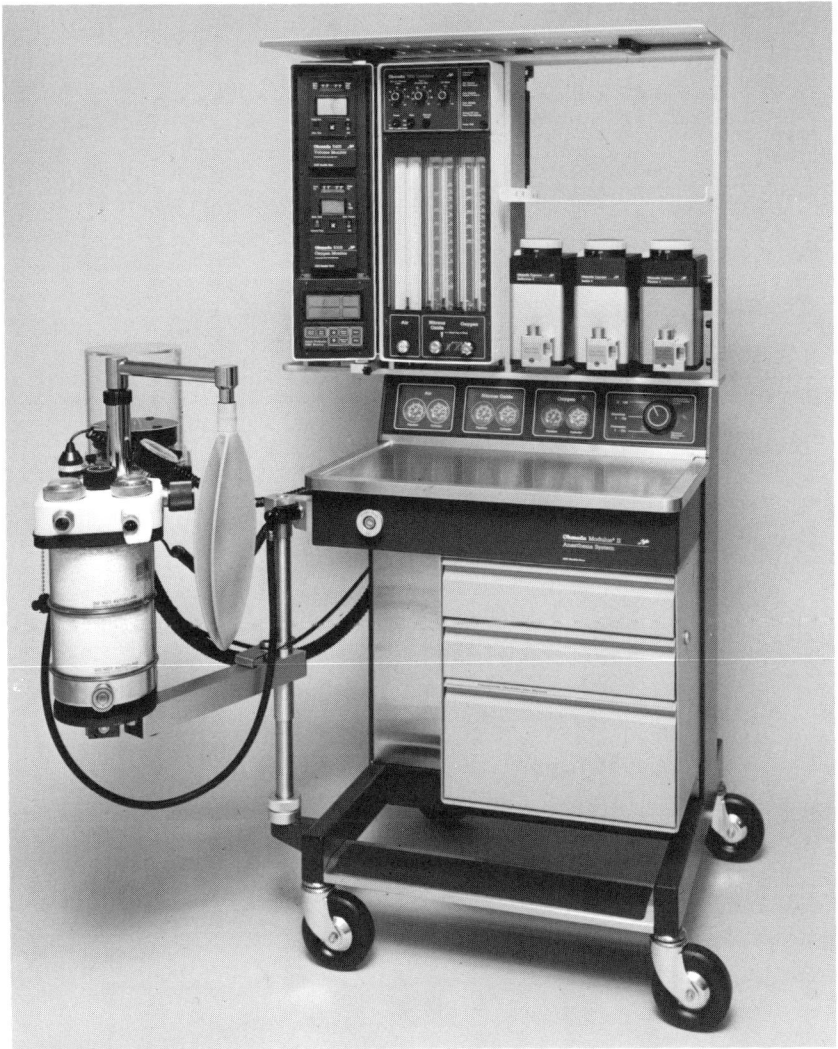

Fig. 2-22 Anesthesia machine assembled at the hospital, inspected, and ready to be turned over to the anesthesiologist. (Courtesy of Ohmeda, The BOC Group, Inc.)

switch to the alternate position and recalibrate. Replace the probe cartridge if the probe will not calibrate.

8. Set the desired "high O_2" and "low O_2" alarm limits.

When certification is completed, the anesthesia machine is placed in the hands of the anesthesiologist (see Fig. 2-22). In-service sessions on the anesthesia machine by the factory service personnel are imperative.

Anesthesia machines are vital to our specialty. They must be accurate, dependable, and safe. Only individuals familiar with the intricacies of anesthesia should attempt to utilize the anesthesia machine. When administering an anesthetic it is reassuring to know the machine has been subjected to quality control and that preventive maintenance is being performed by a factory-certified serviceman.

3

Flowmeters

Flowmeters have been an integral part of anesthesia machines since the advent of mixed gases and vaporizers. The development of accurate, reliable, dry gas flowmeters has been a long process learned through the application of gas laws to clinical requirements. Gas flows are required through a range of 200 ml/min to 15 L/min. Anesthesia machines can presently be purchased with a combination of oxygen, nitrous oxide, air, helium, nitrogen, and carbon dioxide. Each gas requires a specific flowmeter tube and float selected on the basis of the physical characteristics of the gas. Figure 3-1 illustrates a typical flowmeter assembly containing a flow tube, float, flow control knob, and housing.

Dry gas flowmeters are tapered glass tubes which have a larger diameter at the top than at the bottom (see Fig. 3-2). Gas enters the bottom of the tube and emerges at the top. A rotating float, or bobbin, is lifted by the gas until an equilibrium is reached between the upward pressure created by gas escaping around the float and the weight of the float. The higher the float rises in the tube, the greater the gas flow around it.

The annular space between the head of the float and the wall of the tube acts like a circular constriction channel (see Fig. 3-3).[1] When the float lies low in the tube, the circular channel functions as an orifice, with the *viscosity* of the gas the main determinant of gas flow rate. *Density* becomes the major factor in gas flow rate when the float rises to higher levels in the tube, where the circular channel functions as a tubular constriction.[2] Figure 3-4 illustrates the effects of viscosity and density on the flow rate of two gases with very similar viscosities but markedly different densities. Helium first passes through a flowmeter tube and float designed for helium and then into a flowmeter and float designed for oxygen. At a flow rate of 500 ml/min both flowmeters read the same, because helium and oxygen have similar viscosities and the orificelike constriction is viscosity dependent; however, when the flow rate is 20 L/min in the helium flowmeter, the oxygen flowmeter reads only 10 L/min, because high flow rates are density dependent. Gases cannot be interchanged in flowmeters requiring variable flow rates.

The *float,* or bobbin, is usually made of aluminum with a large head, round body, and tapered tip (see Fig. 3-3). Channels are cut in the body of the float so the gas will twirl the float as it rises in the tube. The spinning float rotates in the center of the tube when the tube is perpendicular. A round ball float

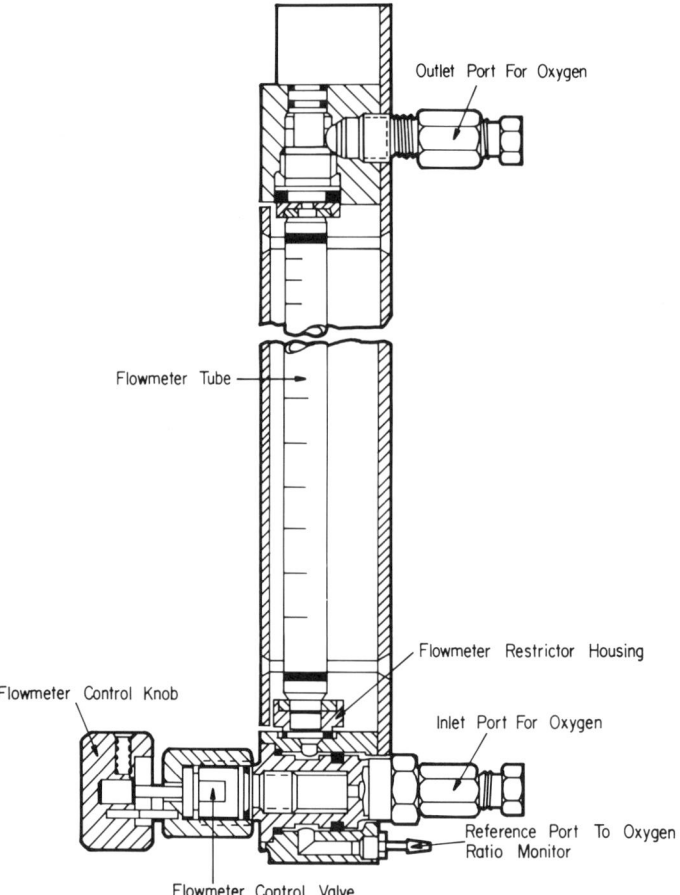

Outlet Port For Oxygen

Flowmeter Tube

Flowmeter Restrictor Housing

Flowmeter Control Knob

Inlet Port For Oxygen

Reference Port To Oxygen Ratio Monitor

Flowmeter Control Valve

Fig. 3-1 Side view of an oxygen flowmeter assembly module. The flowmeter resistor reduces the pipeline pressure from 40 to 48 psig to 15 to 20 psig. (Adapted from Drager IIA Parts Manual, North American Drager, Telford, PA, 1984.)

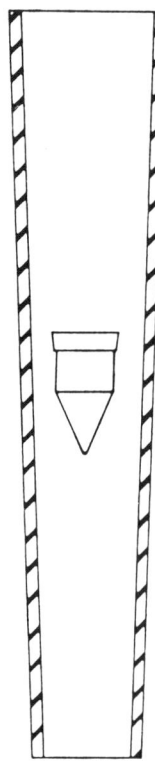

Fig. 3-2 A typical flowmeter tube and float. Note the tapered tube with a larger diameter at the top than the bottom. (Schreiber P: Anaesthesia Equipment: Performance, Classification and Safety. Springer-Verlag, New York, 1972.)

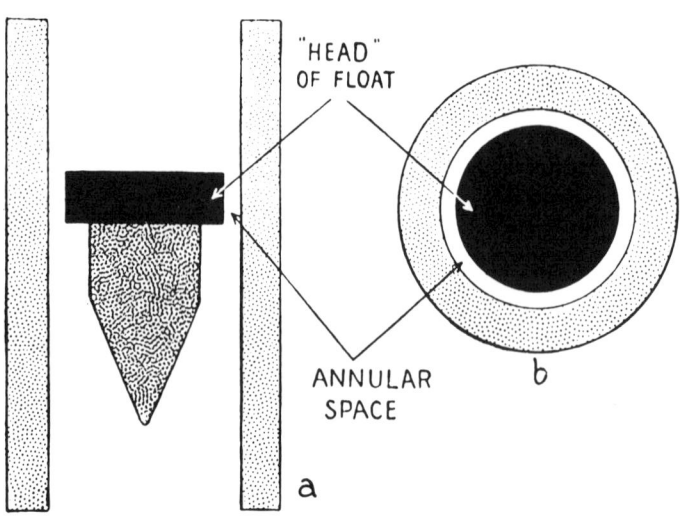

"HEAD" OF FLOAT

ANNULAR SPACE

a

b

Fig. 3-3 Circular constriction channel in the annular space between the float head and the flowmeter tube wall: (a) side view and (b) top view. In a well-functioning flowmeter the float spins effortlessly in the center of the flowmeter tube. (Macintosh R, Mushin WW, Epstein HG: Physics for the Anaesthetist. 3rd Ed. Blackwell, Oxford, 1963.)

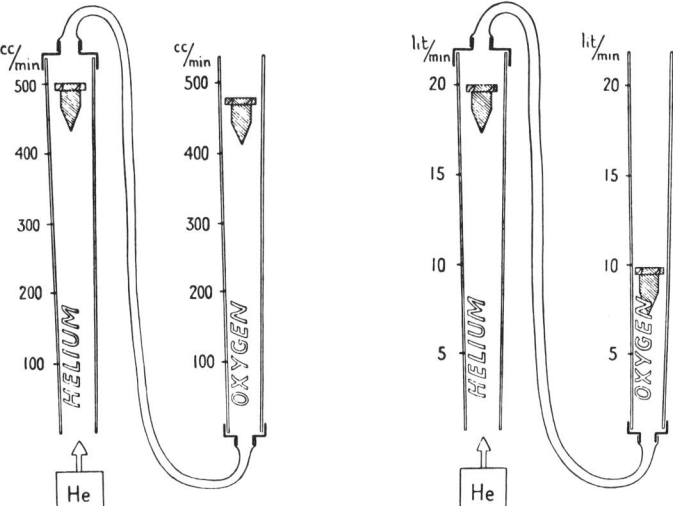

Fig. 3-4 Effects of density and viscosity on the flow rates of helium and oxygen in flowmeters. Helium and oxygen have similar viscosities but very different densities. Viscosity effects predominate at low flow rates while density effects predominate at high flows. The flowmeter on the left illustrates equal flow rates during low-flow settings. The flowmeter on the right shows the marked difference in flow rates at high-flow settings. (Macintosh R, Mushin WW, Epstein HG: Physics for the Anaesthetist. 3rd Ed. Blackwell, Oxford, 1963.)

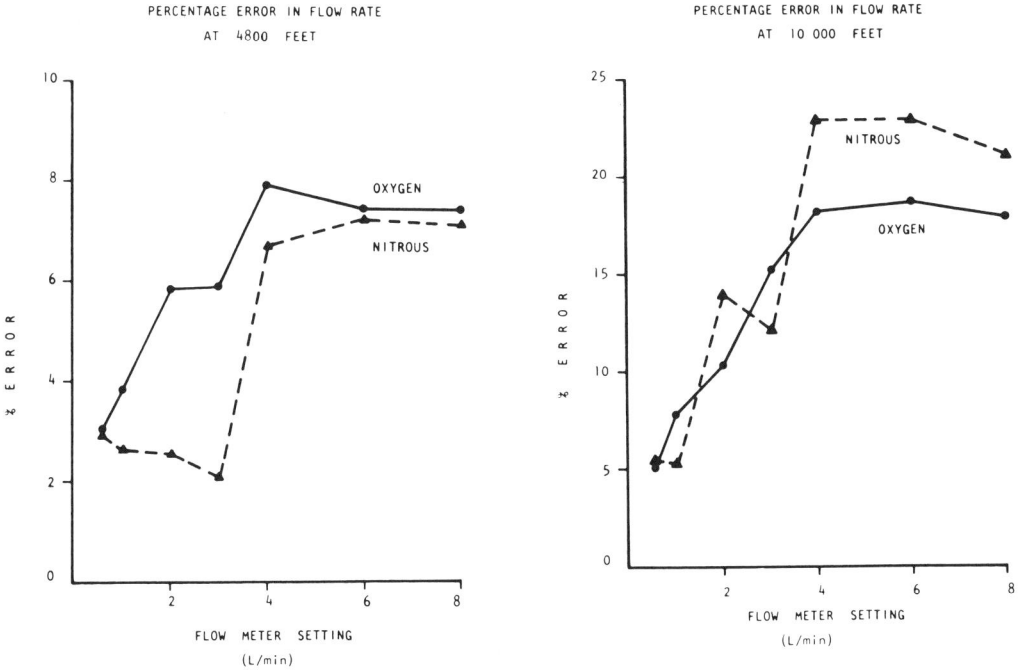

Fig. 3-5 Effect of altitude on flowmeters. At 4,800 ft (barometric pressure of 84.8 kPa, or 643 mmHg) only a small difference is noted between the set and delivered flow rates. In contrast, at 10,000 ft (barometric pressure 69.0 kPa, or 512 mmHg) an error of 22 percent is possible. (James MFM, White JF: Anesthetic considerations at moderate altitude. Anesth Analg 63:1097, 1984. Reprinted with permission, the International Anesthesia Research Society.)

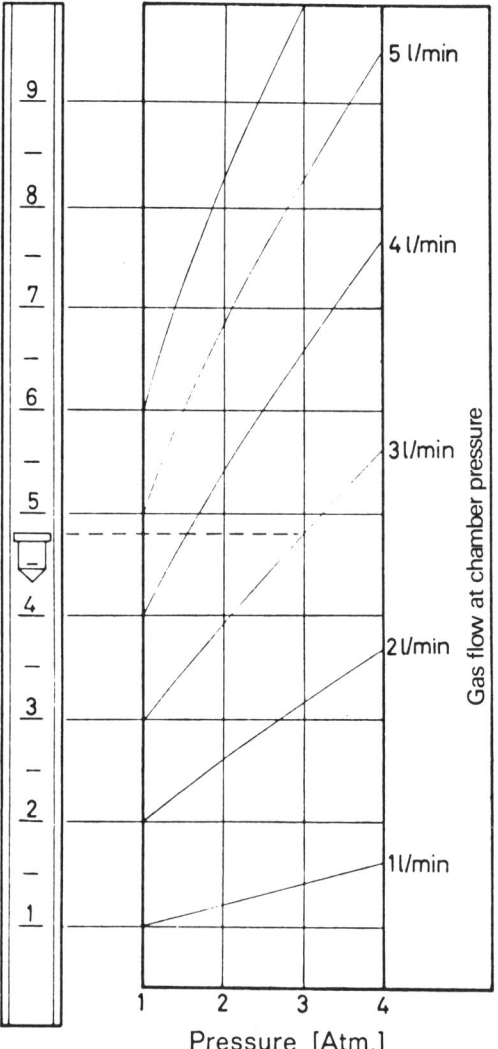

Fig. 3-6 Flowmeter function in a hyperbaric chamber. The top of the float is set to deliver 4.8 L/min but the actual measured flow at a pressure of 3 atm is only 3.0 L/min. (Schreiber P: Anaesthesia Equipment: Performance, Classification and Safety. Springer-Verlag, New York, 1972.)

is less affected by a vertical position.[1] Some ball floats are designed to be used in any flow tube.

Barometric pressure will affect the calibration of the flowmeter. Flowmeters are usually calibrated for 20°C and 760 mmHg. Density is altitude dependent, and viscosity is altitude independent. Indeed, at barometric

pressures below 630 mmHg the delivered flow rate exceeds the set flow rates by 9 to 20 percent (see Fig. 3-5).[3, 4] Conversely, in a hyperbaric chamber the flowmeter will deliver less gas than the flowmeter setting. At a pressure of 3 atm (2280 mmHg) a flowmeter set at 4.8 L/min will deliver only 3 L/min (see Fig. 3-6).[1]

CALIBRATION

A matched flowmeter tube and float are calibrated against a master flowmeter for each specific gas. In turn, master flowmeters are calibrated with a bubble meter[5-8] similar to the one depicted in Figure 3-7. Any burette

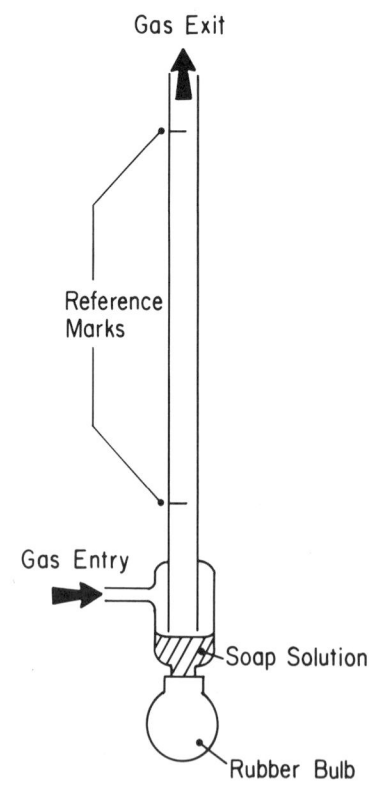

Fig. 3-7 A basic bubble meter used to accurately calibrate a flowmeter. See text for description. (Levy A: The accuracy of the bubble meter method for gas flow measurements. J Sci Instrum 41:449, 1964.)

can be used for the main tube. Etched reference marks in the glass represent the exact water volume, measured by weighing the water displaced between the two marks. A high-sudsing dishwashing detergent is placed in the rubber reservoir bulb.[7] Gas flowing into the bottom of the tube passes over the surface of the soap solution. Once the flow is stabilized, a gentle squeeze of the rubber bulb coats the throat of the upright tube with a soap film bubble which is gently pushed up the tube. As the soap bubble passes the first reference mark a stopwatch is started. The bubble's transit time between the two reference marks is used to calculate the gas flow rate in liters per minute. Meticulous attention to theoretical considerations can result in an accuracy of 0.25 percent for measurements of flow rates[5] between 6 and 6,000 cc/min. A simple bubble burette with an error of less than 2 percent can be constructed from common laboratory parts. Error can be further reduced to less than 0.1 percent by careful repeat measurements and matching the burette volume gas flow rate.[7]

Four to six flowmeters can be calibrated with a homemade bubble burette in 10 to 15 minutes. Such an apparatus could be useful in an anesthesia department where machines are moved constantly. A flowmeter, which flows into a copper kettle, must be drained prior to calibration, because any residual liquid anesthetic will react with the soap bubble and create poor bubbling.[7] Commercial flowmeter devices (Fig. 3-8) similar to master flowmeters are available. These instruments are not accurate enough for precise calibration but can serve to spot-check flowmeters. Measured gas flows are compared against a calibration chart to determine the correct gas flow rate.[9] A rough check of flowmeter accuracy can also be done by testing gas mixtures with a calibrated oxygen sensor. The oxygen and nitrous oxide flowmeters are each set at 2.5 L/min and the oxygen sensor should read 50 percent oxygen. This check does not replace accurate measurements but should show consistent readings at commonly used flow rates.

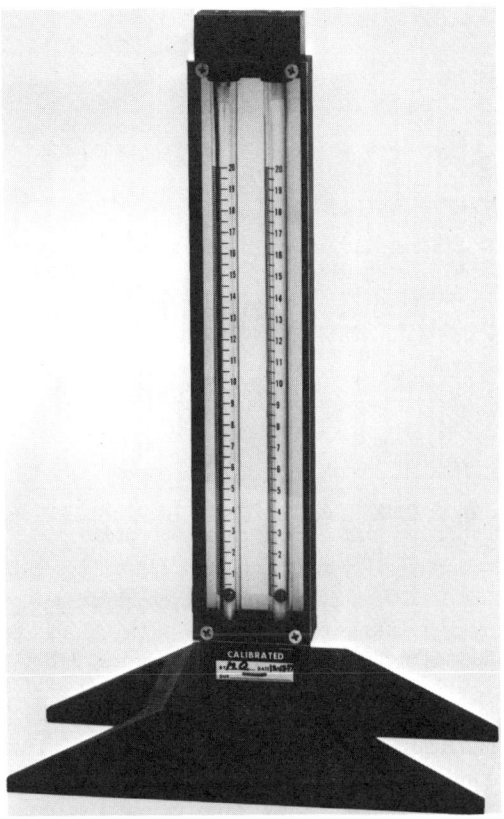

Fig. 3-8 Flowmeter verification device. Accuracy can be checked frequently but the device cannot be used for precision calibration. (Courtesy of Ohmeda, WI. The BOC Group, Inc.)

ACCURACY

Five new flowmeter units were examined by Waaben et al.[8, 10] with the bubble meter method. Measurements were taken from low-flow (0 to 500 cc/min) and high-flow (1 to 10 L/min) oxygen flowmeters. Pronounced deviations, up to 70 percent, were found at oxygen settings of less than 1 L/min (see Fig. 3-9).[8, 11] At flows between 1 and 5 L/min the indicated flow rate was within 5 percent of the measured flow rate. Older oxygen flowmeters were even less accurate (see Table 3-1). A survey[6] of 60 used copper kettle vaporizer flowmeters found an average error of 20 percent.[6] The percent error is indirectly proportional to the flow rate, that is, as the flow

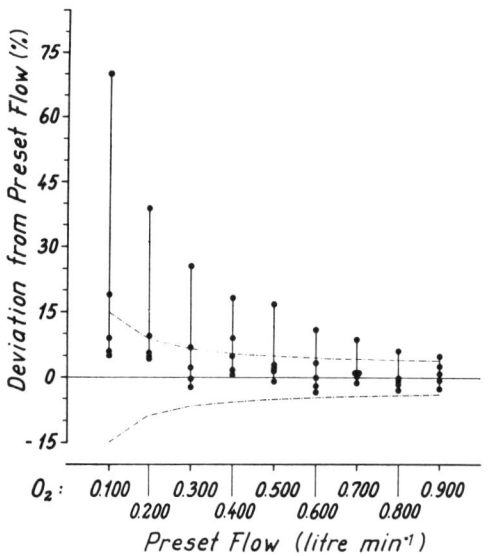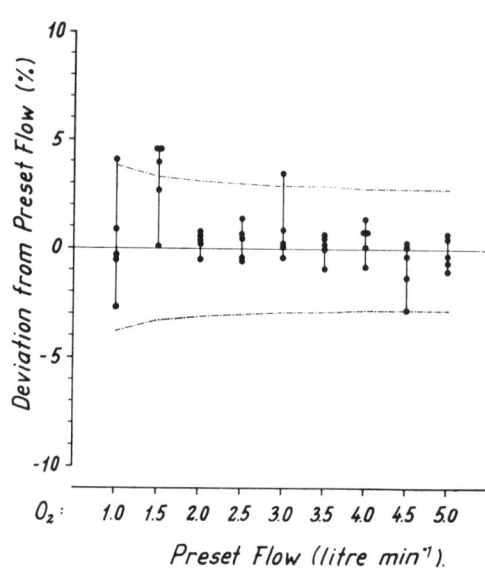

Fig. 3-9 Accuracy of five new oxygen flowmeters. The diagram on the left illustrates the marked deviation from presettings of the low-flow meter. At high flows the flowmeters were within 5 percent of indicated flows. (Waaben J, Brinklov MM, Stokke DB: Accuracy of new gas flowmeters. Br J Anaesth 52:97, 1980.)

increases, the percent error decreases. The clinical significance of flowmeter error[6] becomes evident at flow rates below 1 L/min. During closed-circuit or low-flow anesthesia it is paramount to measure the oxygen concentration in order to avoid hypoxic mixtures from inaccurate flowmeters.[10]

Flowmeter output can be altered by static electricity when a metal float rotameter is used. Static electricity accumulates over a period of days or sometimes in a matter of minutes. Minor movements of the anesthesia machine, that is, during 45 seconds of anesthesia record charting, or ventilator vibration, can

cause build up.[12] Gently rubbing the outside of the flowmeter tube will cause the float to stick and can easily generate a charge of 20,000 V with an energy of 200 μJ. A stoichiometric mixture of cyclopropane and oxygen will ignite at 1 μJ. At least one anesthetic explosion has been attributed to the static electrical charge created in the flowmeter.[13] Spraying the outside and/or inside of the flowmeter tube with an antistatic chemical can stop charge buildup for weeks to months.[12, 14] Natural radiation in the operating room will remove the charge very slowly over a period of days.[12] Sometimes placing a moist fingertip

Table 3-1. Percent of Observations Exceeding the Calibration
Limits for New and Old Oxygen Flowmeters

Gas and Flow Rate	Calibration Limits	Percent of Observations Exceeding Calibration Limits	
		New Flowmeters	Old Flowmeters
Oxygen, 100-900 cc/min	5% indicated flow	35.5	71.9
Oxygen, 1.5 L/min	5% indicated flow	0.0	12.6

(Waaben J., Brinklov M. M., Stokke D. B.: Accuracy of new gas flowmeters. Br J Anaesth 52:97, 1980.)

on the flow tube and the anesthesia machine metal at the same time will provide provisional grounding of the charge.[14] Ball floats made of sapphire or glass do not seem to build up static electrical charge.

Dirt in the flow tube can easily cause inaccuracies. A small filter placed in the restrictor housing of the flowmeter assembly will help alleviate this problem. Compressed air is especially prone to have small particles of dirt in the gas.

Mistakes in the replacement of flowmeter tubes and floats can cause large errors in flow rates. One replacement for a flowmeter tube, scale, and float was found to deliver 1,500 cc/min when set to deliver only 250 cc/min; this flowmeter was connected to the Vernitrol and could have easily resulted in a serious anesthetic overdose.[15] Fortunately, the mistake was discovered just prior to the administration of the first anesthetic from the repaired machine.

Flowmeter accuracy and safety can be maintained by making sure the flowmeters are perpendicular, the floats are spinning freely, only qualified service personnel maintain the anesthesia machine, and circuit oxygen is analyzed during low-flow techniques.

FEATURES

Separate flowmeters for high- and low-flow oxygen resulted in an anoxic death when the low-oxygen flowmeter was used with the high-nitrous oxide flowmeter in a circuit without an oxygen analyzer.[16] One interim solution to this problem is to make guards for the low-flow meters.[17] However, the best solution is to arrange the flowmeters in tandem as illustrated in Figure 3-10, with one flowmeter knob controlling the flow through both tubes.

Flowmeter knobs are needle valves (see Fig. 3-11) which allow the gas entering the flowme-

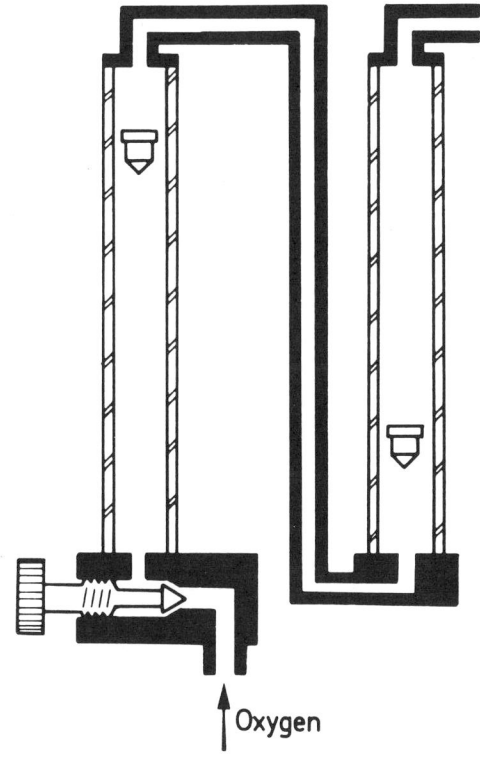

Fig. 3-10 Low- and high-oxygen flowmeters arranged in tandem. A single flowmeter knob controls the oxygen flow rate. (Schreiber P: Anaesthesia Equipment: Performance, Classification and Safety. Springer-Verlag, New York, 1972.)

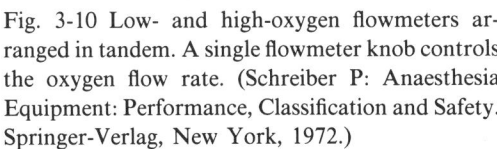

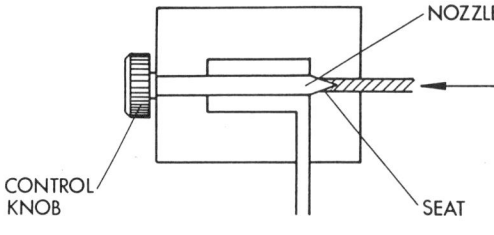

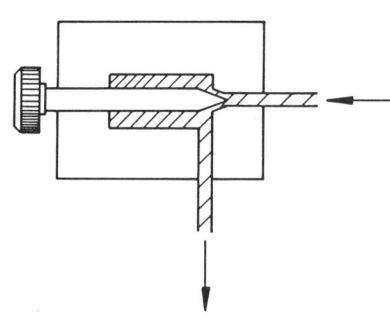

Fig. 3-11 Flowmeter knob needle valve. (Courtesy of North American Drager, Telford, PA.)

ter tube to be precisely controlled. Each knob is color coded for the gas it controls, for example, green for oxygen and blue for nitrous oxide. The oxygen knob has a distinct shape (see Fig. 3-12) which sets it apart from all other knobs. This touch identification safety feature can alert the anesthesiologist when oxygen flow rates are being changed.[18-20] Gas flow is increased by turning the flowmeter knob clockwise. Flowmeter control knobs are delicate instruments which can be easily damaged if excessive force is applied when shutting off the gas flow.

The oxygen flowmeter is always the first gas on the right side of the flowmeter bank as the anesthesiologist faces the machine. Identical positioning of the critical oxygen flowmeter on all anesthesia machines is another attempt to eliminate factors contributing to human error.

Flowmeters can even be pin-indexed in a manner similar to the system used for the cyl-

inder yokes. Figure 3-13 shows the pin index as described by the American National Standards Institute (ANSI)[18] for single and double flowmeters. This eliminates the possibility of installing a flowmeter calibrated for nitrous oxide in place of an oxygen flowmeter.

Minimal oxygen flow is provided by an adjustable stop on the oxygen flowmeter control knob. An oxygen flow of 200 to 300 cc/min is maintained when the flowmeter control knob is turned completely counterclockwise. Provision of a low oxygen flow is an attempt to meet the requirements for the minimal oxygen consumption of the patient. On the Drager Narkomed IIA anesthesia machine the minimal oxygen flow feature is disabled when the air flowmeter is activated.

Flowmeter lights are featured as a option on the anesthesia machine. Safety is increased in those cases which require the operating room lights to be dimmed or turned off. The hazards and inconvenience of checking the flowmeters in a dark room with only a flashlight are eliminated.

Flowmeter tubes are protected by a plastic shield. Individual flowmeter knob controls can also be protected with a bar extending in front of the knobs but still allowing access.

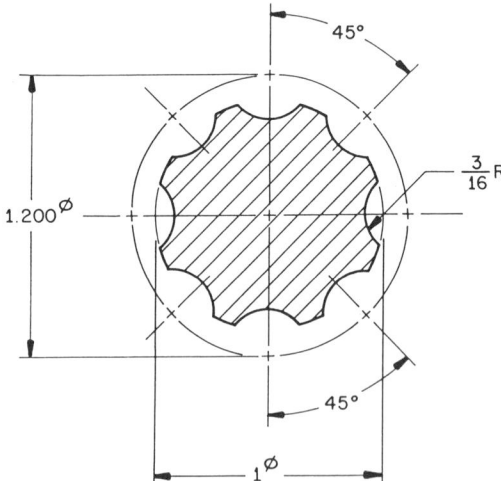

Fig. 3-12 Design of the oxygen touch-control flowmeter knob. (Schreiber P: Safety Guidelines—Anesthesia Systems. North American Drager, Boston 1984.)

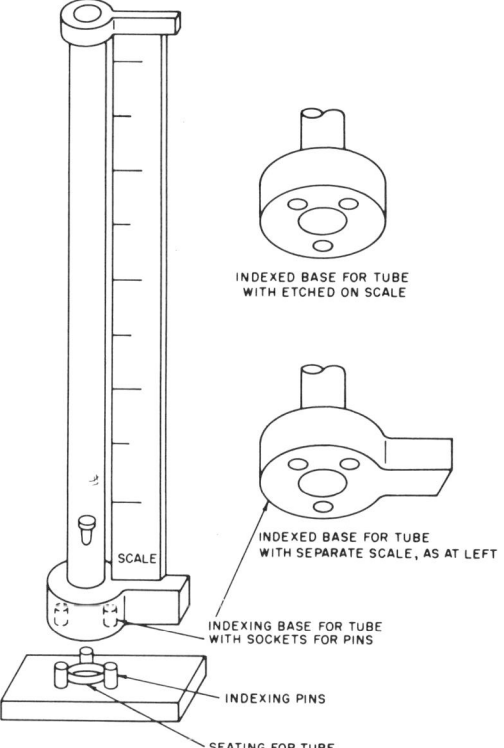

INDEXED BASE FOR TUBE
WITH ETCHED ON SCALE

INDEXED BASE FOR TUBE
WITH SEPARATE SCALE, AS AT LEFT

SCALE

INDEXING BASE FOR TUBE
WITH SOCKETS FOR PINS

INDEXING PINS

SEATING FOR TUBE

Fig. 3-13 Pin index system for flowmeters. Each gas is assigned a specific matching sequence for index pins and sockets. (This material is reproduced with permission from American National Standard Z79.8-1979, © 1979 The American National Standards Institute. Copies of this standard may be purchased from ANSI, 1430 Broadway, New York NY 10018.)

REFERENCES

1. Schreiber P: Anaesthesia Equipment: Performance, Classification and Safety. Springer-Verlag, New York, 1972
2. Macintosh R, Mushin WW, Epstein HG: Physics for the Anaesthetist. 3rd Ed. Blackwell, Oxford, 1963
3. Friedman J, Lightstone PJ: The effect of high altitude on flowmeter performance. Anesthesiology 55:A117, 1981
4. James MFM, White JF: Anesthetic considerations at moderate altitude. Anesth Analg 63:1097, 1984
5. Levy A: The accuracy of the bubble meter method for gas flow measurements. J Sci Instrum 41:449, 1964
6. Sadove MS, Thomason RD, Thomason CL, Ries M: An evaluation of flowmeters. J Am Assoc Nurse Anesth 45:162, 1976
7. Smith TC: Calibration of gas flowmeters with the bubble burette. Anesthesiology 33:553, 1970
8. Waaben J, Stokke DB, Brinklov MM: Accuracy of gas flowmeters determined by the bubble meter method. Br J Anaesth 50:1251, 1978
9. Flowmeter verification device. Operation maintenance manual. Stock #178-1652-001. Ohio Medical Products (Ohmeda), Madison, 1981
10. Waaben J, Brinklov MM, Stokke DB: Accuracy of new gas flowmeters. Br J Anaesth 52:97, 1980
11. Hodge EA, Waaben J, Stokke DB et al: Accuracy of anaesthetic gas flowmeters. Br J Anaesth 51:907, 1979
12. Clutton-Brock J: Static electricity and rotameters. Br J Anaesth 44:86, 1972
13. Masson AHB: Anaesthetic explosions. Anaesthesia 20:95, 1965
14. Hagelsten JO, Larsen OS: Inaccuracy of anaesthetic flowmeters caused by static electricity. Br J Anaesth 37:637, 1965
15. Kelley JM, Gabel RA: The improperly calibrated flowmeter—another hazard. Anesthesiology 32:467, 1970
16. Mazze RI: Therapeutic misadventures with oxygen delivery systems: the need for continuous in-line oxygen monitors. Anesth Analg 51:787, 1972
17. Rendell-Baker L, Klein OL, Charles P: Hazard of separate low and high flow O_2 flowmeters: an interim solution. Anesthesiology 56:155, 1982
18. American National Standard: Minimum performance and safety requirements for components and systems of continuous-flow anesthesia machines for human use. Z79.8-1979. American National Standards Institute, New York, 1979
19. Calverley RK: A safety feature for anaesthetic machines—touch identification of oxygen flow control. Can Anaesth Soc J 18:225, 1971
20. Schreiber P: Safety Guidelines—Anesthesia Systems. North American Drager, Telford, PA, 1984

4

Vaporizers

A vaporizer is required to accurately enrich the gas mixture with the vapor of a liquid anesthetic agent. Precise concentrations of liquid anesthetic agents can be delivered over a wide range of carrier gas flows. Anesthetic agents which achieve the anesthetic state at a very low brain partial pressure and yet have a high atmospheric partial pressure must be administered to the patient in a precise fashion or else overdosage will occur very rapidly. Halothane, for instance, has a vapor or partial pressure of 243 mmHg at 20°C but requires only a brain partial pressure of less than 7 mmHg to establish the anesthetic state.

Technological advances in agent-specific vaporizers allow the anesthesiologist to administer a precise, predictable concentration of anesthetic vapor to the patient with ease. A brief overview of the fundamental principles of vaporizers will enable us to understand how they function. The Drager Vapor 19.1 and Cyprane Tec 4 (see Fig. 4-1) vaporizers will serve as examples for discussion. Detailed information regarding gas laws, heat of vaporization, and other physical characteristics of anesthetic agents can be found in physics texts devoted to anesthesia.[1, 2]

VAPORIZATION

The molecules in a liquid are in constant movement and stay together because of the bonding characteristics of closely packed molecules. The rate of molecular movement is directly proportional to the temperature of the liquid. Molecules near the surface which develop enough speed or energy to overcome the force of the attracting molecules of the undersurface layer enter the atmosphere and become vapor.

Molecules in the vapor state collide with each other and the walls of the containing vessel creating a pressure called the *saturated vapor pressure* or partial pressure. The vapor pressure is a state of equilibrium in which the number of molecules in a closed container leaving the surface is equal to the number entering the liquid at any given temperature. The vapor pressure is dependent on only the temperature and nature of the liquid over a wide range of barometric pressures.[3-6] It is calculated by multiplying the volume concentration (percent v/v) of vapor by the barometric pressure. At 20°C the vapor pressure of halothane is 243 mmHg; thus the concen-

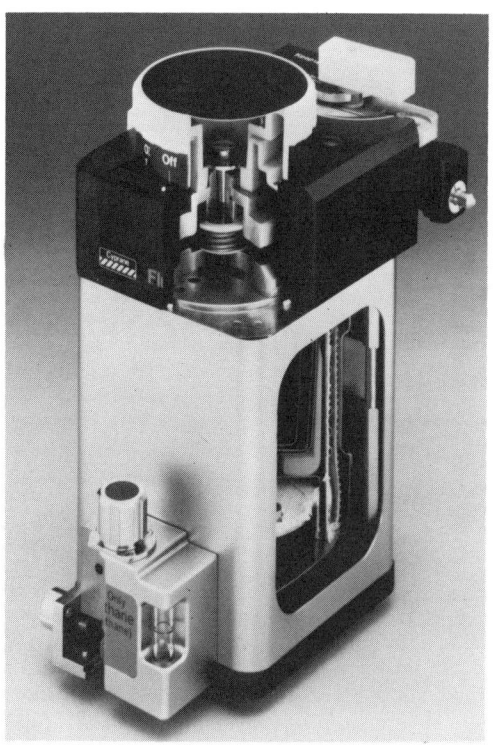 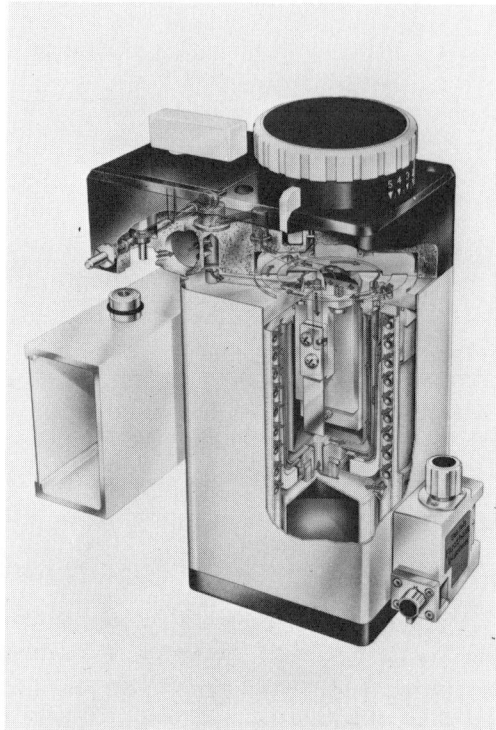

Fig. 4-1 Cutaway view of a Cyprane Tec 4 vaporizer. On the left hand is a cut vaporizer; on the right is a schematic cutaway view. The wicks are against the outside wall of the vaporizer to provide maximal heat exchange. A bimetallic plate can be seen in the center of the schematic drawing. Note the complexity of the concentration dial. (Courtesy of Ohmeda, The BOC Group, Inc.)

tration of halothane at a barometric pressure of 650 mmHg is 37 percent and that at 760 mmHg is 32 percent. At low (high altitude) and high (hyperbaric chamber) barometric pressures the concentration of the anesthetic is dependent on the barometric pressure and the vapor pressure is dependent on the temperature.[4, 5]

Increasing the temperature of the liquid increases molecular speed and causes greater numbers of molecules to leave the surface. Heat is extracted from the liquid as the molecules leave the surface. As the liquid cools, the remaining molecules lose speed or energy. In order to continue vaporization the molecules require heat from an external source. You can feel the heat needed to convert a liquid into a vapor by spraying the back of your hand with ethyl chloride: As the liquid rapidly vaporizes, heat is extracted from the skin and a cold sensation is experienced. In fact, a white, frosty area may appear which is caused by the transient condensation and freezing of water vapor from the air surrounding the hand.

The rate and efficiency of vaporization can be improved by increasing surface area and controlling temperature. The surface area can be increased by bubbling the carrier gas through the liquid anesthetic. The surface area of molecular exchange is then dependent on the size of the bubbles, that is, the greater the number of small bubbles the greater the surface area. Numerous small bubbles passing quickly through a liquid can cause the temperature to decrease very rapidly. For instance, when oxygen is bubbled through ether in a glass vaporizer, the temperature drops so fast that water vapor condenses and ice forms on the outside of the glass. Continued

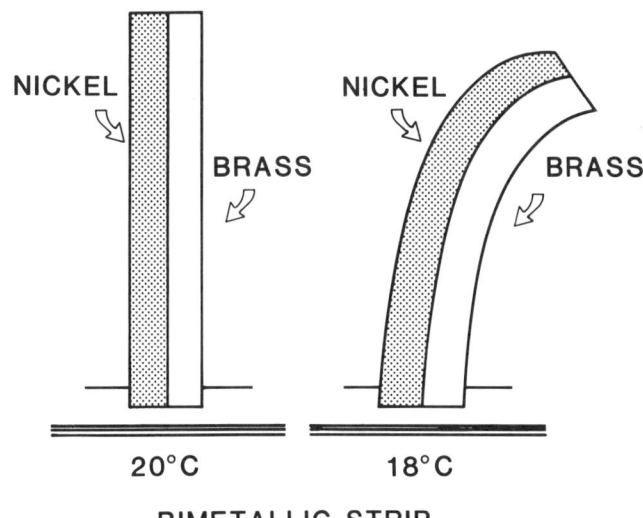

Fig. 4-2 A bimetallic strip made by welding brass to nickel. Bending of the bimetallic strip is dependent on differences between the linear expansion coefficients of brass and nickel. Temperature fluctuations occur during vaporization of the anesthetic liquid. Output concentration is controlled by the bimetallic strip, which changes the carrier gas splitting ratio through the bypass and the vaporizing chamber.

NICKEL

BRASS

20°C

NICKEL

BRASS

18°C

BIMETALLIC STRIP

high concentrations of ether can be maintained only by surrounding the glass vaporizer with a constant-temperature water jacket.[7] The copper kettle vaporizer is an excellent example of an efficient bubble vaporizer. Multiple tiny bubbles are formed as the carrier gas passes through a sintered bronze disk at the entrance to the liquid. Temperature is maintained over a wide range of flow rates by the addition of heat from the room through the copper and into the liquid.[8]

Vaporization can also be improved by placing *wicks* against the walls of the vaporizing chamber. Wicks provide additional temperature control and ensure maximal vapor saturation. The wicks function like plant capillary tubes to raise the liquid anesthetic agent above the fluid level. The surface area for vaporization is increased (see Fig. 4-1). Locating the wicks directly against the metal wall of the vaporizer provides for maximal heat exchange. Maintaining maximum vapor saturation in the vaporizing chamber ensures that (1) no initial burst of high vapor concentration will occur when the vaporizer is turned on and (2) the output of the vaporizer will not be affected by movement of the anesthesia machine.[9] The Drager Vapor 19.1 wick system holds 60 ml and the Cyprane Tec 4 wicks

hold 35 ml of anesthetic liquid.[10, 11]

Temperature compensation in accurate specific-agent vaporizers is assisted by a temperature-sensitive valve or an expansion member. These devices control the amount of carrier gas which flows into the vaporization chamber and that which completely bypasses the vaporizer.[10, 11] Each device, in principle, is really a bimetallic plate with one side of brass and one side of nickel (see Fig. 4-2). Each metal has a specific coefficient of linear expansion; temperature alterations thus result in predictable linear dimension changes. Two different expansion rates cause the plate to bend and change the orifice opening, controlling the proportions of carrier gas going to and bypassing the vaporizing chamber.

VAPORIZER OUTPUT

Specific agent vaporizers can be very accurate over a wide range of flow rates. Figure 4-3 shows the output of the Drager Vapor 19.1 halothane vaporizer. The concentration output of the Drager Vapor 19.1 vaporizer is independent of the fresh gas flow rate from 300 cc/min to 7 L/min. Concentration decreases slightly at the highest percentage set-

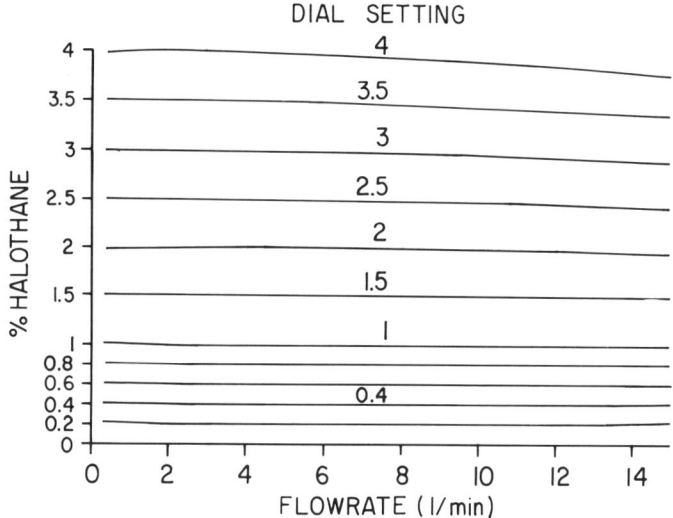

Fig. 4-3 Output performance curves for the Drager Vapor 19.1 halothane vaporizer. The carrier gas is air. (Redrawn from data, courtesy of North American Drager, Telford, PA.)

ting as fresh gas flows reach 7 to 15 L/min. Output studies are carried out at the factory, using air or oxygen as the carrier gas. Each vaporizer is individually tested and the concentration dial calibrated and etched.[10-12]

Vaporizer output is altered when the carrier gas contains mixtures of oxygen and nitrous oxide.[13-23] Changing the carrier gas from 100 percent oxygen to 100 percent nitrous oxide gives rise to a biphasic pattern in the output of the vaporizer.[20] Figures 4-4 and 4-5 illustrate the initial decrease in concentration output, which lasts about 45 seconds before the establishment of a new plateau at 3 minutes. Initially, differences in gas viscosity or density were thought to be responsible for the rapid fall in concentration output. However, the solubility of nitrous oxide (4 ml of N_2O per milliliter of halogenated anesthetic) in the liquid anesthetic was found to be the mechanism.[14, 16, 18, 20] Following the use of a mixed carrier gas, changing to 100 percent oxygen causes a slight increase in output concentrations as nitrous oxide leaves the liquid anesthetic.[16] Oxygen and nitrous oxide establish different plateaus during steady-state performance because of inherent flow-splitting characteristics of the vaporizer which are unrelated to gas density differences.[20] Rapid transient changes are not clinically important during high-flow anesthesia but caution may be necessary during low-flow anesthesia when changes in output concentrations may be prolonged.[13, 14]

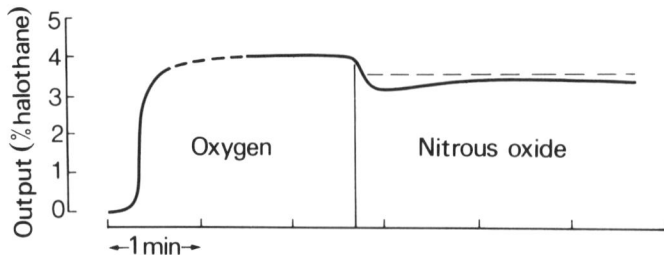

Fig. 4-4 Transient effect on output concentration of halothane due to changing the carrier gas from oxygen to nitrous oxide in the Fluotec Mk III: flow rate 5 L/min and dial setting 4 percent. (Redrawn from Palayiwa E, Sanderson MH, Hahn CEW: Effects of carrier gas composition on the output of six anaesthetic vaporizers. Br J Anaesth 5:1025, 1983.)

MATERIALS

Metals used in the fabrication of vaporizer chambers must have acceptable thermal conductivity and specific-heat characteristics. Thermal conductivity is measured by observing the rate at which heat flows through a cross section of a substance under known temperature gradients (units are calories per second-cm per degree Celsius).[24] Low thermal conductivity means the substance is a poor conductor of heat but a good insulator; for example, air has a thermal conductivity value of 0.000054 and is an excellent insulating material. Metals have high conductivities and dissipate heat rapidly; for example, silver has a value of 0.99. Specific heat is defined[24] as the number of calories needed to raise the temperature of a unit mass by 1°C. The specific heat of water is the same as the calorie, namely, the quantity of heat required to raise 1 g of water by 1°C. For copper, however, (specific heat 0.093) 0.09 calorie and for platinum (specific heat 0.032) 0.03 calorie will raise 1 g of the substance by 1°C.

Copper was chosen for the copper kettle

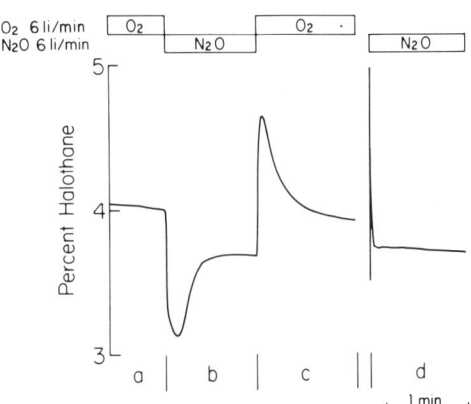

Fig. 4-5 Effect of changing the carrier gas on the output concentration of halothane. (Drager Vapor 19.1 vaporizer). In the gap between (c) and (d) halothane is drained from the vaporizer, presaturated with nitrous oxide, and refilled. (Redrawn from Gould DB, Lampert BA, MacKrell TN: Effect of nitrous oxide solubility on vaporizer aberrance. Anesth Analg 61:938, 1982. Reprinted with permission, the International Anesthesia Research Society.)

because of a low specific heat, a relatively high thermal conductivity, and a reasonable cost.[8, 25] Platinum and silver have more desirable specific heat and thermal conductivity characteristics but are very expensive. Today vaporizer chambers are constructed of brass coated with copper and nickel, and then chromium-plated.[12] The choice of the construction metal is not as critical in agent-specific vaporizers, since the vaporizer has excellent temperature compensation mechanisms.

FLOW OF CARRIER GAS THROUGH THE VAPORIZER

Mixtures of carrier gas exit the flowmeters and enter the fresh gas inlet of the vaporizer. When the vaporizer is in the off position, the fresh gas bypasses the vaporizer and enters directly into the vaporizer gas outlet. Turning the concentration knob counterclockwise opens the control port, thus allowing the carrier gas to enter the vaporizer (see Figs. 4-6 and 4-7). A bypass mechanism splits the gas stream, sending a portion to the vaporizing chamber and the remaining portion to the vaporizer gas outlet. Fresh gas entering the vaporizing chamber picks up the saturated vapor of the liquid anesthetic and carries it to the vaporizer gas outlet. Temperature compensation devices control either the amount of carrier gas exiting the vaporizing chamber or the ratio of vaporizing chamber gas to bypass gas. The net result is the precise addition of anesthetic vapor to the fresh gas with predictable accuracy over a wide range of fresh gas flows and temperature modulations.

EVOLVING SAFETY FEATURES

Overfilling the Vaporizer

Liquid anesthetic was accidentally delivered to a patient when a high gas flow passed through an overfilled vaporizer.[26] Each vaporizer should have a liquid-level indicator with maximal filling limited by the filling port being lower than the maximal filling level in the sump of the vaporizing chamber. Figures 4-

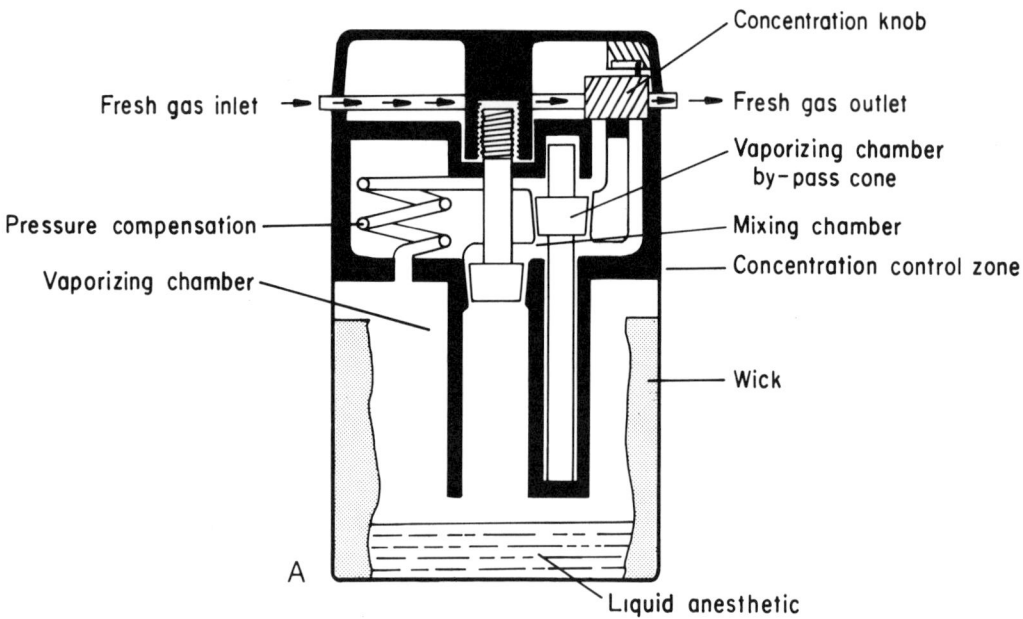

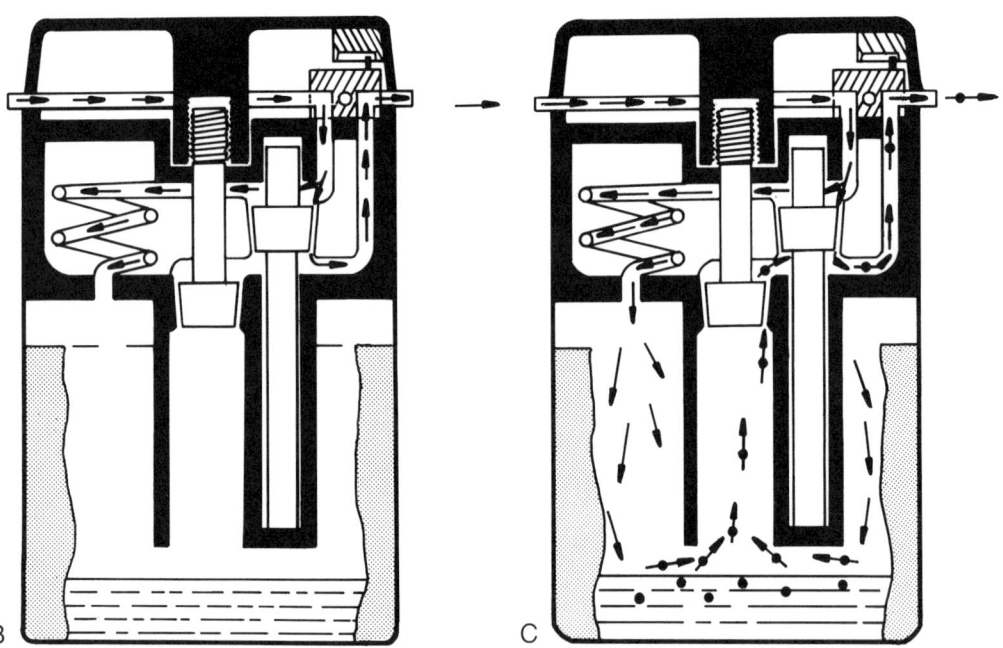

Fig. 4-6 Gas flow through a vaporizer. (A) Fresh gas flow completely bypasses the vaporizer. (B) The concentration dial has been turned counterclockwise, which opens the port for fresh gas inflow. Gas flows into the vaporizing chamber and the fresh gas outflow port. (C) Fresh gas enters the vaporizing chamber and acts as a carrier for the liquid anesthetic vapor into the fresh gas outflow port. (Redrawn from Drager Vapor 19.1, System Features. Instruction Manual. North American Drager, Telford, PA, 1984.)

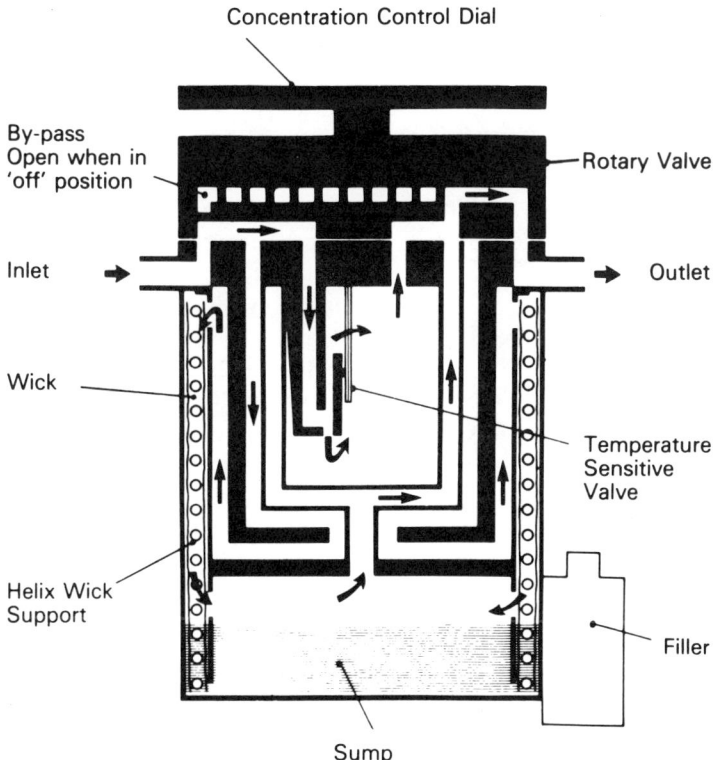

Concentration Control Dial

By-pass
Open when in
'off' position

Rotary Valve

Inlet

Outlet

Wick

Temperature
Sensitive
Valve

Helix Wick
Support

Filler

Sump

Fig. 4-7 Schematic of a Cyprane Tec 4 single agent vaporizer. The arrows indicate the flow of the carrier gas thru the vaporizer. Each major component is labeled for clarity. (Courtesy of Ohmeda, The BOC Group, Inc.)

1 and 4-7 show the liquid-level indicators for the Cyprane Tec 4 series vaporizer below the maximal liquid level of the vaporizing chamber sump.

Reversed Flow

Reversed flow of carrier gas[27] through a vaporizer can increase the vaporizer output by a factor of 2. Portable and free-standing vaporizers should be eliminated from the practice of anesthesia. Vaporizers on quality anesthesia machines are mounted on fixed vaporizer interlock brackets which do not allow the reversed flow of fresh gas. Should the anesthesiologist desire to have rapid interchangeability of single-agent vaporizers, the Cyprane Tec 4 series can be removed, stored on a rack, and replaced on demand.

Tipping the Vaporizer

A free-standing vaporizer knocked to the floor was responsible for a cardiac arrest.[28] Output concentrations can be extremely high after a vaporizer is tipped and then used immediately. Drager Vapor 19.1 vaporizers have small legs which provide a standing base, but when the vaporizer is tipped by more than 45°, it must be flushed out by running 10 L/min of carrier gas with the concentration dial wide open.[11] Cyprane Tec 4 vaporizers have an internal baffle system which allows the vaporizer to be tipped by up to 180° without changing the initial output concentration. However, anytime a vaporizer is found in a nonvertical position, caution must be exercised during the initial use of the instrument.

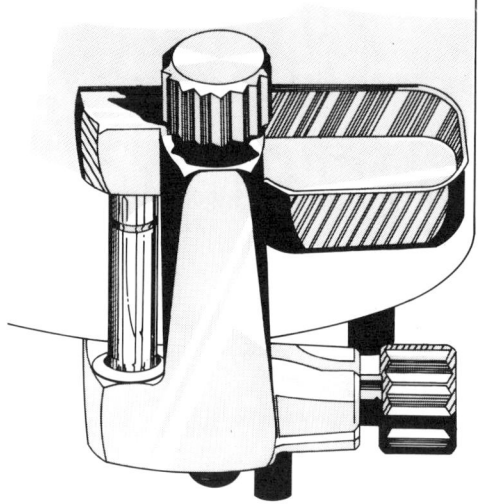

Fig. 4-8 Simple funnel filler for an agent-specific vaporizer. (Redrawn from Drager Vapor 19.1, System Features. Instruction Manual. North American Drager, Telford, PA, 1984.)

Filling with the Wrong Anesthetic

The American National Standard Institute (ANSI) recommends a permanently attached, standard, agent-specific keyed filling mechanism.[29] Many anesthesiologists find these keyed or pin safety filling devices to be a nuisance because of spilling and leakage.[30, 31] Vaporizers are sold with options of a pin safety filling system or a common funnel filler (see Fig. 4-8). Anesthetic agents are packaged in bottles with a keyed bottle collar. Figure 4-9 shows a filling spout with one end keyed to the bottle collar and the other end keyed to the filling mechanism of the vaporizer. In addition, the anesthetic agents are provided in color-coded bottles—for example, red for halothane and purple for isoflurane—which correspond to the colors of the agent-specific vaporizers. Despite color codes and warnings, however, anesthetic agents have been put in the wrong vaporizer.[31]

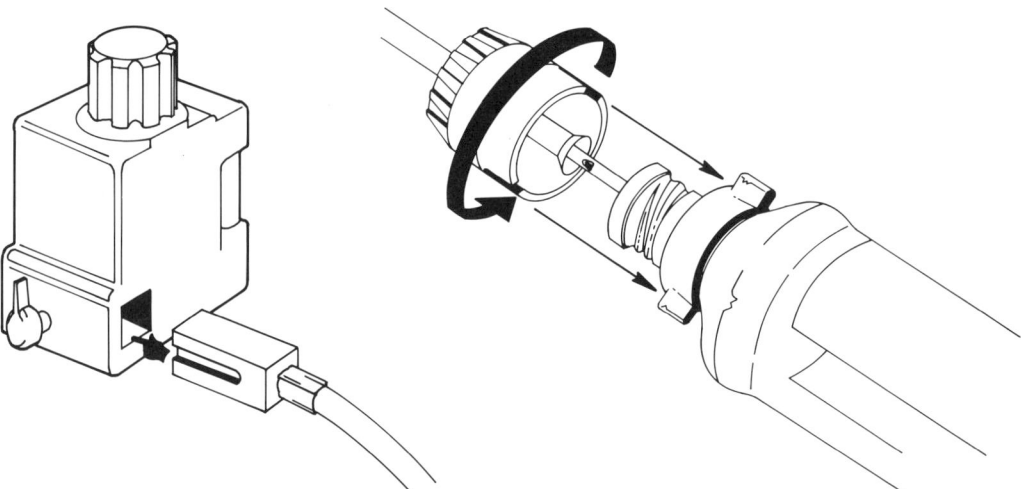

Fig. 4-9 An agent-specific keyed vaporizer filling system is permanently attached to the vaporizer, and shown on the left. An adapter with a small, indented trough in the side of its block inserts into the appropriately keyed vaporizer port. The right diagram shows the bottle attachment of the keyed filling adapter. Two slots, particularly spaced for each individual anesthetic agent must match two prongs mounted on the neck of the anesthetic agent bottle. Keyed continuity between bottle and vaporizer is established when both the bottle end and vaporizer end of the keyed filling device match. (Redrawn from illustration, courtesy of Ohmeda, The BOC Group, Inc.)

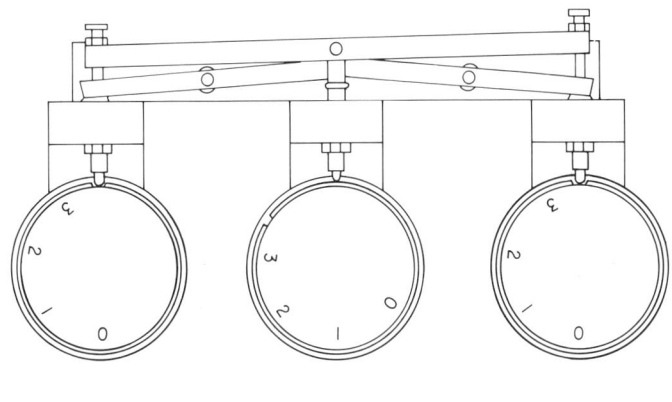

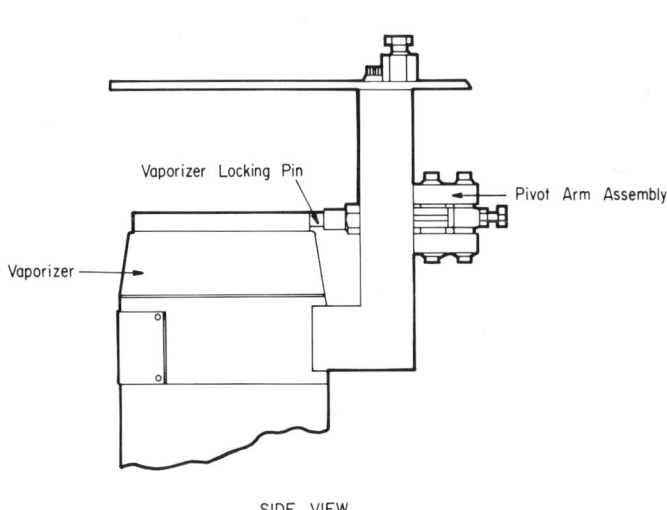

Fig. 4-10 Vaporizer exclusion system. The pins protruding from the back bar allow only one vaporizer to be turned on during the administration of an anesthetic. The diagram on the top is the top view. (Redrawn from Drager Vapor 19.1, System Features. Instruction Manual. North American Drager, Telford PA, 1984.)

Simultaneous Administration of Multiple Agents

Unfortunately, there are anesthesia machines still in use which allow the administration of two or more volatile anesthetics at the same time. Exclusion systems (Fig. 4-10) are available which will eliminate the possibility of administering more than one agent at a time. A cam-activated pin device limits operation to only one vaporizer. Agent-specific vaporizers and vaporizer exclusion systems have certainly contributed to the safety of administering potent volatile anesthetics.

Pumping Effect

Pressure fluctuations transmitted to the vaporizer during intermittent positive-pressure ventilation or oxygen flushing can increase the vaporizer output concentration.[32, 33] In most vaporizers the pumping or pressurizing effect can be disregarded at flow rates above 3 L/min but must be given consideration during closed-circuit or low-flow anesthesia.[3, 6, 33]

Figure 4-11 illustrates the pumping effect principle in a noncompensated vaporizer. Inflation pressure from the ventilator is trans-

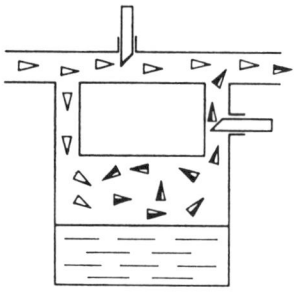

Increasing pressure

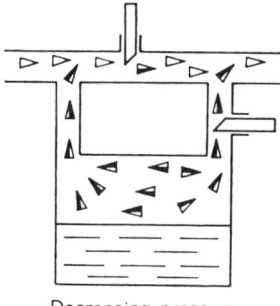

Decreasing pressure

Fig. 4-11 Pumping effect in a noncompensated vaporizer. As the pressure in the vaporizer chamber fluctuates, a mixture of gas and vapor leaves the chamber. A continuation of the fluctuation results in waves of vapor being pumped into the exit orifice. (Schreiber P: Anaesthesia: Performance, Classification and Safety. Springer-Verlag, New York, 1972).

mitted up the fresh gas pipe, increasing the pressure in the vaporizing chamber. Additional fresh gas molecules enter the chamber in accordance with Boyle's law and increased numbers of anesthetic molecules leave the container as the pressure is reduced. Fresh gas and anesthetic molecules leave in waves during each pressure fluctuation. Continued pumping results in a progressive rise in volatile anesthetic concentration at the vaporizer outlet. The highest output concentration is achieved when the concentration dial setting and fresh gas flows are low.[3, 6, 12]

Flowmeter-controlled universal vaporizers, for example, the copper kettle, can be protected by (1) insertion of a pressurizing valve downstream from the vaporizer, (2) placement of a unidirectional valve and reservoir bag between the patient and the vaporizer, or (3)

inserting a check valve in the vaporizing chamber outlet.[6, 34-36] Practical solutions for safer agent-specific vaporizers include a combination of (1) reduction in the volume of the vaporizing chamber, (2) direction control of the entry pressure surge into the vaporizing chamber, (3) provision of a small annular expansion chamber adjacent to the vaporizing chamber, (4) insertion of a long, narrow annular tube or passageway into the inlet of the vaporizing chamber (see Fig. 4-12), and (5) pressurizing the vaporizer.[6, 12, 33] The hissing noise encountered when the Drager Vapor 19.1 vaporizer is turned off is caused by the release of up to 200 mbars of pressure in the vaporizing chamber.[1] No wonder the liquid anesthetic agent gushes all over the room when someone opens the filler port with the vaporizer turned on!

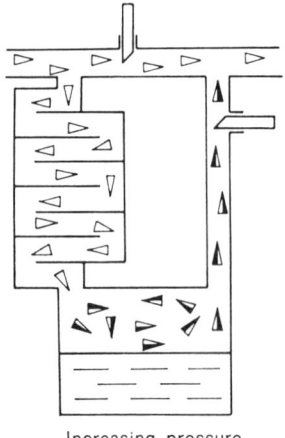

Increasing pressure

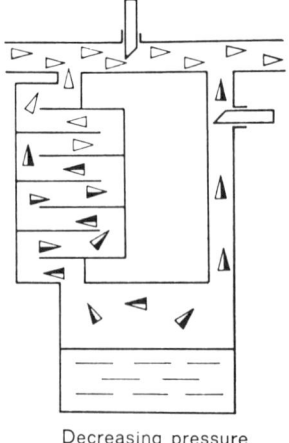

Decreasing pressure

Fig. 4-12 Prevention of the pumping effect in the vaporizer by insertion of a long mazelike pipe into the inlet of the vaporizing chamber. Fluctuating pressures are blunted, thus ensuring accurate vaporization. (Schreiber P: Anaesthesia:Performance,Classification and Safety. Springer-Verlag, New York, 1972.)

Miscellaneous Factors

Liquid halothane can turn brown after sitting for about 2 months. Initially the discoloration was thought to be due to thymol but halothane-free radicals produced by ultraviolet light irradiation and ionizing radiation in the atmosphere now provide the most likely explanation.[37, 38] Discoloration of enflurane and isoflurane in vaporizers has been noted without associated malfunction of the vaporizer.[39, 40] The source of the discoloration is thought to be residual hydrocarbons leached from the plastic wick spacers of the vaporizer.

Thymol at 0.01 percent is used to promote the stability of halothane. Thymol does not vaporize readily because it has a high boiling point (233°C) so it accumulates during successive fillings of halothane. High concentrations of thymol may coat the rotary valve, causing stickiness, or affect the accuracy of the vaporizer by an action on the flow control unit.[12, 38] Vaporizer manufacturers have reduced the sticking phenomenon by making the bearing surface of the rotary valve flat and reducing the surface area of the machined ducts and control channel in the upper disk. Thymol residues can be removed by either (1) draining the vaporizer, refilling it with halothane, gently rotating it for 1 hour, and then discarding the halothane or (2) draining the vaporizer and then cleaning the spindle and rinsing the vaporizing chamber with diethyl ether.[11, 41] Problems with thymol can be completely eliminated by draining the halothane vaporizer on a regular basis.

CALIBRATION OF VAPORIZERS

Vaporizers should be tested for performance after a shipment, any major service repair, or equipment modification. A number of instruments are available that can satisfactorily test the vaporizer in the operating room and/or factory.

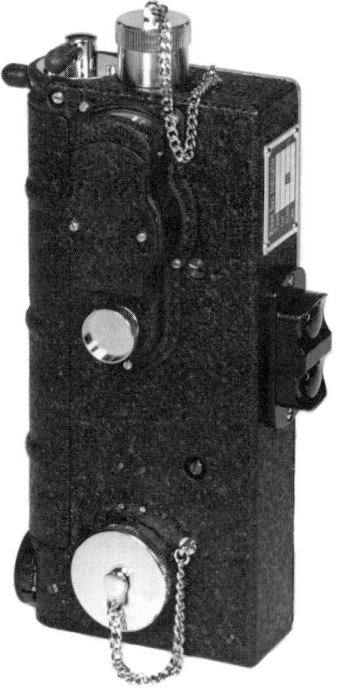

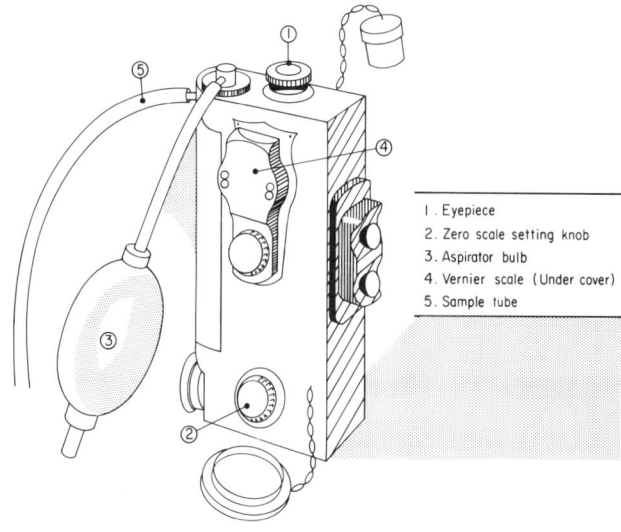

1 . Eyepiece
2 . Zero scale setting knob
3 . Aspirator bulb
4 . Vernier scale (Under cover)
5 . Sample tube

Fig. 4-13 Riken portable anesthetic gas analyzer. The schematic diagram on the right identifies instrument's features. (Photo and schematic [redrawn] courtesy of Riken. Portable Anesthetic Gas Indicator Model 18. AM Bickford, Wales Center, NY, 1984.)

Refractometers

Interference refractometers (see Fig. 4-13) measure the refractive power of the anesthetic agent against the refractive power of oxygen. The refractive power is calculated from the refractive index times 10^6. For example, oxygen[42] has a refractive power of 271.5 and a refractive index of 1.0002715. The refractive index of a gas is found by dividing the velocity of light in a vacuum by the velocity of light in the gas. The refractive power of a gas is directly proportional to its density or molecular concentration. Method sensitivity for a binary gas mixture is dependent on the differences in the refractive powers of the two components.[42, 43] A refractometer has two chambers, as shown in Figure 4-14. One cham-

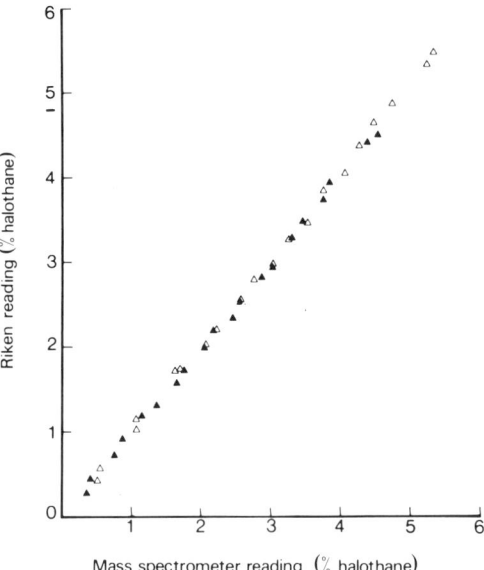

Fig. 4-15 Comparison of halothane concentration analyses by the Riken refractometer and the mass spectrometer. Carrier gas was either oxygen (open triangles) or nitrous oxide (solid triangles). (Adapted from Palayiwa E, Sanderson MH, Hahn CEW: Effects of carrier gas composition on the output of six anaesthetic vaporizers. Br J Anaesth 5:1025, 1983.)

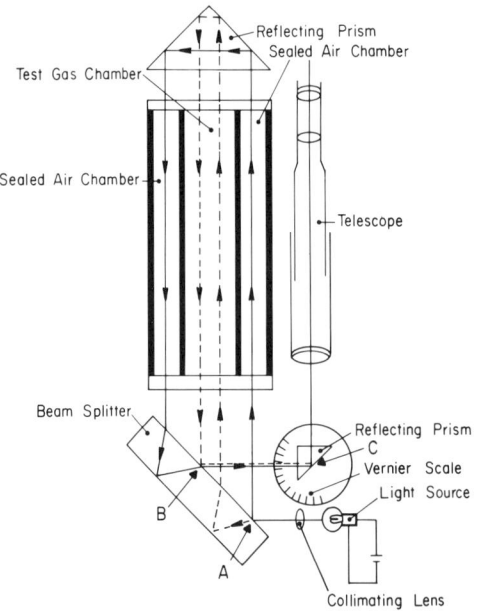

Fig. 4-14 Design of the optical pathway in the portable interference refractometer which analyzes anesthetic concentrations. The light beam is split at point A and recombined at point B. At point C a prism reflects the interference bands to the telescope. (Redrawn from Riken. Portable Anesthetic Gas Indicator Model 18. AM Bickford, Wales Center, NY, 1984.)

ber is sealed and contains air. The other chamber is used for introduction of the anesthetic gas mixture. A beam of light is collimated and passed through an assembly of glass prisms. Two beams pass through the sealed chamber in different directions. Two reflected beams pass through the test gas chamber. All light beams are combined by the beam splitter and reflected to the prism adjusted by the vernier scale. Through the telescope the operator sees interference bands superimposed on a 0 to 6 percent scale.[42, 44] Zero calibration is achieved by measuring oxygen against air. A known anesthetic gas in oxygen is then aspirated into the chamber and a reading obtained from the vernier scale. Factory calibration is done with halothane, and vernier readings will reflect the percent concentration of halothane. Vernier readings for isoflurane, enflurane, and nitrous oxide are multiplied by a conversion factor of 1.07, 1.08, and 5.76, respectively.[44] Prisms in the portable refractometer units fold the light path to make the unit compact, robust, and self-contained (see Fig. 4-14). Calibration, linearity, and stability (see Fig. 4-15) have been excellent.[42] Excellent correlation between the Riken refractometer and the mass spectrometer has been made (see Fig. 4-15). At present the best method available for the calibration of vaporizers uses the refractometer.

Mass Spectrometers

The use of mass spectrometers to measure the concentration of anesthetic agents has been very limited in the past because of overlap in the spectra of anesthetic agents and respiratory gases.[45] For instance, nitrous oxide and carbon dioxide both have a molecular weight of 44 and the fragmented charged par-

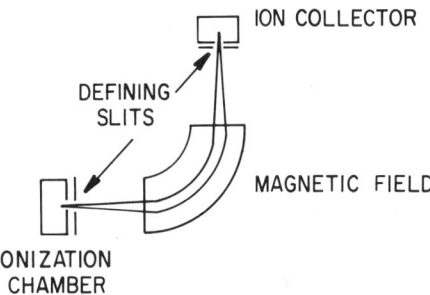

Fig. 4-17 A magnetic sector mass spectrometer. Ions are deflected through an arc of 90° by a magnetic field to refocus at the ion collector. The process reduces cost and improves resolution. (Adapted with permission from Leck JH: The evolution of mass spectrometers. p. 1. In Payne JP, Bushman JA, Hill DA (eds): The Medical and Biological Application of Mass Spectrometry. Copyright by Academic Press, London, Ltd. 1979.)

ticles of halothane can have a molecular weight close to 44. The spectrum overlap problem has been solved by the spectrum overlap eraser, which "allows quantitative measurement of individual gases in a mixture when several contribute to the signal detected at one or more of the mass numbers."[46] The response time for mass spectrometers is rapid, 0.080 to 0.350 second, which makes breath-by-breath measurements of respirations possible.

Figures 4-16 and 4-17 outline the principles of the mass spectrometer. A vacuum is essential to eliminate the influence of molecular collisions. Positive ions of the sample gas are created in the ionization chamber through electron bombardment and then accelerated through the same potential difference. The ions are then projected as a slightly convergent beam into a magnetic field. Lightweight ions have short trajectories while heavier ions have large radii. Only ions which focus at the defining slit can pass through the opening to be concentrated in the Faraday cage or ion collector. An ion current, proportional to the ion beam intensity, is created by the passage of ions into the collector. The magnetic field

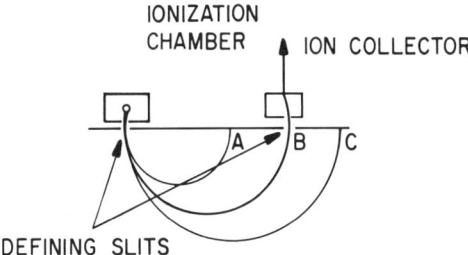

Fig. 4-16 Basic principles of a Dempster mass spectrometer. Gas molecules are ionized by electron bombardment in the vacuum of the ionization chamber. Ions leave the defining slit of the ionization chamber and may enter the defining slit of the ion collector, depending on their circular trajectories (A,B,C). At the ion collector the entering ions create a current proportional to the ion beam intensity. (Adapted with permission from Leck JH: The evolution of mass spectrometers. p. 1. In Payne JP, Bushman JA, Hill DA (eds): The Medical and Biological Application of Mass Spectrometry. Copyright by Academic Press, London, Ltd. 1979.)

strength is controlled by increasing or decreasing the trajectory radius. Ion beams differing in mass by as little as 1 part in 10,000 can be separated.[47] Commercial mass spectrometers are available for routine measurements of respiratory and anesthetic gases in the operating room. One central access point can monitor 10 to 12 operating rooms. Cost effectiveness under clinical conditions will have to be determined through long-term application.

Quartz Crystal Detector

A quartz crystal oscillates when placed in a resonance circuit at a frequency determined by crystal thickness and mass.[48] An electronic system has been devised in which two piezoelectric quartz crystals are connected by oscillator circuits. One crystal serves as a reference crystal and the other crystal, coated with silicon oil, is the detector crystal. Silicon oil serves as a lipophilic layer into which the halogenated anesthetic can enter. As the mass of halogenated anesthetic in the lipophilic layer increases, the natural resonant frequency of the crystal decreases in direct proportion to the partial pressure of the anesthetic gas.[49] An electronic signal is generated between the detector and reference crystal and is proportional to the partial pressure of the anesthetic.[50, 51]

The Engstrom crystal anesthetic gas analyzer will reproducibly measure dry anesthetic vapor concentrations in a response time of less than 0.75 second at a carrier gas flow of over 5 L/min. A transducer containing the two crystals is placed in the breathing circuit. Analysis of a specific halogenated agent is chosen by the selector switch. Errors in analyzer

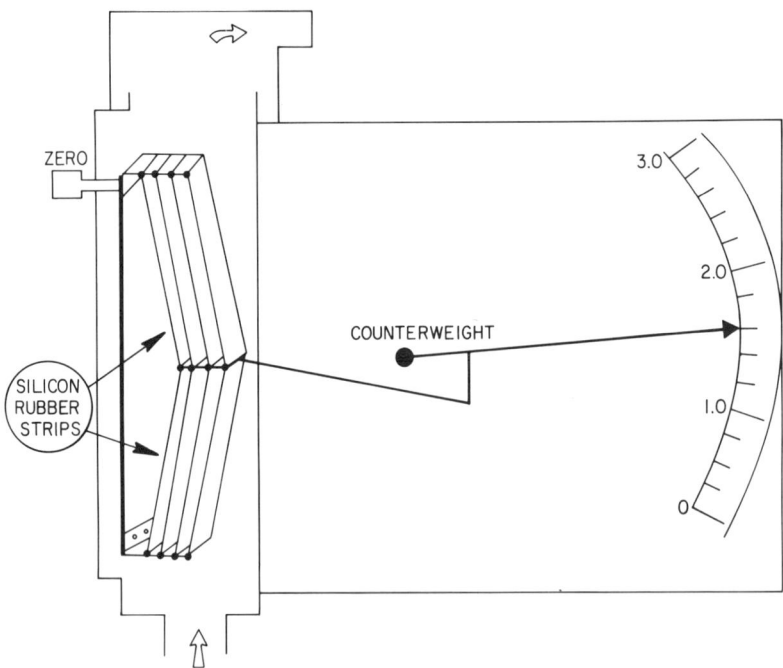

Fig. 4-18 Schematic of the Narko-test instrument, which operates on the principle of the elasticity of silicon rubber strips. Rubber strip tension changes in direct proportion to anesthetic agent rubber solubility. (Redrawn from Lowe HJ, Hagler K: Clinical and laboratory evaluation of an expired anesthetic gas monitor (Narko-test). Anesthesiology 34:378, 1971.)

output measurements against anesthetic gas standards for enflurance and halothane were 0.9 and 1.87 percent of readings, respectively.[50] Analyzer response is usually a linear function of the vapor concentration of halothane; however, a major decrease in accuracy can occur during use.[51] Nitrous oxide (100 percent) causes only a 0.11 percent offset in the measurement of halothane. Water vapor decreases the response time and shifts the crystal's natural response time.[50, 51] Once the instrument has been calibrated, it can satisfactorily measure the output concentrations of a number of vaporizers. Continuous in-line analysis of halogenated agents is possible.[50]

Infrared Analysis

Halothane, enflurane, and isoflurane can be analyzed by infrared instruments. Each agent must be measured at a specific wavelength.[52] A discussion of how infrared analysis works can be found in Chapter 7.

Elasticity of Silicon Rubber Strips

The absorption of anesthetics diminishes the elasticity of silicon rubber. A series of counterweighted silicon rubber bands under tension can be configured to respond to changing concentrations of anesthetics (see Fig. 4-18).[6, 53, 54] The linear response time for all anesthetics varies with the rubber solubility of the anesthetic agent. For instance, for 1 percent halothane at 4 L/min the plateau is reached within 90 seconds. Temperature compensation is provided by a built-in bimetallic strip. The commercial Narko-test is believed to be suitable for measuring concentrations inside a low-flow circle system.[54] The Narko-test is felt useful for the routine testing of large numbers of vaporizers but, because of inherent mechanical properties, it must not be regarded as a primary standard for vaporizer calibration.[53]

MAINTENANCE AND REPAIR OF VAPORIZERS

The repair of any vaporizer should not be attempted by anyone except a factory-trained serviceman. Mechanical tolerances within the vaporizer are measured by microns and do not lend themselves to adjustment by amateurs. Any adjustment, no matter how trivial, requires testing the output concentration of the vaporizer. All vaporizers requiring repair must be sent to the factory to ensure the maintenance of the highest standard of excellence.[10, 11]

The routine maintenance and recalibration of agent-specific vaporizers are *recommended* annually for the Cyprane Tec 4 vaporizers.[10, 55] A field check by a refractometer confirms the concentration accuracy over a limited range of temperature and pressure conditions. An annual checklist includes such items as (1) complete disassembly of components, (2) thorough cleaning, (3) inspection for damage and wear, (4) renewal of wicks, seals and worn items, (5) necessary lubrication, and (6) adjustments made after testing the vaporizer over a wide range of temperature and pressure conditions.[11] North American Drager states the Vapor 19.1 vaporizer "requires no costly annual re-calibration."[11] They recommend a yearly in-house verification of the vaporizer with a refractometer. The buyer has the option to disregard the recommendation of the manufacturer. However, it would be prudent to have some kind of on-going field tests performed at least once or twice annually by authorized service personnel.

Remember: Vaporizers are sensitive, accurate, scientific instruments involved directly in critical life support. Treat them with great care.

REFERENCES

1. Hill DW: Physics Applied to Anaesthesia. Butterworths, London, 1971
2. Macintosh R, Mushin WW, Epstein HG: Phys-

ics for the Anaesthetist. 3rd Ed. Blackwell, Oxford, 1963

3. Hill DW: The design and calibration of vaporizers for volatile anaesthetic agents. Br J Anaesth 40:648, 1968

4. James MFM, White JF: Anesthetic considerations at moderate altitude. Anesth Analg 63:1097, 1984

5. McDowall DG: Anaesthesia in a pressure chamber. Anaesthesia 19:321, 1964

6. Schreiber P: Anaesthesia Equipment: Performance, Classification and Safety. Springer-Verlag, New York, 1972

7. Epstein HG: Principles of inhalers for volatile anaesthetics. Br Med Bull 14:18, 1958

8. Morris LE: A new vaporizer for liquid anesthetic agents. Anesthesiology 13:587, 1952

9. Hill DW: Halothane concentrations obtained with a Drager "vapor" vaporizer. Br J Anaesth 35:285, 1963

10. Cyprane Tec 4 Continuous Flow Vaporizer. Operators Instructions. Ohmeda, West Yorkshire, England 1983

11. Drager Vapor 19.1, System Features. Instruction Manual. North American Drager, Telford, PA, 1984

12. Paterson GM, Hulands GH, Nunn JF: Evaluation of a new halothane vaporizer: the Cyprane Fluotec Mark 3. Br J Anaesth 41:109, 1969

13. Diaz PM: The influence of carrier gas on the output of automatic plenum vaporizers. Br J Anaesth 48:387, 1976

14. Gould DB, Lampert BA, MacKrell TN: Effect of nitrous oxide solubility on vaporizer aberrance. Anesth Analg 61:938, 1982

15. Knill R, Prins L, Strupat J et al: Nitrous oxide and vaporizer outputs: Transient or continuous effect? Anesth Analg 59:808, 1980

16. Lampert BA, Gould DB, MacKrell TN, et al: The influence of N_2O solubility in volatile anesthetics. Anesthesiology 57:A164, 1983

17. Latto IP: Administration of halothane in the 0-0.5% concentration range with the Fluotec Mark 2 and Mark 3 vaporizers. Br J Anaesth 45:563, 1973

18. Lin C: Enflurane vaporizer accuracy with nitrous oxide mixtures. Anesth Analg 58:1979

19. Nawaf K, Stoelting RK: Nitrous oxide increases enflurane concentrations delivered by ethrane vaporizers. Anesth Analg 58:30, 1979

20. Palayiwa E, Sanderson MH, Hahn CEW: Effects of carrier gas composition on the output of six anaesthetic vaporizers. Br J Anaesth 5:1025, 1983

21. Prins L, Strupat J, Clement J et al: An evaluation of gas density dependence of anaesthetic vaporizers. Can Anaesth Soc J 237:106, 1980

22. Stoelting RK: The effect of nitrous oxide on halothane output from Fluotec Mark 2 vaporizers. Anesthesiology 35:215, 1971

23. Stoelting RK, Nawaf K: Enflurane vaporizer accuracy with nitrous oxide mixtures. Anesth Analg 58:441, 1979

24. Hausmann E, Slack EP: Physics. 4th Ed. D. Van Nostrand, Princeton, 1957

25. Morris LE, Feldman SA: Considerations in the design and function of anesthetic vaporizers. Anesthesiology 19:642, 1958

26. Rendell-Baker L, Milliken RA: Vaporizer overflow a preventable hazard. Anesthesiology 50:478, 1979

27. Marks WE, Jr, Bullard JR: Another hazard of free-standing vaporizers, increased anesthetic concentration with reversed flow of vaporizing gas. Anesthesiology 45:445, 1976

28. Munson WM: Cardiac arrest: Hazard of tipping a vaporizer. Anesthesiology 26:235, 1965

29. American National Standard: Minimum performance and safety requirements for components and systems of continuous flow anesthesia machines for human use. 279.8-1979. American National Standards Institute, New York, 1979

30. Davies JM, Strunin L, Craig DB: Leakage of volatile anaesthetics from agent-specific keyed vapourizer filling devices. Can Anaesth Soc J 29:473, 1982

31. Karis JH, Menzel DB: Inadvertent change of volatile anesthetics in anesthesia machines. Anesth Analg 61:53, 1982

32. Greenhow DE, Barth RL: Oxygen flushing delivers anesthetic vapor: a hazard with a new machine. Anesthesiology 38:409, 1973

33. Hill DW, Lowe HJ: Comparison of concentration of halothane in closed and semiclosed circuits during controlled ventilation. Anesthesiology 23:291, 1962

34. Karl WF: Valve and bag assembly for halothane. Anesthesiology 23:584, 1962

35. Keenan RL: Prevention of increased pressures in anesthetic vaporizers with a unidirectional valve. Anesthesiology 27:734, 1963

36. Keet JE, Valentine GW, Riccio JS: An arrange-

ment to prevent pressure effect on the Vernitrol vaporizer. Anesthesiology 24:734, 1963

37. Bosterling B, Trevor A, Trudell JR: Binding of halothane-free radicals to fatty acids following UV irradiation. Anesthesiology 56:380, 1982

38. Rosenberg PH, Alila A: Accumulation of thymol in halothane vaporizers. Anaesthesia 38:581, 1984

39. Gandolfi AJ, Blitt CD, Weldon S: Discoloration and impurities in isoflurane vaporizer. Anesth Analg 62:366, 1983

40. Wald A: Switchover valve failure. Anesth Analg 60:843, 1981

41. Noble WH: Accuracy of halothane vaporizers in clinical use. Can Anaesth Soc J 17:135, 1970

42. Hulands GH, Nunn JF: Portable interference refractometers in anaesthesia. Br J Anaesth 42:1051, 1970

43. Edmonson W: Gas analysis by refractive index measurement. Br J Anaesth 29:570, 1957

44. Riken. Portable Anesthetic Gas Indicator Model 18. AM Bickford, Wales Center, NY, 1984

45. Gillbe CE, Henneghan CPH, Branthwaite MA: Respiratory mass spectrometry during general anaesthesia. Br J Anaesth 53:103, 1981

46. Davis WOM, Spence AA: A modification of the MGA 200 mass spectrometer to enable measurement of anaesthetic gas mixtures. Br J Anaesth 51:987, 1979

47. Leck JH: The evolution of mass spectrometers. p. 1. In Payne JP, Bushman JA, Hill DA (eds): The Medical and Biological Application of Mass Spectrometry. Academic Press, London, 1979

48. King WH: Piezoelectric sorption detector. Anal Chem 36:1735, 1964

49. Cooper JB, Edmondson JH, Joseph DM et al: Piezoelectric sorption anesthetic sensor. IEEE Trans Biomed Eng 28:459, 1981

50. Hayes JK, Westenskow DR, Jordan WS: Monitoring anesthetic vapor concentrations using a piezoelectric detector: evaluation of the Engstrom EMMA. Anesthesiology 59:435, 1983

51. Kay B, Cohen AT, Wheeler MF: A laboratory investigation of a multigas monitor for anesthesia (EMMA). Anaesthesia 37:446, 1982

52. Chenoweth MB: Spectrophotometric fluorometric techniques. p. 279. In Bellville JW, Weaver CS (eds): Techniques in Clinical Physiology—A Survey of Measurements in Anesthesiology. Macmillan, Ontario, 1969

53. Lowe HJ, Hagler K: Clinical and laboratory evaluation of an expired anesthetic gas monitor (Narko-test). Anesthesiology 34:378, 1971

54. White DC, Warley-Smith B: the "Narcotest" anaesthetic gas meter. Br J Anaesth 44:1100, 1972

55. Waddell J: Vaporizer Servicing Policy. Letter, 1 October 1984. Ohmeda, Madison, WI

5

Carbon Dioxide Absorption

Carbon dioxide was classified as "gas sylvester" (of the wood) by Van Helmont in 1700. He prepared carbon dioxide by either heating charcoal or reacting calcium carbonate with distilled vinegar.[1] In 1727 the pneumatic chemist Steven Hales recognized the difference between exhaled and inhaled gases. He was "persuaded that the air separated from bodies . . . was not different from that of the atmosphere . . . only on account of its being infected and rendered noxious by vapours which were foreign to its nature."[2] He successfully removed carbon dioxide from expired respiratory gases by passing it through a filter containing a solution of salt of tartar. A candle burned longer in the presence of the filtered respiratory gas. By 1772 Lavoisier controlled the carbon dioxide content of inhaled gases through the absorption of carbon dioxide by caustic alkali. He recognized the toxic effects of carbon dioxide and determined the carbon dioxide output of man.[1]

Absorption of carbon dioxide as it relates to the development of the carbon dioxide canister for the anesthesia machine has been described in Chapter 1. Bubbling the expired gas through a container of alkali proved to be cumbersome. Granules of soda lime proved to be the most practical and inexpensive process for carbon dioxide absorption.

Pioneers of World War I spent a great deal of time in choosing the best mixture of carbon dioxide absorbents for gas masks. In 1915 Robert E. Wilson fused a mixture of ingredients necessary for carbon dioxide absorption into a solid mass by the incorporation of an inert silicate binder. The fused mass could be crushed, screened through a mesh, and used for carbon dioxide absorption.[3] The rapid acceptance of carbon dioxide absorption canisters in the specialty of anesthesia followed the clinical introduction of cyclopropane in 1933. Absorber design has been flexible enough to accommodate the physical characteristics of the absorbent granules and the requirements of the patient's respirations.

ABSORBENT GRANULES

Two major commercial sources of carbon dioxide absorbent granules are available: Sodasorb (originally called Wilson Soda Lime; Dewey and Almy Chemical Co., Division of W. R. Grace & Co., Lexington, MA 02173) and Baralyme (barium hydroxide octahydrate; Allied Healthcare Products, Inc., 1720 Sublette Avenue, St. Louis, MO 63110). Table 5-1 compares some of the characteristics of Sodasorb and Baralyme. Through a slow

Table 5-1. Comparison of Baralyme and Sodasorb

Characteristics	Baralyme	Sodasorb
Moisture content	11-16%	14-19%
Mesh	4-8	4-8
Regeneration	Minimal	Minimal
Indicator dye	Ethyl violet	Ethyl violet
Hardness	75	80
Reaction with tissues	Irritant	Irritant
Inert binder	Yes	Yes
Disposable packaging	Yes	Yes

continuum absorbent granules improved in quality and character. Lever-lock containers, disposable containers, improved granule uniformity, and increased absorbency capacity are some of the changes which have made absorption granules safer and more efficient.

Chemical Reaction

Absorbent granules interact with carbon dioxide in an irreversible chemical reaction to eventually form calcium carbonate. Chemically soda lime (a mixture of sodium and calcium hydroxide) in the presence of water and carbon dioxide reacts in the following manner:

$$2CO_2 + 2H_2O \rightleftarrows 2H_2CO_3 \rightarrow \quad 4H^+ + 2CO_3^{2-}$$
$$+ \qquad +$$
$$2NaOH \rightarrow 2OH^- + 2Na^+$$
$$+ \qquad +$$
$$Ca(OH)_2 \rightarrow 2OH^- + Ca^{2+}$$
$$\downarrow \qquad \downarrow$$
$$4H_2O + Na_2CO_3$$
$$+ CaCO_3$$

The reaction proceeds in three phases: gaseous, liquid, and solid. Carbon dioxide obviously represents the gaseous phase. The liquid phase is the very thin film of water containing the hydroxides which surrounds the granule. The solid phase consists of undissolved sodium, calcium, potassium, inert silicate, and diatomaceous earth (Sodasorb) or undissolved barium, calcium, and potassium (Baralyme)[3-6] Conversion of hydroxides to

carbonates begins on the surface of the granule and proceeds inward.[7]

Size of Granules

Carbon dioxide is absorbed by oxides, peroxides, and hydroxides. Hydroxides are favored because they are stable and easily handled in granule form. Hydroxides of cesium, rubidium, lithium, magnesium, and strontium are excellent absorbents but expensive and highly toxic. Barium, calcium, potassium, and sodium hydroxides are inexpensive, have a low toxicity, and are relatively effective. Granule size is of utmost importance in exposing a maximum surface area for chemical interaction. The standard granule size of 4 to 8 mesh has been accepted through trial and error. An 8-mesh granule is one which will pass through a screen with eight wires per linear inch in each direction. Each granule is poxed with pores to increase the surface exposure area. Brown,[8,9] using an entity called the bulk mass transfer coefficient, $K_g a$, to measure the effectiveness of pores in the absorption of carbon dioxide, predicted an active surface area of 4- to 8-mesh particles as 5 to 6 cm^2/cc. He found the actual active surface area for the absorption of 4- to 8-mesh particles to be greater than 100 cm^2/cc. The typical pore volume for soda lime is between 25 and 32 cc/100g dry weight with a packed density of 86 to 92 g/100 cc. Pores are important in allowing the carbon dioxide molecules to diffuse deeper into the granule as activity on the surface decreases. "The amount of carbon dioxide diffusing into the granule depends on the area of the pore mouths opening on the external surface of the granule and is inversely related to the average distance carbon dioxide diffuses into the pore."[8] The irregular granule surface means there is little probability of interdigitation between granules. Moisture is retained very well by the highly permeable mass of granules.[3] Three of the most important factors for absorbent granules are size, porosity, and the nature of the granule surface.

Moisture Content

Soda lime absorbs most efficiently[7,10] when the granule moisture content is between 10 and 22 percent. The upper acceptable limit for Sodasorb[11] is 19 percent. Baralyme contains eight molecules of water of crystallization in the barium hydrate, with additional water being added to achieve the desired U.S. Pharmacopeia (USP) level.

Heat Generation

The overall exothermic carbon dioxide absorption reaction releases approximately 14,000 cal for every 22.2 L of carbon dioxide absorbed.[12] Temperatures[12] within the soda lime[12] can reach 45 to 50°C. Since the exothermic reaction continues after the granules are exhausted, a warm carbon dioxide canister does not guarantee functional granules.[3] The condensation ring which forms at the reaction interface is sometimes used to monitor the reaction rate or degree of absorbent usage.[11]

Resistance

Mesh of size 4 to 8 is the best combination for low resistance and adequate surface area. Size 4 to 8 mesh has 25 to 35 granules per cubic centimeter with about 65 percent air.[12] The specific resistance K of 4 to 8 mesh is 1 mm H_2O per liter per minute.[13] The resistance R to airflow within a filled canister is dependent upon the velocity V of the airflow, the length L, and the cross-sectional area A of the absorber. Resistance is $R = KLV/A$, which means that a 2-L canister with a chamber less than 18 cm long and a diameter greater than 12 cm has a resistance of less than 1 cmH_2O at a flow rate of 60 L/min.

The resistance in 500- and 1250-g canisters during rigid experimental conditions was, respectively, 3.0 and 3.2 cmH_2O during expiration and −3.0 and −3.2 cmH_2O during inspiration.[14] Resistance in the circle absorber can be virtually eliminated when gases in the circuit are circulated by mechanical circulators. However, with large double canisters and quality absorbent granules the resistance in the canister is clinically negligible.

Dust

Dust from soda lime has been implicated as the cause of facial burns and bronchospasm.[15] All current carbon dioxide absorbents can cause irritation to mucus tissue. Friability of the granules may be decreased by increasing hardness with inert silicate. This must be done carefully, since an excess of silicate will eliminate the granules ability to absorb carbon dioxide. The addition of diatomaceous earth (kieselguhr) will reduce clogging of granule pores by excess silicates.[4] During the manufacture of Sodasorb the granules are coated by a patented method to further reduce dust formation.[3] The soda lime slurry of years gone by has been replaced by a granule made of sodium hydroxide, calcium hydroxide, and potassium hydroxide combined with inert silica and diatomaceous earth. The entire manufacturing process is designed to produce absorbent granules with durability, consistent quality, and a uniform mesh size.

The hygroscopic properties of sodium or barium hydroxide and sodium carbonate caused a "caking" or binding phenomenon in the past. The paths between granules were obliterated, resulting in increased resistance in the canister and reduced absorption efficency.[12,16] Methods now incorporated in granule manufacture have successfully eliminated the binding problem.

Routine testing of the rebreathing bag by overfilling the bag and checking for leaks was found to be hazardous because of dust contamination of the breathing circuit.[17] However, Ribak[18] was unable to duplicate the finding when using disposable tandem carbon dioxide absorber canisters at inflation pressures of 50 to 60 cmH_2O.

Regeneration

The apparent resurrection of expended absorbent granules is attributed to the chemical reaction

$$Na_2CO_3 + Ca(OH)_2 \rightarrow 2NaOH + CaCO_3$$

The sodium carbonate is causticized by excess calcium hydroxide, as was shown by Forreger[19] in 1948. Figure 5-1 shows that 30 minutes of regenerative cycling does not appreciably change the time efficiency of the carbon dioxide canister.[20] Regeneration may be an interesting phenomen, but it does not extend the life of the soda lime or contribute to the practical use of the absorbent granules.

Barium hydrate granules do not regenerate but will appear to rejuvenate if left, because the violet color will lighten through simple migration of chemical by-products. After 15 minutes of exposure to expired respiratory gases the color will return to the original one noted at the end of the previous use period.[6,11]

Sterility

Carbon dioxide canisters have been universally used for a long time. To date no study has been able to conclusively demonstrate that patients become infected during exposure to the anesthesia circuit. Under experimental conditions nebulized suspensions of bacteria have been shown to pass through soda lime and barium hydroxide lime, but cross-infection by this source has not been demonstrated clinically.[21] Adriani and Rovenstine[12] exposed the inhalation and exhalation gases of the circle system to the contents of a Petri dish. The Petri dish was actually placed in the circle

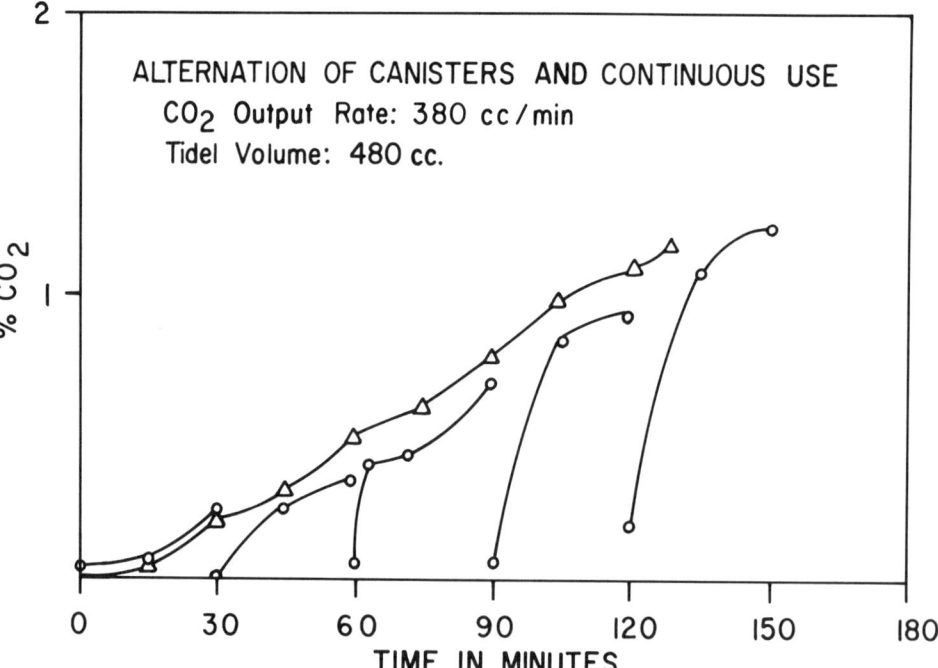

Fig. 5-1 Regeneration of soda lime does not change the time efficiency of the absorbent granules. The solid line shows the continuous use of a carbon dioxide absorption canister. Interruptions on the lower line represent 30-minute regenerative cycling of a two-canister system. (Reprinted by permission from Brown ES, Elam JO: Practical aspects of carbon dioxide absorption. NY State J Med 55:3436. Copyright 1965, The Medical Society of the State of New York.)

in place of the patient's face to simulate contamination from an infected patient. *Bacillus coli* and tubercule bacilli were placed in the Petri dish. Glass beads embedded in the soda lime were removed immediately after exposure to the Petri dish and showed the bacteria were passing into the canister. No growth was found on any plate exposed to air currents exiting the canister immediately after contamination, 2 hours later, and after 24 hours. The possibility of cross-contamination from a carbon dioxide absorber canister is very remote. Bacteria may pass through the absorbent beds but the absorbent granules will not sustain bacterial growth.

A few investigators warn of possible bacterial contamination from the circle system.[22,23] Disposable bacterial filters were developed for the circle system.[24] In 1980 anesthesiologists spent approximately $50 million on these single-use devices designed to prevent the potential transmission of bacteria.[25] Recent prospective clinical studies support the concept that the circle system is an unlikely source of bacterial contamination.[26-28] These prospective clinical studies recommended we "stop using bacterial filters for breathing circuits."[29]

Reactivity with General Anesthetics

Absorbent granules do not chemically react with any of the general anesthetics in wide use today. However, as absorbent granules dry the pores open and halothane, enflurane, and isoflurane can be absorbed in a manner similar to the reaction of small organic molecules with molecular sieves.[30,31] The absorption process is reversible, thus, theoretically, induction could be slowed and a subsequent patient given an inadvertent exposure to the anesthetic agent. Trichloroethylene reacts with soda lime or barium lime in the presence of heat to form hydrochloric acid, dichloroacetylene, phosgene, and carbon monoxide.[32,33] Fortunately, trichlorethylene is not in widespread use in the United States.

Testing

Standards for the composition and performance of medical soda lime have been established by the USP.[3,34,35] Absorbent granules must be tested for (1) moisture, (2) mesh size distribution, (3) hardness, and (4) absorption capacity. The testing methods employed for Sodasorb will be discussed. Each company may test differently but still comply with the USP standard.[3]

Moisture testing

A total of 20 g of absorbent granules are taken from the final stage of batching, placed in a drying oven, and reweighed after drying. Water loss is calculated as a percentage of the original weight and must be between 14 and 19 percent for high-moisture Sodasorb.

Mesh size distribution

A 200-g sample of granules is agitated in a Ro-Tap machine at 1,750 rpm for 5 minutes using no. 4, no. 6, and no. 8 screens and "fines" pan. A maximum of 7 percent oversized particles (retained by a no. 4 screen) and 7 percent undersized particles (retained by a no. 8 screen) is allowed. Less than 65 percent must be in the proportion retained by no. 6 and no. 8 screens.

Hardness

A sample of 50 g of absorbent granules from the no. 6 and no. 8 screens are subjected to 45 lb of hydraulic pressure in a steel cylinder for 1 minute. The resultant contents are placed on a no. 10 screen in the Ro-Tap agitator machine. The material left on the no. 10 screen must weigh over 40 g. The minimum desirable hardness is 80 on a hardness scale of 100. The hydraulic pressure test replaces the slower common abrasion test method.

Absorption capacity

A USP apparatus similar to the one shown in Fig. 5-2 assays the chemical properties of the absorbent granules. A 10-g sample is placed in the U-tube containing $CaCl_2$, which traps any moisture produced during the neutralization reaction. After the U-tube is weighed, carbon dioxide is run through at 75 cc/min. After 20 minutes the carbon dioxide flow is stopped and the U-tube cooled and reweighed. The minimum permissible quantity of carbon dioxide absorbed by the granules means a minimum increase in weight of 22 percent.

The Dewey and Almy Chemical Division (manufacturer of Sodasorb) perform an additional "simulated clinical test."[3] Absorbent granules are placed in an in vitro circuit designed to simulate the conditions found in the operating room. A spirometer fitted with a piston imitates tidal volume and rate of respiration (see Fig. 5-3). Carbon dioxide is volumetrically monitored at the input end of the apparatus. At the output end a carbon dioxide analyzer analyzes the carbon dioxide concentration.

Indicator Dye

Dye has long been incorporated in the granules to signal lack of absorbent capacity. A patent for self-indicating soda lime was granted to John R. Ruhoff of the Mallinckrodt Chemical Works of St. Louis on January 13,

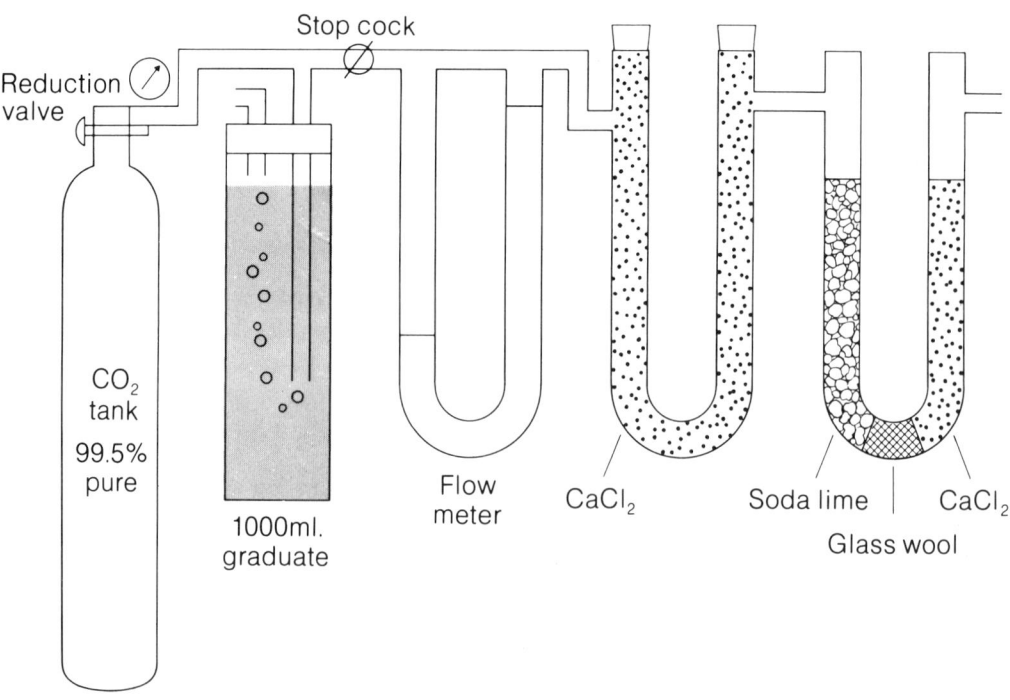

Fig. 5-2 The USP test apparatus for determining the chemical characteristics of absorption granules. Moisture is trapped by the calcium chloride through a neutralization reaction. The U-tube is weighed before and after a known quantity of carbon dioxide is passed through the system. The minimum permissible quantity of carbon dioxide absorbed will give at least a 22 percent weight increase. (The Sodasorb: Manual of Carbon Dioxide Absorption. Dewey and Almy Chemical Division, WR Grace & Co., Indianapolis, 1980.)

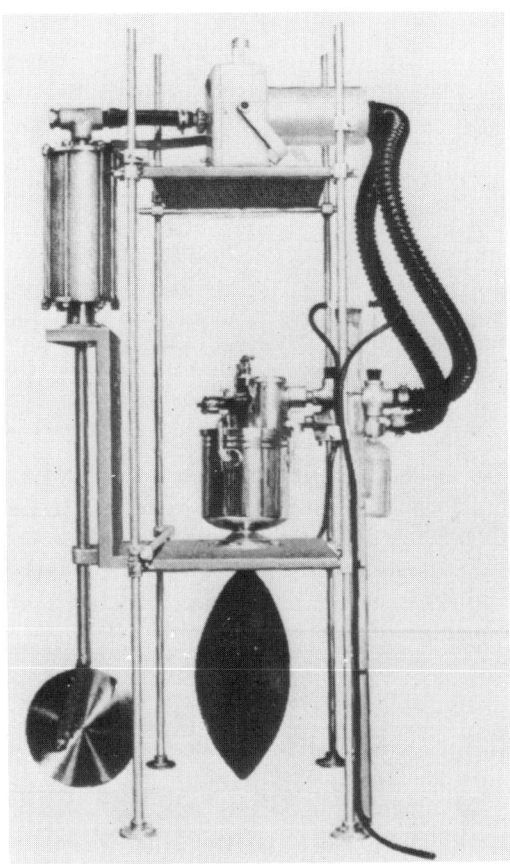

Fig. 5-3 Spirometer designed for the simulated clinical test for Sodasorb absorption. The input of carbon dioxide is volumetrically monitored and the output of carbon dioxide is measured by infrared analysis. Sodasorb granules are tested over a wide range of simulated tidal volumes and respiratory rates. (The Sodasorb: Manual of Carbon Dioxide Absorption. Dewey and Almy Chemical Division, WR Grace & Co., Indianapolis, 1980.)

1942. Indicator dyes are not completely reliable but have certainly increased the safety of using absorbent granules.[4,14,20,36] Many dyes have been used with granules: Mimoza Z dye concentrate, Clayton Yellow, Peeramine Brilliant Yellow, MN extra dye concentrate, and ethyl violet.[4,6] Baralyme and Sodasorb presently use ethyl violet as the indicator dye.[6,11] Ethyl violet {N-[4-[bis[4-(diethylamino) phenyl]methylene]-2,5-cyclohexadien-1-ylidene]-

N-ethyl chloride; $C_{31}H_{42}N_3Cl$} is a weak organic insoluble base with a critical pH of 10.3 which is converted by carbonic acid to a soluble violet salt (see Fig. 5-4).[3,35,37] A deep violet (purple) color in the granule indicates complete exhaustion. The color change usually parallels the falling absorption capacity of the granules. In 1944 Adriani cautioned anesthesiologists not to rely entirely on the indicator dye color change but, in addition, to use the three clinical signs of hypercarbia. He defined these signs as (1) hyperpnea, (2) hypertension, and (3) lack of heat production in the canister.[35] The presence of these clinical signs should make one think of obtaining an arterial blood gas or monitoring the end-tidal carbon dioxide level.

Indicator dyes in the granules are helpful to warn us of changes in the absorber. Color changes indicate that a chemical reaction is underway, even though we do not know the exact extent. Indicator dyes are especially valuable in the in-series double canisters presently employed.[38]

Absorption Efficiency

Absorbers have the highest efficiency when the space between the granules is equal to or greater than the tidal volume of the patient.[12,14,20,39] Under usual clinical conditions fresh soda lime can reduce the concentration of carbon dioxide from 5 to 0.5 percent in only 0.16 second of contact time. Fresh Baralyme requires 0.32 second under similar conditions.[20]

Each 100 g of soda lime will give 1 hour of useful life[20] at a tidal volume of 500 cc, a respiratory rate of 15 per minute, and a carbon dioxide production rate of 280 cc/min. Measurements of carbon dioxide absorption capacity will vary according to the packing of the canister and the channeling phenomenon. Soda lime absorbs 14 to 23 L of carbon dioxide per 100 g of granules and barium lime absorbs 9 to 18 L of carbon dioxide per 100 g of granules.[3,20] A total of 100 g of absorbent has

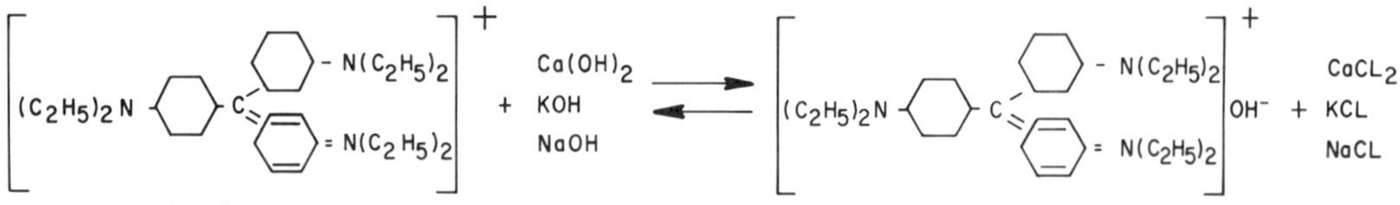

$$\left[(C_2H_5)_2N \bigcirc C \overset{- N(C_2H_5)_2}{\underset{= N(C_2H_5)_2}{\bigcirc}} \right]^+ \begin{matrix} Ca(OH)_2 \\ + KOH \\ NaOH \end{matrix} \rightleftharpoons \left[(C_2H_5)_2N \bigcirc C \overset{- N(C_2H_5)_2}{\underset{= N(C_2H_5)_2}{\bigcirc}} \right]^+ OH^- + \begin{matrix} CaCL_2 \\ KCL \\ NaCL \end{matrix}$$

Dye salt (blue)   Dye base (colorless)

Fig. 5-4 Chemical structure of ethyl violet. As ethyl violet is mixed with a new absorbent, the blue dye salt is converted to a colorless dye base by reaction with hydroxyl groups. Carbon dioxide consumes base during absorption, which causes the chemical reaction to shift toward the left. The resultant blue or violet color thus "indicates" the absorbent granule is becoming or is already exhausted. (Redrawn from Kinsel EA, technical superintendent. Dewey and Almy Chemical Division, WR Grace & Co., Atlanta, 1985.)

been quoted to absorb as much as 50 L of carbon dioxide.[40] On a practical basis, if the tidal volume is between 0.5 and 1.0 L and the carbon dioxide output 12 to 18 L/hour, the expected total load during an 8-hour period would be between 100 and 150 L of carbon dioxide. A well-designed canister with 870 g of absorbent granules would absorb the carbon dioxide and ensure an outlet concentration of less than 1 percent carbon dioxide.[41]

The interstitial space of absorbent granules is approximately 47 percent of the gross volume. As the granules react with the expired carbon dioxide, the pores in the granules and the intergranular space begin to fill with water, thus reducing the void space. Reduction in void space below the tidal volume of the patient reduces the efficiency of absorption. Addition of a second canister in series allows the ideal void volume to be maintained and preserves absorption efficiency. The best arrangement is two 1-L canisters in series.

In an effort to save money one hospital purchased a supply of soda lime which did not contain indicator dye. The anesthesiologists were not informed of the purchase and were used to changing the soda lime when the indicator dye turned the appropriate color. A patient was eventually exposed to a low-flow circle system with exhausted absorbent granules and developed a high arterial carbon dioxide level. Fortunately the fresh gas inflow rates were increased and the problem investigated.

The incident was inappropriately labeled "unusual failure of anesthetic equipment," even though it was human error.[42] Carbon dioxide granules are used in circle systems every day and constant vigilance is necessary to avoid repetition of such an incident.

Present Granules

Absorbent granules are presently 4 to 8 mesh, have low dust, contain 14 to 19 percent water, use ethyl violet indicator dye, are inert to the majority of anesthetic agents, are stable in use, and meet the standards of the National Formulary and USP.[34,35]

Packaging of absorbed granules is available as large bulk containers, individual single-canister packages, and completely disposable containers (see Fig. 5-5 and 5-6). Each anesthesiologist must determine the most economical and convenient packaging to meet his needs.

CANISTER

The large, round double canister with transparent sides has evolved over the years. The physical characteristics of the canister derived from experimental as well as trial-and-error processes have determined the most efficient canister design for absorbing carbon dioxide.

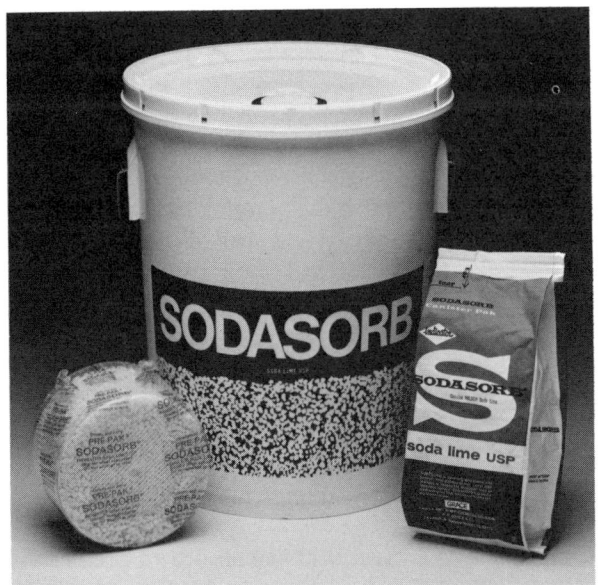

Fig. 5-5 Packaging of Sodasorb granules: a disposable container, a large bulk container, and a single-canister refill size. (Courtesy of Dewey and Almy Chemical Division, WR Grace & Co., Atlanta, 1985.)

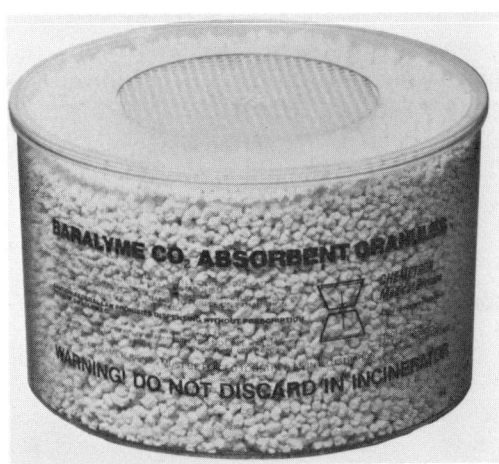

Fig. 5-6 A disposable container of Baralyme carbon dioxide absorbent granules. Each container must be unwrapped and placed in the canister correctly for proper function. (Courtesy of Allied Healthcare Products, St. Louis, 1984.)

Shape and Size

The to-and-fro canister designed by Waters has proven to be very close to the best design for the circle absorber.[43] Adriani and Byrd[39] studied the effect of shape on the efficiency of absorption. A number of absorber shapes with various configurations (cylindrical, spherical, oval–flat, oblong, and conical) were studied. A constant cubic volume of 500 g of granules in 425 cc of air space was maintained for each shape. Efficiency was not changed by canister shape but was optimal when the air space between the granules was equivalent to the tidal volume of the patient.

The double canister is recommended as being the most efficient and practical method for carbon dioxide absorption.[13,10,44] A double canister used in 1876 in a respiratory apparatus served as the model for the double-canister anesthesia machine[45] designed in Germany in 1906. A double canister can be reversed, easily replaced when using a disposable unit, and it provides a backup for proper carbon dioxide absorption.

Transparent canisters became important with the advent of indicator dyes. Initially the material in the canisters was easily degraded by chemical reaction, but the walls of present-day canisters appear to resist chemical degradation effectively.

Channeling

Channeling occurs in a loosely packed canister or when the canister design allows the gases to pass along the sides. A small space at the top of the canister allows the gases to mix and distribute more evenly. In a vertical canister the gases must pass from the top to the bottom to avoid carrying dust into the circuit. Annular rings or baffles placed at intervals increase the path of peripheral airflow and partially compensate for the reduced resistance along the sidewall.[3,13,41,46]

All canisters have some element of channeling. Figure 5-7 shows a standard canister exposed to 10 hours of continuous use and then analyzed to observe the pattern of carbon dioxide absorption. The majority of the chemical reaction occurred in the upper half of the chamber. Theoretically the first seventh of the canister absorbs 90 percent of the carbon dioxide.[16] Two paths of intermittent absorption are identified along each side. Many absorbent granules are not used during the administration of the anesthetic. Change of the indicator dye in the upper one-half of the top canister means the bottom canister should be moved to the top position, a new canister placed in the bottom position, and the absorbent granules in the exhausted canister discarded.

Flow Rate

The efficiency of the absorbent granules is affected by the rate of flow into the canister. Tidal volume, respiratory rate, and peak flow rate have been shown to adversely affect efficiency in single canisters.[47] Large tidal volumes reduce the efficiency of small canisters rapidly but have only minor effects on large canisters. Increasing tidal volume and reducing respiratory rate will decrease small canister efficiency. Changes in tidal volume and respiratory rate have little effect on the overall effective absorption capacity of the large absorbers. Increased peak flows will rapidly decrease canister efficiency.

Present Design

Anesthesia circle system carbon dioxide absorber canisters are presently cylindrical, are usually used in a series of two, have transparent sides, have baffles or annular rings, have a volume of 900 to 1,200 cc, contain approximately 850 to 1,300 g of absorbent granules, and are available in disposable self-contained units.

An adult patient with a carbon dioxide production of 300 ml/min under general anesthesia via a circle system with a fresh gas flow of 2 L/min will have carbon dioxide successfully removed by a 600 to 700 g soda lime

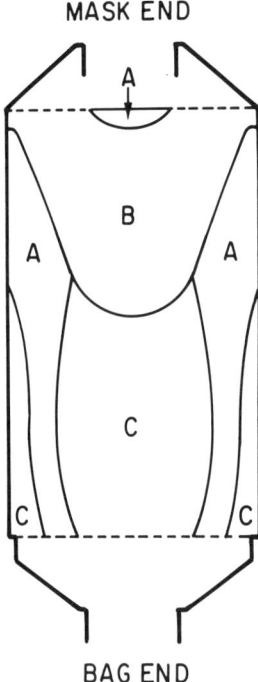

MASK END

BAG END

Fig. 5-7 Channeling in the carbon dioxide canister. Areas marked A show partial color change, area B has turned dark purple, and areas marked C show no color change after 10 hours of intermittent use. (Conroy WA, Seevers MH: Studies in carbon dioxide absorption. Anesthesiology 4:160, 1943.)

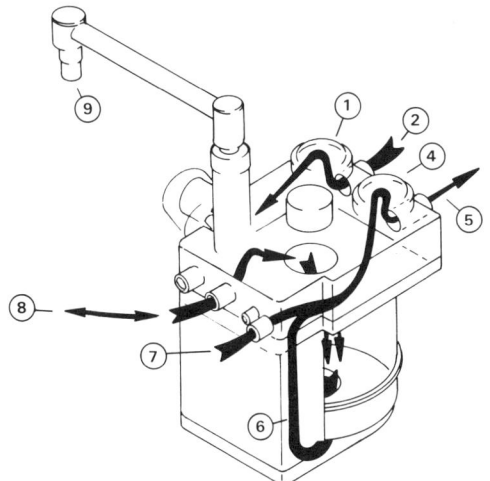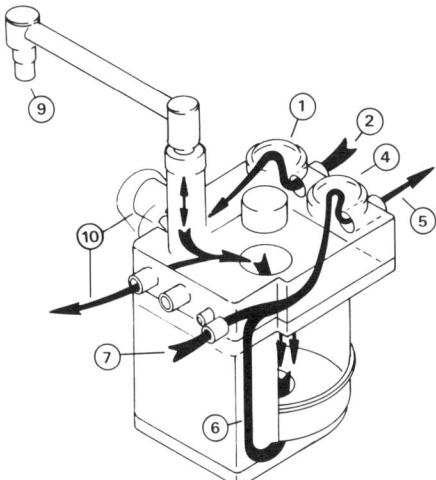

Fig. 5-8 Flow diagram through the GMS absorber of the Modulus II anesthesia machine. BAG/APL mode has been selected in the bottom diagram and VENTILATOR mode selected in the top diagram: (1) exhalation check valve, (2) exhaled gases from patient, (4) inhalation check valve, (5) to patient, (6) exhaled gases with CO_2 removed, (7) fresh gas mixture from anesthesia machine, (8) ventilator, (9) reservoir bag, and (10) APL ("pop-off") valve with excess gas to scavenging interface valve. (Courtesy of Ohmeda, The BOC Group, Inc.)

compartment over a period of at least 5 hours.[23] Figure 5-8 shows the flow diagram through a carbon dioxide absorber. Absorbers can be purchased with a bypass mechanism. A survey in Canada found that 53 percent of 313 anesthesiologists felt the bypass should not be removed and 79 percent felt the bypass should have clearer labeling.[48] Some anesthesiologists have recommended the prohibition of a bypass on the absorber owing to potentially hazardous hypercarbia. Faulty assembly of the carbon dioxide absorber can result in high levels of inspired and expired carbon dioxide.[49] Anesthesiologists using gas flows greater than 5 L/min during anesthesia convert the circle system to a nonrebreathing system.

REFERENCES

1. Foregger R: Lavoisier's research on carbon dioxide and its control. Anesthesiology 23:662, 1962

2. Oeuvres de Lavoisier: 1, p. 458, 1864.

3. Sodasorb: Manual of Carbon Dioxide Absorption. Dewey and Almy Chemical Division, W. R. Grace & Co, Indianapolis, 1980

4. Hale DE: The rise and fall of soda lime. Anesth Analg 46:648, 1967

5. Kilborn MG: Preliminary clinical report on a new carbon dioxide absorbent—Baralyme. Anesthesiology 2:621, 1941

6. Michaely CE, engineering manager. Letter, 11 November 1984. Allied Healthcare Products, St Louis

7. Adriani J: The effect of varying the moisture content of soda lime upon the efficiency of carbon dioxide absorption. Anesthesiology 6:163, 1945

8. Brown ES: The activity and surface area of fresh soda lime. Anesthesiology 19:208, 1958

9. Brown ES: Voids, pores and total air space of carbon dioxide absorbents. Anesthesiology 19:1, 1958

10. Mousel LH, Weiss WA, Gilliom LA: A clinical study of carbon dioxide absorption during anesthesia. Anesthesiology 7:375, 1946

11. Anapole VI, plant manager. Letter, 22 March 1985. Dewey and Almy Chemical Division,

W. R. Grace & Co., Atlanta

12. Adriani J, Rovenstine EA: Experimental studies on carbon dioxide absorbers for anesthesia. Anesthesiology 2:1, 1941
13. Elam JO: The design of circle absorbers. Anesthesiology 19:99, 1958
14. Conroy WA, Seevers MH: Studies in carbon dioxide absorption. Anesthesiology 4:160, 1943
15. Lauria JI: Soda-lime dust contamination of breathing circuits. Anesthesiology 42:628, 1975
16. Brown ES: Certain physical properties and reaction kinetics of carbon dioxide absorbents. USAF School of Aviation Medicine, Brooks AFB, San Antonio, 1954
17. Debban DG, Bedford RF: Overdistention of the rebreathing bag: a hazardous test for circle-system integrity. Anesthesiology 42:365, 1975
18. Ribak B: Reducing the soda-lime hazard. Anesthesiology 43:277, 1975
19. Foregger R: The regeneration of soda lime following absorption of carbon dioxide. Anesthesiology 9:15, 1948
20. Brown ES, Elam JO: Practical aspects of carbon dioxide absorption. NY State J Med 55:3436, 1965
21. Stark DCC, Green CA, Pask EA: Anaesthetic machines and cross-infection. Anaesthesia 17:12, 1962
22. Dryden GE: Risk of contamination from the anesthesia circle absorber: an evaluation. Anesth Analg 48:939, 1969
23. Jorgensen B, Jorgensen S: Carbon dioxide elimination from circle systems. Acta Anaesthesiol Scand 53:86, 1973
24. Martin JT, Ulrich JA: A bacterial filter for an anesthetic circuit. Anesth Anal 48:944, 1969
25. Du Moulin GC, Hedley-Whyte J: Bacterial interactions between anesthesiologists, their patients, and equipment. Anesthesiology 57:37, 1982
26. Du Moulin GC, Saubermann AJ: The anesthesia machine and circle system are not likely to be sources of bacterial contamination. Anesthesiology 47:353, 1977
27. Feeley TW, Hamilton WK, Xavier B et al: Sterile anesthesia breathing circuits do not prevent postoperative pulmonary infection. Anesthesiology 54:369, 1981
28. Garibaldi RA, Britt MR, Webster C et al: Failure of bacterial filters to reduce the incidence of pneumonia after inhalation anesthesia. Anesthesiology 54:364, 1981
29. Mazze RI: Bacterial air filters. Anesthesiology 54:359, 1981
30. Grodin WK, Epstein MAF, Epstein RA: The mechanism of halothane absorption by dry soda lime. Br J Anaesth 54:561, 1982
31. Grodin WK, Epstein MAF, Epstein RA: Soda lime absorption of isoflurane and enflurane. Anesthesiology 62:60, 1985
32. Firth JB, Stuckey RE: Decomposition of trilene in closed circuit anaesthesia. Lancet p 814, June 30, 1945
33. Wylie WD, Churchill-Davidson HC: A Practice of Anesthesia. Lloyd-Luke Medical Books, Bucks, England, 1972
34. Barium Hydroxide Lime. United States Pharmacopeia. 21st Ed. United States Pharmacopeial Convention, Rockville, 1985
35. Soda Lime. National Formulary. United States Pharmacopeial Convention, Maryland, 1985
36. Adriani J: Soda lime containing indicators. Anesthesiology 5:45, 1944
37. Ethyl violet. Registry Handbook. Chemical Abstracts Service Registry Handbook. Ohio State University, Columbus, 1965–1971
38. Adriani J: Disposal of carbon dioxide from devices used for inhalational anesthesia. Anesthesiology 21:742, 1960
39. Adriani J, Byrd ML: A study of carbon dioxide absorption appliances for anesthesia: the canister. Anesthesiology 2:450, 1941
40. Schreiber P. Anaesthesia Equipment: Performance, Classification and Safety. Springer-Verlag, New York, 1972
41. Elam JO: Channeling and overpacking in carbon dioxide absorbers. Anesthesiology 19:403, 1958
42. Detmer MD, Chandra P, Cohen PJ: Occurrence of hypercarbia due to an unusual failure of anesthetic equipment. Anesthesiology 52:278, 1980
43. Waters RM: Clinical scope and utility of carbon dioxide filtration in inhalation anesthesia. Anesth Analg 3:20, 1924
44. Kappesser RC: Modification of double canister circle filter. Anesthesiology 14:415, 1953
45. Foregger R: Respiratory apparatus of Theodor Schwann. Anesthesiology 27:187, 1966
46. Ten Pas RH, Brown ES, Elam JO: Carbon dioxide absorption: the circle versus the to-and-fro. Anesthesiology 19:231, 1958

47. Brown ES: Factors affecting the performance of absorbents. Anesthesiology 20:198, 1959

48. Neufeld PD: Results of the Canadian Anaesthetists Society opinion survey on anaesthetic equipment. Can Anaesth Soc J 30:469, 1983

49. Luich RJ: CO_2 absorber malassembly. Anesthesiology 59:598, 1983

50. Kinsel EA, technical superintendent. Letter, 1 February 1985. Dewey and Almy Chemical Division, W. R. Grace & Co., Atlanta

6

Anesthesia Circuits

Numerous circuits have been designed for the anesthesia machine but only a few are actually used by anesthesiologists in private practice. This chapter will address those circuits which are usually utilized with the Ohmeda Modulus II and the Narkomed IIA anesthesia machines. Multiple sources review other anesthesia circuits of interest.[1-6]

"Closed circuit" and "Bain circuit" (modified Mapleson D) anesthesia systems have stirred up a great deal of controversy. Both sides have fanatics who see only what they wish to see in relationship to anesthesia circuits. Somewhere in the middle ground stands the true value of closed-circuit anesthesia and the modified Mapleson D circuit in the practice of anesthesia.

Present-day utilization of anesthesia circuits is based on a conglomeration of scientific facts, clinical observation, instilled habits, pseudo-economics, and long-standing prejudices. Even today we do not understand the exact physical mechanisms which occur in the anesthesia circuit with altered fresh gas flow rates, lung compliance changes, and spontaneous or controlled ventilation. Additions to the circuits, such as a scavenging system and bacterial filters, are also in question and have usually been added without scientific forethought but instead on the basis of such things

as threats to malpractice. Scavenging, for instance, has not been shown to be a necessity in the operating room but still remains an additional hazard to the patient. Intermittently using the circle and Bain systems can be complex and during switchovers serious errors can be made by the anesthesiologist.

CIRCLE SYSTEM

Circle systems have been incorporated in anesthesia machines for a long time in the United States. The introduction of cyclopropane in 1933 made the circle system absolutely necessary.[7] Closed-circuit anesthesia became widespread because of the expense and explosive nature of cyclopropane. Anesthesiologists used low-flow techniques without the use of oxygen analyzers, mass spectrometers, end-tidal carbon dioxide monitors, or the host of other instruments presently advocated for use in closed-circuit anesthesia.

Following the introduction of halothane in 1956 an increase was seen in the use of higher flows ("semiclosed," "semiopen") in anesthesia.[8,9] A number of factors seemed to combine to foster the use of higher flows in anesthesia. First, the Vernitrol and copper kettle created the environment for a typical 5-L gas flow.[10]

The vapor pressure of halothane made it easy to set the total gas flow at 5 L and mentally convert the milliliters of flow through the copper kettle or Vernitrol into the percent of halothane being delivered to the circle system.[11] Second, initial agent-specific vaporizers were inaccurate at low flow rates, functioning best at fresh gas flows from 3 to 5 L/min. Third, the introduction of the minimum alveolar concentration (MAC) concept caused many anesthesiologists to equate the concentration of the anesthetic agent delivered in a high-flow system with the alveolar concentration.[9] High-flow anesthesia habits were persistently taught to generations of anesthesiologists. Today many anesthesiologists set induction flow rates at 5 L/min and do not reduce the maintenance flow rates to 1 L/min in the circle system despite the introduction of specific-agent vaporizers capable of accurate outputs at low flow rates.[12]

A flow of 5 L/min in the circle system almost negates the need for carbon dioxide absorption granules, because the system is converted to a semiclosed system.[13] At flow rates above 3 L/min the Bain or CPRAM circuit could be substituted for the circle system. The problems of the circle system would be eliminated and the advantages of a Mapleson D system introduced. Perhaps the introduction of mass spectrometers into the operating room and the formation of the Closed Circuit and Low Flow Anesthesia Systems Society[14] will educate the anesthesiologist to the economical and practical use of lower flow rates during the maintenance of anesthesia.

Design and Function

Figure 6-1 illustrates the components of the circle system: a carbon dioxide absorber, an inspiratory valve, an expiratory valve, an adjustable pressure-limiting valve (APL valve, "pop-off valve," or "relief" valve), a reservoir (rebreathing) bag, circuit hoses, and a fresh gas hose inlet. The pop-off valve is connected to a scavenging system for exiting excess anesthesia gases. A ventilator hose replaces the reservoir bag when controlled ventilation is introduced.

Different configurations of the basic components of the circle system have emerged.[1] The

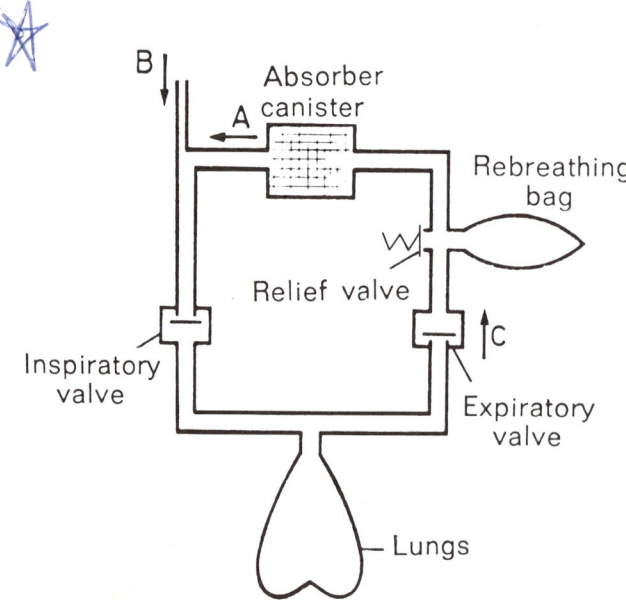

Fig. 6-1 Basic components of a circle system. Fresh gas flow enters the circle at B and flows directly through the inspiratory valve to the lungs. Expired gases pass through the expiratory valve at C to either enter the rebreathing bag, exit the circuit at the relief valve, or stay in the circuit and pass on through the absorber canister at A. (Schreiber P: Anaesthesia Equipment: Performance, Classification and Safety. Springer-Verlag, New York, 1972.)

design in Figure 6-1 incorporates the majority of positive features desired in a circle system.[1] The pop-off valve is positioned between the exhalation valve and the carbon dioxide canister to allow the discharge of low-concentration anesthetic gases during the induction phase and the discharge of high-concentration gases during the emergence phase.[1,16] Venting excess exhaled gases just prior to the carbon dioxide canister conserves considerable amounts of carbon dioxide absorbent granules.[1,16-18] Fresh gas flows directly through the inhalation valve to the patient, ensuring a direct route for the anesthetic gases and emergency oxygen administration.[16,17] Changes in anesthetic gas concentrations are reflected immediately in the inspiratory limb of the circuit. Location of the absorber between the pop-off valve and the fresh gas inlet assists in reducing the respiratory resistance in the circle.[1] The reservoir bag can be located anywhere in the circuit, but it is usually placed in the expiratory limb for convenience. In this position expiratory limb resistance is slightly reduced.[17] During a deep breath the gas in the reservoir bag flows through the carbon dioxide absorber, the inspiratory valve, and into the lung. Continual rebreathing is prevented by controlling unidirectional flow with expiration and inhalation valves. During inspiration the patient inhales a mixture of fresh and rebreathed gas. During expiration the patient's breath joins the fresh gas at the T-junction of the corrugated tube.[19]

Removing the carbon dioxide absorbent granules from the circle system and ventilating the patient with a minute ventilation of 120 to 150 ml/kg (using a fresh gas flow between 50 and 60 ml/kg per minute and a respiratory rate of 10 to 12 per minute) will allow the $PaCO_2$ to be controlled[13,20,21] at 33 to 45 mmHg. When the circle system inflow rate equals the patient's minute volume, the system converts to a nonrebreathing system, during both spontaneous and controlled ventilation.[17] Carbon dioxide absorption is not justified or necessary[15] when the fresh gas flow exceeds 4 L/min.

Advantages

Maximum efficiency of the circle system is utilized with a closed-circuit technique. Benefits of closed-circuit anesthesia are purported to be (1) increased humidification, (2) decrease in operating room pollution, (3) decreased heat loss, (4) closer observation of the patient, and (5) increased understanding of uptake and distribution.[9,22] Quantitative pharmacokinetics necessary to use and understand closed-circuit techniques have been developed.[23]

Low arterial carbon dioxide levels can be achieved with the circle system. The Mapleson D system is not suitable for intentional hypocarbia.[24] Closed-circuit anesthesia requires the presence of the carbon dioxide canister. However, the absorbent granules make it very difficult to increase the arterial concentration of carbon dioxide during emergence from anesthesia. In addition to the anesthetic depth being changed, sometimes the tidal volume and/or respiratory rate must be markedly decreased.

Accurate out-of-circuit vaporizers (Drager 19.1 or Cyprane Tec 4) or direct injection of liquid anesthetic into the circuit can be used for closed-circuit anesthesia.[12] The simple technique of 500 ml/min of nitrous oxide and 500 ml/min of oxygen combined with halothane, enflurane, or isoflurane seems to be a practical approach for closed-circuit anesthesia.[25] Whenever closed circuit is employed, the problems outlined by Bushman et al.[26] must be remembered: (1) Nitrogen can accumulate and dilute inspired oxygen, (2) inspired gas concentrations are unpredictable if nitrous oxide, oxygen, and uncalibrated vaporizers are used, (3) $PaCO_2$ may increase secondary to ventilatory depression, (4) high oxygen concentrations may have deleterious effects, and (5) difficulty may be encountered in producing rapid emergence without pollution of the operating room.

Economic considerations have been proposed as a major reason to reinstitute closed-circuit anesthesia.[27-30] Many hospitals are justifying the purchase of expensive mass spectrometry systems by citing the "savings" in cost for halothane, enflurane, isoflurane, and nitrous oxide. However, the contribution of closed-circuit anesthesia to the overall cost savings in anesthesia has been questioned.[2,22] Are complicated monitoring systems, dosage schedules, and computations really worth the questionable marginal economic advantage? Perhaps a more realistic approach would be to realize the cost potential of using lower flows during the maintenance of anesthesia following an induction with high flows.

Disadvantages

Unfortunately the circle system is the most complex anesthetic system.[6] Many fittings and connections can leak or even disconnect. Figure 6-2 shows a number of places in the circle system found to disconnect. In fact, disconnections in anesthesia circuits are thought to account for the majority of serious accidents in anesthesia. Using "minimal flows" of 500 ml/min in closed-circuit anesthesia requires a no-leak system.[8,25] Leaks in present-day anesthesia machines can be detected using the

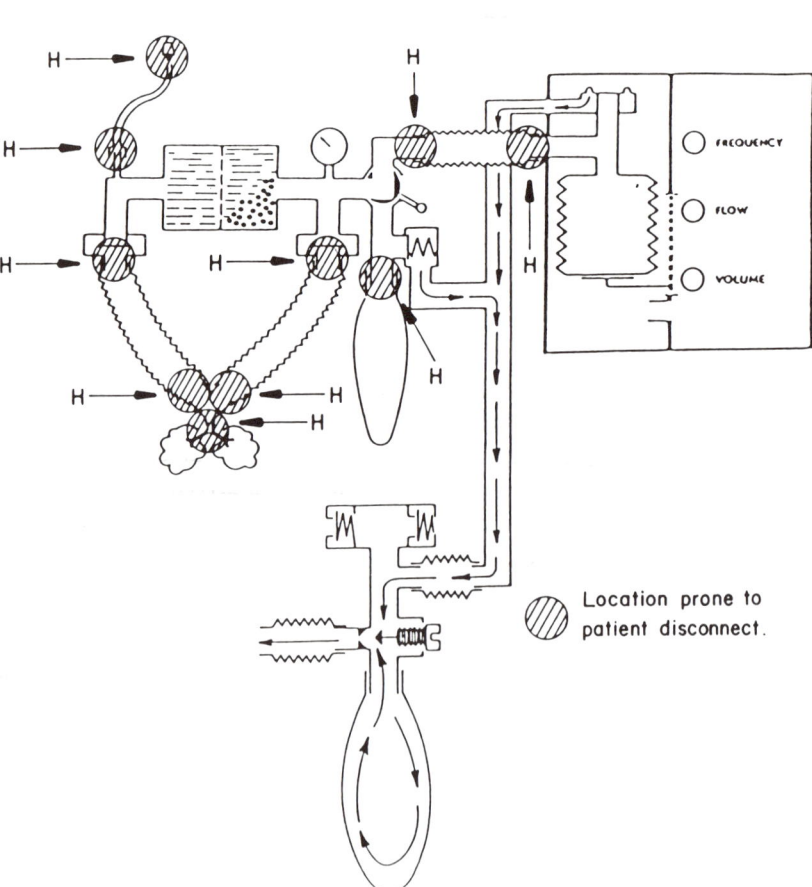

Fig. 6-2 Schematic of the circle system, ventilator attachment, and scavenger system. Connecting points with potential for disconnects are emphasized by the striped circles. (Schreiber P: Anesthesia Systems. North American Drager, Telford, PA, 1985.)

low-and high-pressure leak tests outlined in the instruction and operational manuals.[31,32] A simple test has been outlined to detect a leak when using a ventilator with bellows which rise during filling. Set the fresh gas flow at 300 ml/min and cycle the ventilator four to five times.[33] If the bellows fail to fill each time, a leak is present somewhere in the anesthesia system. The anesthesiologist can also monitor gas composition, that is, end-tidal carbon dioxide levels, in the circuit to detect the presence of a disconnection. However, instruments can fail and the anesthesiologist must continue to monitor the patient by the usual clinical signs. When closed-circuit anesthesia is not required and moderate to high flows of gases are to going be used, it would be appropriate to substitute another breathing system for the circle system.

A circle system is less versatile than a Bain system. Two corrugated tubes attached to a large canister are not as flexible as the thin, lightweight tube of the Bain circuit. Long breathing tubes are available for the circle system but are not as adaptable as one long single tube.

SEMICLOSED SYSTEMS

Mapleson[4] classified the semiclosed anesthesia systems (see Fig. 6-3) according to the position of the pressure relief valve, the fresh gas flow input, and the position and/or presence of the reservoir bag. The most practical and popular system is the Mapleson D. Placing the fresh gas flow tube inside the corrugated tubing of the Mapleson D system by Bain and Spoerel[34] began a long and sustained controversy in anesthesia. Commercial modified Mapleson D anesthesia circuits, such as the Bain and the Controlled Partial Rebreathing Anesthesia Method (CPRAM) breathing systems (see Figs. 6-4 and 6-5), are available that can be adapted to any anesthesia machine.[34,35] Totally nonrebreathing systems

are not practical in the adult because of the inordinately high flows required to prevent rebreathing. For all practical purposes semiclosed systems used in adults are partial rebreathing systems and will henceforth be referred to as Mapleson D or Bain circuits. Even at normal tidal volumes in the adult the minimum fresh gas flow to prevent rebreathing is at least twice the patient's minute volume.[3] If the tidal volume during controlled ventilation is set higher than during the preceding spontaneous ventilation, the fresh gas flow must be increased accordingly.[3]

Partial rebreathing systems for special applications, for example, modified Ayre's T-piece (Mapleson E; Fig. 6-3) for pediatrics, are available and usually require only the attachment of the fresh gas hose from the anesthesia machine. These systems have been discussed and reviewed in a number of publications.[3-5,35-41]

Bain and Spoerel[8] postulate that closed-circuit anesthesia was abandoned because "anesthesiologists were uncomfortable with the complete rebreathing technique and turned up the flow rates for practical reasons." Following the widespread use of muscle relaxants, two additional problems made anesthesiologists uneasy about closed-circuit anesthesia: First, the paralyzed patient required a leak-free circuit and, second, in the paralyzed patient it is virtually impossible to determine the depth of anesthesia. Switching to a partial rebreathing system eliminates both problems. The higher flows compensate for small leaks in the system and sophisticated instruments are not required to monitor the anesthetic concentration in the circuit. Thus paralyzed patients can be ventilated at a constant level of anesthesia.[8]

Resistance to flow in the Bain circuit and the conventional circle system is less than the recommended maximum permissible resistance to breathing (below 3 cmH$_2$O) without an endotracheal tube in adults.[42] The size of the endotracheal tube is the most important

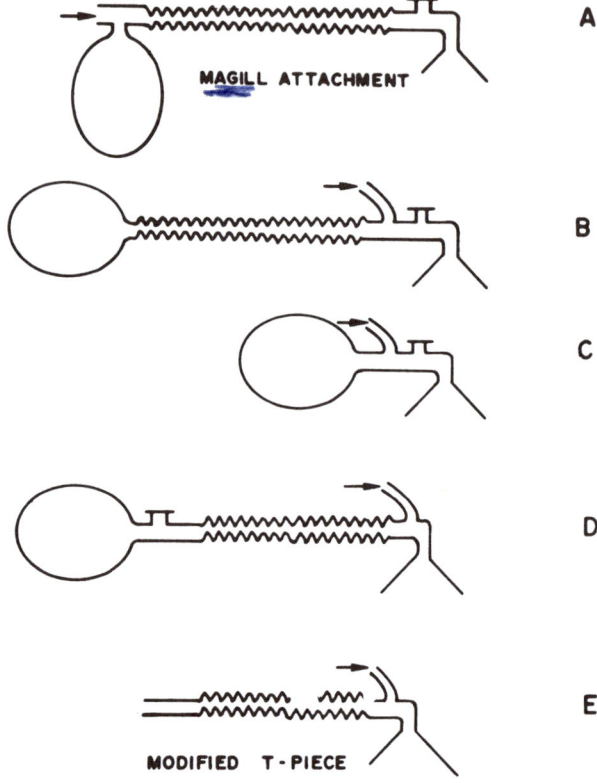

MAGILL ATTACHMENT   A

B

C

D

MODIFIED T - PIECE   E

➤ FRESH GAS INFLOW FROM ANAESTHETIC MACHINE

Fig. 6-3 The classification of rebreathing systems by Mapleson. (Bain JA, Spoerel WE: A streamlined anaesthetic system. Can Anaesth Soc J 19:426, 1972.)

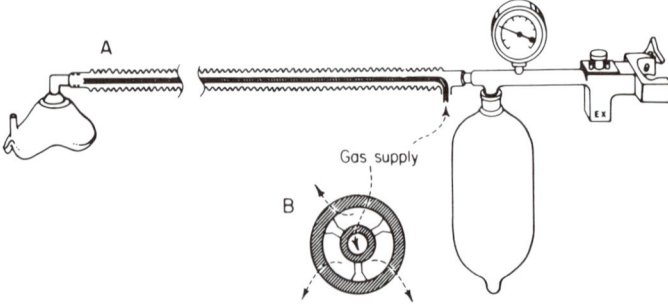

Fig. 6-4 Modified Mapleson D breathing circuit connected to a simple adapter, which has a pressure manometer, a pop-off valve, and a reservoir bag mount. The insert (B) illustrates the fresh gas inflow through the inner tube and outflow via the outer tube. (Chu YK, Rah KH, Boyan CP: Is the Bain breathing circuit the future anesthesia system? An evaluation. Anesth Analg 56:84, 1977. Reprinted with permission, The International Anesthesia Research Society.)

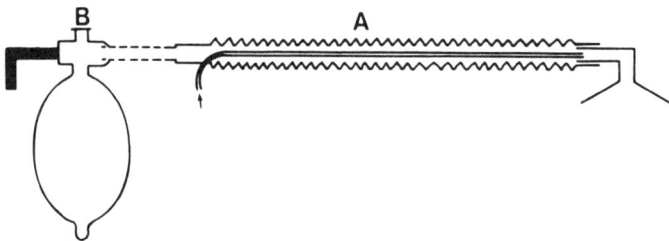

Fig. 6-5 A Bain circuit: (A) corrugated tube with the inner fresh gas hose and (B) bag mount with the pop-off valve. (Bain JA, Spoerel WE: Flow requirements for a modified Mapleson D system during controlled ventilation. Can Anaesth Soc J 20:629, 1973.)

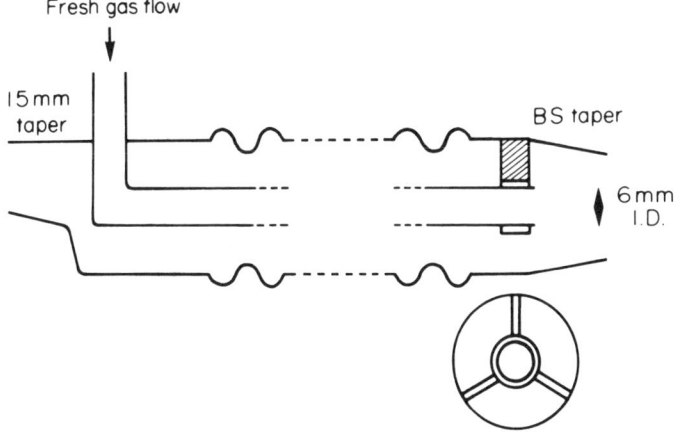

Fig. 6-6 Illustration of the fresh gas inlet and outlet of the Bain circuit. The patient end of the fresh gas hose is mounted in the middle of the single corrugated tube. (Henville JD, Adams AP: The Bain anaesthetic system: an assessment during controlled ventilation. Anaesthesia 31:247, 1976.)

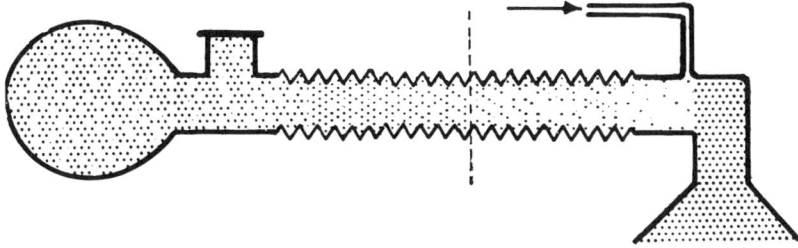

Fig. 6-7 Schematic of expiration in the Mapleson D system. Gas to the right of the dotted line, together with fresh gas entering at the arrow, will enter the patient during the next inhalation. Gas to the left of the dotted line will exit the circuit. (Waters DJ, Mapleson WW: Rebreathing during controlled respiration with various semiclosed anaesthetic systems. Br J Anaesth 33:374, 1961.)

factor in determining resistance in breathing circuits. Other less significant factors include gas density, humidity, and spontaneous versus controlled ventilation. Even in the presence of an endotracheal tube, circuit resistance must not exceed 7 cmH₂O. Differences in resistance between circuits are less than 1.4 cmH₂O and is considered to be of little clinical significance.[42]

Design and Function

Bain and Spoerel[34] introduced the Bain circuit (modified Mapleson D system) in 1972. The fresh gas hose enters the single corrugated tubing at the machine end and travels inside the lumen to the patient end, as shown in Figures 6-5 and 6-6. An expiratory valve and a reservoir bag are placed conveniently at the anesthesia machine.[43] Expiratory gases enter the corrugated tubing from the endotracheal tube or face mask and flow around the fresh gas hose inside the corrugated tubing and eventually out the expiratory valve. Expiratory gas is distributed in the corrugated tube of the Mapleson D circuit as depicted in Figure 6-7. During inhalation, fresh gas is delivered directly to the patient and mixed with gas from the corrugated tubing. All the gas near the face mask (right of the dotted line in Fig. 6-7) will go to the patient.[40] The remainder of the gas will eventually exit via the expiratory valve.

The Mapleson D system was found to involve the least rebreathing during controlled respiration. Ventilation of patients[40] with 500 ml, at 16 times a minute, with an estimated dead-space ventilation of 1.8 L/min, gave a total ventilation of 7.9 L/min with an end-tidal carbon dioxide concentration of 4.3 percent.

Elimination of carbon dioxide from the Bain circuit is dependent on the fresh gas flow, the tidal volume, and to some extent the pattern of breathing.[43,44] Carbon dioxide is eliminated from the circuit in direct proportion to the fresh gas flow according to predictable expo-

nential washout curves.[35] Changes in circuit carbon dioxide levels are reflected in alveolar and blood carbon dioxide levels. A comparison of four independent studies in Figure 6-8 shows a direct correlation between fresh gas flow and PaCO₂. If the fresh gas flow is less than the total minute volume of ventilation, good mixing of gases[45] becomes the main determinant of PaCO₂. The delivery tube of the Bain system projects directly into the stream of expired gas and is thought to be an advantage in creating homogeneous mixtures of gases. Tidal volume and respiratory rate[44-47] can be set over a wide range without affecting the predictability of the PaCO₂.

A completely satisfactory mathematical description of the Mapleson D circuit function is yet to be devised.[48,49] An excellent experimental and theoretical study in 1984 proposed a theoretical formula for the Bain circuit.[50] Rebreathing was found to be governed by the expiratory time fraction and the ratio of the fresh gas flow to the expired total ventilation. Whenever the patient has a prolonged expiration, the fresh gas flow must be increased to prevent excessive rebreathing. Halothane was found to be a better anesthetic during spontaneous respiration because of less depression of the breathing center. A minute ventilation two to three times the fresh gas inflow will give rise to the homogeneous mixing of expired gases and fresh gas inflow at the machine end[3,4,24,51] of the circuit and perhaps throughout the entire length of the circuit at low tidal volumes.[35,37] Nunn[52] stated, "Anaesthetists show astonishing ingenuity in 'improving' gas circuits. While some of these often appear harmless, it sometimes proves that the effects are surprisingly complex and it may become almost impossible to determine the composition of the gas which the patient is inhaling."

Rebreathing occurs in the Bain circuit at all conventional flow rates.[36,53-55] Normocarbia can be maintained during partial rebreathing in the circuit.[45,56] Alexander[55] found that patients anesthetized with halothane and allowed to breath spontaneously required a fresh gas flow of at least 150 ml/kg per minute to

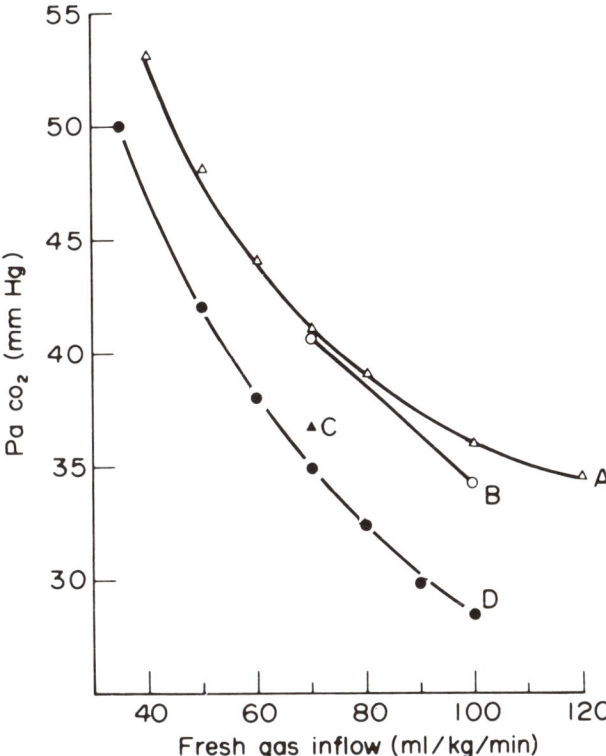

Fig. 6-8 Relationship between fresh gas inflow and $PaCO_2$ using the Bain circuit during controlled ventilation. Points A to D represent four different studies. (Henville JD, Adams AP: The Bain anaesthetic system: an assessment during controlled ventilation. Anaesthesia 31:247, 1976.)

avoid hyperventilation secondary to carbon dioxide retention. Others[36,57,58] have found the minimum fresh gas flow required to prevent rebreathing in the Bain circuit during spontaneous ventilation to be in the range of 100 to 120 ml/kg per minute. A favorable comparison of oxygenation and carbon dioxide elimination was found between the Bain circuit and the semiclosed breathing circuit with a carbon dioxide absorber.[59] Controlled ventilation in the Bain and the semiclosed circle breathing circuits at a tidal volume of 10 ml/kg and a rate of 10 to 17 per minute resulted in mean $PaCO_2$ values of 40.8 and 34.3 mmHg at fresh gas flows of 70 and 100 ml/kg per minute, respectively.[45]

Fresh gas flow rates can be calculated on a weight basis for normal and obese patients but in patients with thyrotoxicosis, fever, or those receiving intravenous hyperalimentation the flow rate must be increased or, better still, the carbon dioxide levels monitored.[46,56]

The theoretical behavior of the Bain circuit does not always follow the clinical behavior owing to (1) inequality between the effective volume of the apparatus dead space and the determination of volumetric displacement, (2) the variation of the size of the anatomic dead space, and (3) the dependence of alveolar gas composition on the pattern of ventilation and lung blood flow.[43]

Advantages

Advantages of the Bain circuit are listed as (1) a single tube goes to the patient, (2) it is lightweight, (3) all unidirectional valves are eliminated, (4) it is useful in all age groups, (5) no carbon dioxide absorption is required, (6) sterilization of the circuit is easy, (7) it is adaptable to all kinds of anesthetic procedures, and (8) it is ideal for head and neck procedures.[34,45,58] Over the ensuing years the

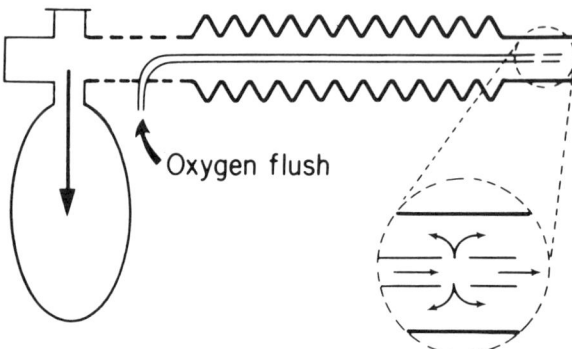

Oxygen flush

Fig. 6-9 A diagram of the CPRAM (Controlled Partial Rebreathing Anesthesia Method) breathing system. Fresh gas entering the oxygen flush port of the circuit exits at the patient end through the side and end holes of the inner tube, as shown in the insert drawing. Vortex dynamics are claimed to be improved by the sideholes, thus improving both humidification and the removal of carbon dioxide. (Robinson S, Fisher DM: Safety check for the CPRAM circuit: to the editor. Anesthesiology 59:488, 1983.)

Bain circuit has been commercially developed with some slight variations made by entrepreneurs to compete in the marketplace. For instance, the CPRAM breathing system has basically the same design as the Bain circuit except for the construction of the distal port of the fresh gas hose inside the corrugated tubing. The inner hose patient end is cone shaped. Two sideholes (see Fig. 6-9) allegedly provide "vortex dynamics" which improve both the humidification of fresh gases and the efficient removal of carbon dioxide.[60]

The Bain circuit has been used in a wide variety of anesthetic techniques and clinically has proven to be safe and reliable.[56,61] Mapleson D circuits have been shown to have the lowest compression volume and to be the most efficient.[62] Perhaps the circuit "will play a major role in the design of future anesthesia machines" and eventually "qualify as a universal breathing system."[45,59]

Disadvantages

Complications related to the inside tube or fresh gas hose of the Bain circuit have occurred. Initially the outside corrugated tube was black, making the inside tube impossible to visualize. Now the outside tube is transparent and the inside tube is colored, which allows the anesthesiologist to check the inside tube

for kinking,[63] inappropriate connections of the fresh gas hose,[64] disconnections at the machine end,[65] and perhaps total absence.[66] Disconnecting the inside tube at the machine end and attaching the anesthesia machine fresh gas hose to the pressure manometer site will convert the Bain circuit from a partial rebreathing circuit into an almost total rebreathing circuit. Under these circumstances a high $PaCO_2$ and a possibly low PaO_2 can be expected.[64,65] Testing the Bain circuit by the usual method of obstructing the endotracheal tube end and pressing the oxygen flush valve is not sufficient. A Pethick[67] test should be done in addition. The oxygen flush valve is activated with the endotracheal tube end open. If the patient end of the inside tube is properly positioned, a Venturi effect is created by the high flow and the reservoir bag completely collapses. When performing this test with the CPRAM circuit, it is necessary to insert a mask elbow or endotracheal tube connector at the patient end.[60,68] Prudent inspection of the circuit, high-flow inflation of the circuit, and the Pethick test will certainly eliminate the majority of problems associated with the Bain circuit.

Using both the circle system and the Bain circuit on the same anesthesia machine can be cumbersome. Utilization of the Bain circuit on the circle system requires an adaptor (see Figs. 6-10 and 6-11). Switching from the circle

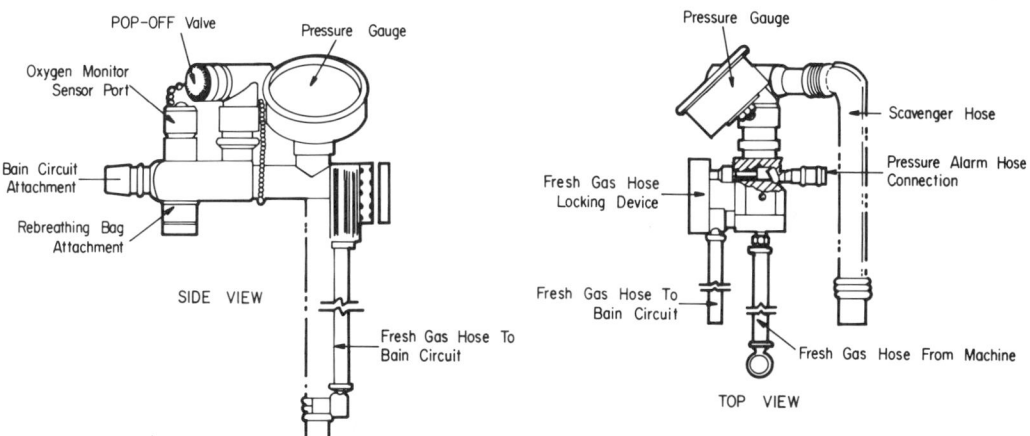

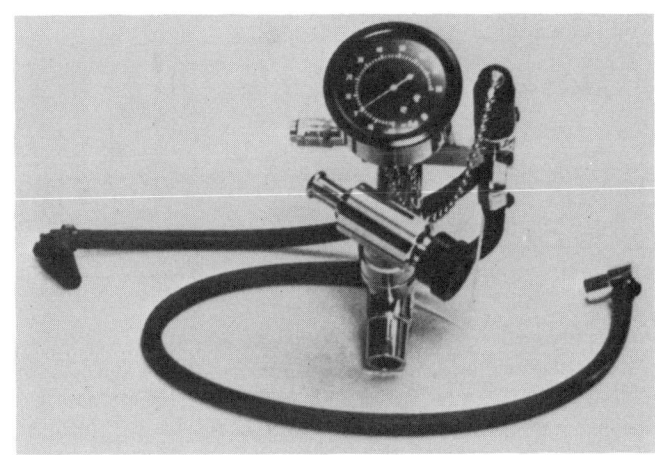

Fig. 6-10 A North American Drager Bain circuit adapter. The oxygen monitor, scavenger hose, fresh gas hose, and alarm devices must be transferred from the circle system to the Bain circuit. (Photo and schematic [redrawn] courtesy of North American Drager, Telford, PA.)

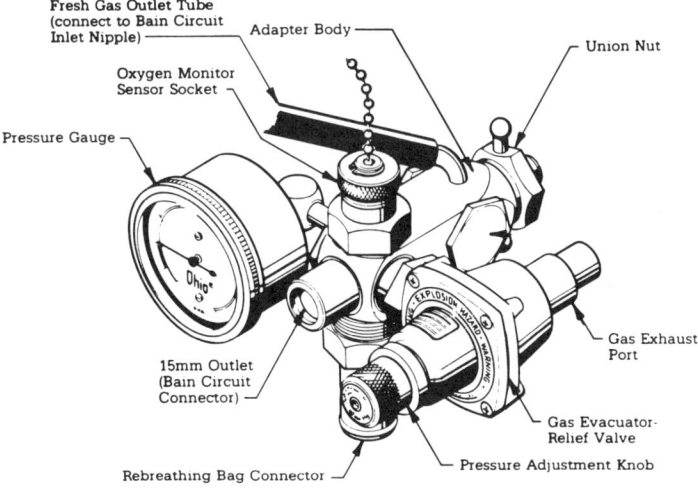

Fig. 6-11 An Ohmeda Bain circuit adapter. The outlet where the patient circuit attaches has a 15 mm inside diameter, and a 22 mm outside diameter. It is a coaxial connector. (Courtesy of Ohmeda, The BOC Group, Inc.)

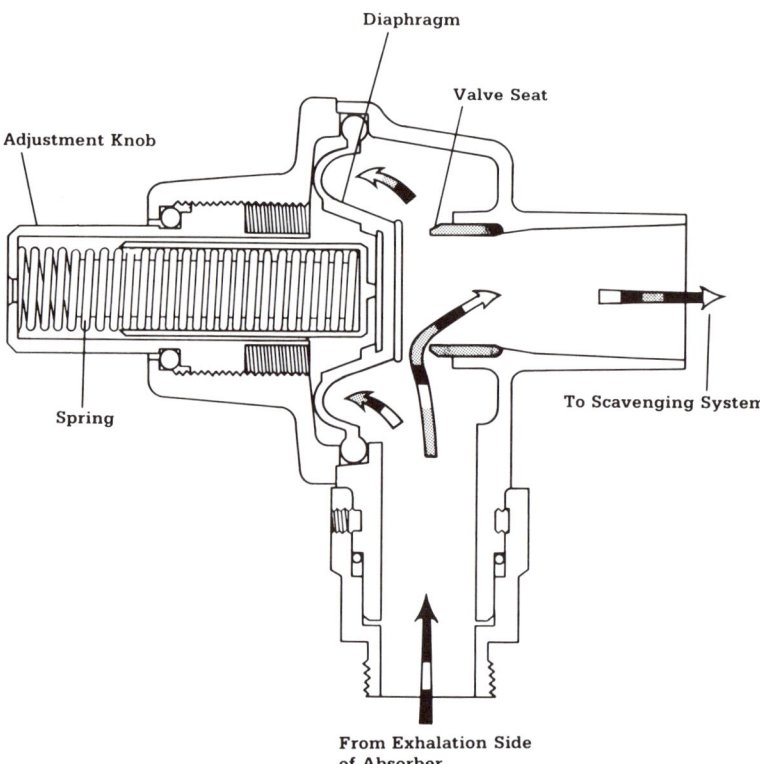

Fig. 6-12 Schematic of an adjustable pressure-limiting (APL) or pop-off valve. The force on the diaphragm is controlled by the spring and adjustment knob. Exhaled gases exit to the scavenging system when the system pressure on the diaphragm forces it from contact with the valve seat. (Reproduced with permission from Bowie E, Huffman LM: The Anesthesia Machine: Essentials for Understanding. Ohmeda, The BOC Group, Inc., 1985.)

system to the Bain adapter on the Narkomed IIA anesthesia machine requires moving (1) the pressure alarm hose, (2) the scavenging hose, (3) the oxygen analyzer, and (4) the fresh gas hose. In addition, the Bain adapter requires a special mount on the anesthesia machine and when the Bain is in use the ventilator safety switchover mechanism (which excludes the pop-off valve during ventilator function) is excluded. These steps are essential and require a mental or written checklist by the anesthesiologist to ensure compliance.

One group of investigators[24,69] considers the Bain circuit unsafe because (1) it assumes but does not measure the carbon dioxide excretion or production and (2) rebreathing can alter the alveolar gas relationship and the composition of inspired gas. They recommend a fresh gas flow of 8 L/min for all adults in order to "cover all eventualities" and avoid rebreathing. Widespread application of the Bain circuit at flows which allow partial rebreathing certainly does not support such an extreme cautionary opinion.

VALVES

Three valves, the APL or pop-off valve (Fig. 6-12), the expiration valve (Fig. 6-13), and the inspiration valve (Fig. 6-14), are necessary in the circle system. Only the pop-off valve is necessary in the Bain circuit. Absence of

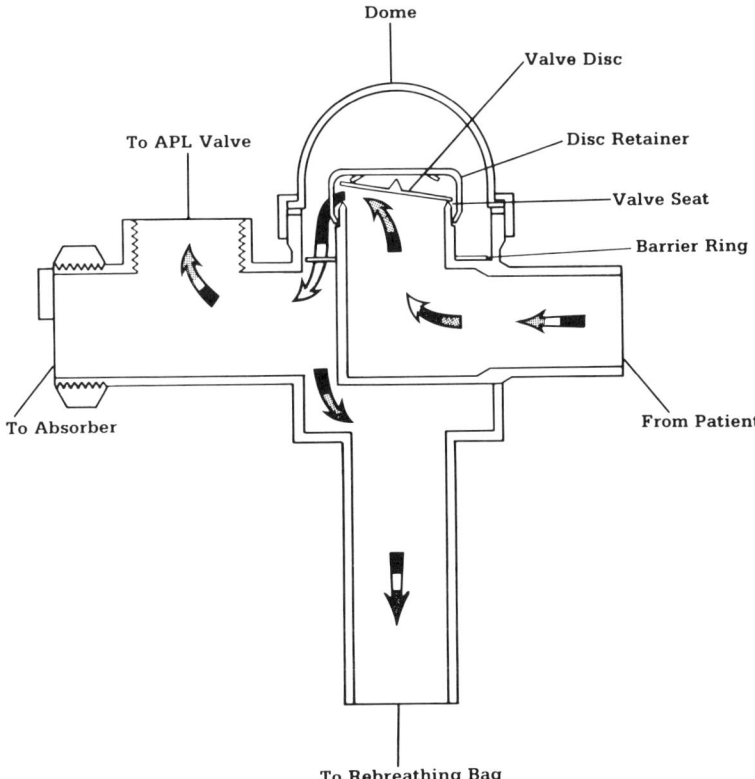

Fig. 6-13 Schematic of the exhalation check valve in the circle system. The valve disk is lifted by the exhaled gas that flows from the patient. The disk rests on the valve seat during inhalation. (Reproduced with permission from Bowie E, Huffman LM: The Anesthesia Machine: Essentials for Understanding. Ohmeda, The BOC Group, Inc., 1985.)

both the expiration and inspiration valves in the circle system will allow almost total rebreathing from the circuit. Profound respiratory acidosis with a pH of 6.71 and a $PaCO_2$ of 234 mmHg has been documented during valve absence.[70] Expiration and inspiration valves can also malfunction by failing to open or close properly.[16] Wetting, especially of the expiratory valve, causes sticking. In one instance, an expiratory valve was lost during the routine cleaning of an anesthesia machine. One year later the expiratory valve had worked its way directly over the inlet for the reservoir bag. Functioning as a one-way flutter valve, it allowed excessive pressures to build up within the circuit and bilateral tension pneumothorax occurred.[71]

Combination of unidirectional valves in the absorber and in the Y-piece presents the hazard of inadvertently opposed valves. Use of the oxygen flush in this situation has resulted in bilateral tension pneumothorax, pneumomediastinum, and pneumoperitoneum.[72]

In a prospective study involving 55 institutions and 715 anesthesia machines Kim et al.[73] found either one or both unidirectional valves incompetent in 15 percent of the machines. Foregger machines had the highest frequency of incompetency at 25 percent, Ohmeda (Ohio) machines at 15 percent, and North American Drager machines at 5 percent. Warping of the valve was found to be the most common cause of incompetency. The anesthesia machines with incompetent valves

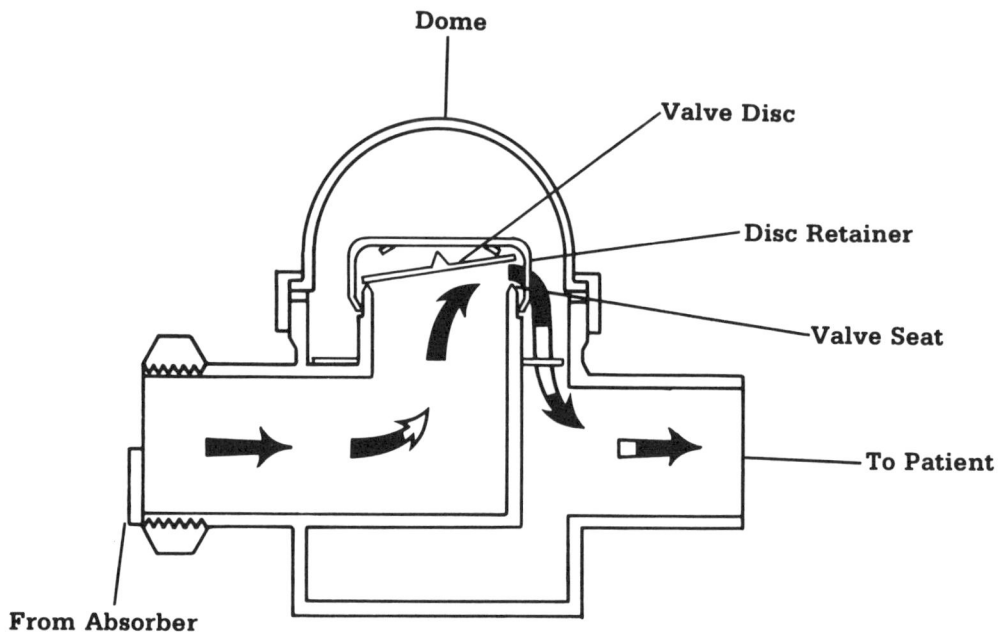

Fig. 6-14 Schematic of the inhalation valve in the circle system. The valve disk is lifted up by the fresh gas flow from the common gas outlet through the absorber. The disk rests on the valve seat during exhalation. (Reproduced with permission from Bowie E, Huffman LM: The Anesthesia Machine: Essentials for Understanding. Ohmeda, The BOC Group, Inc., 1985.)

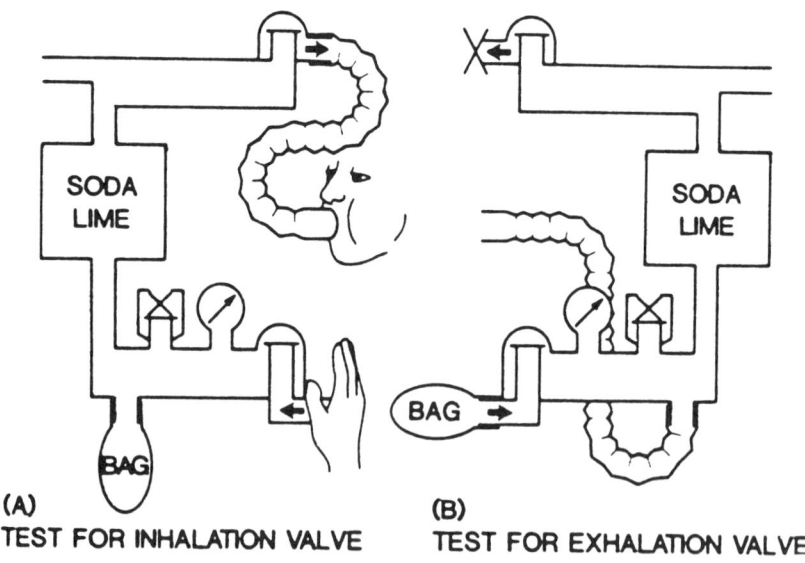

Fig. 6-15 Competency test for the inhalation and exhalation valves of the circle system. See text for details. (Kim J, Kovac AL, Mathewson HS: A method for detection of incompetent unidirectional dome valves: a prevalent malfunction. Anesth Analg 64:745, 1985. Reprinted with permission, The International Anesthesia Research Society.)

would be capable of producing serious hypercapnia in children and spontaneously breathing adults. A 1-minute test for the expiration and inspiration dome valve is outlined[73]:

1. Preparation. Close the pop-off valve, disconnect the breathing tubes, and turn off all gas flow.
2. Inhalation valve check. Attach the reservoir bag to the bag connector site, place a corrugated tube on the inhalation outlet, and cover the exhalation outlet with the palm of the hand (Fig. 6-15A). Gently blow into the corrugated tubing.
3. Exhalation valve check. Attach the reservoir bag to the exhalation inlet, place a corrugated tube on the reservoir bag connector site, and cover the inhalation outlet with the palm of the hand (Fig. 6-15B). Gently blow into the corrugated tubing.
4. Interpretation of results. The reservoir bag will not fill if the valve is competent. If the reservoir bag fills after replacement of the suspected valve, inspect the annular seat for irregularities.

The procedure seems simple, fast, and does not require any special equipment. Perhaps the test should be introduced as a part of the daily checkout routine for the anesthesia machine.

HUMIDIFICATION

In 1961 Toremalm[74] found the mucociliary transport system to be interrupted by exposure to dry gases. Anesthetic gases were later shown to have detrimental effects on the respiratory mucous membrane.[75] Ciliated epithelial cells obtained from bronchial lavage in patients exposed to only 3 hours of dry anesthetic gases were found[76] to have damaged cilia and endplates in 39 percent, cytoplasmic changes in 39 percent, and nuclear changes in 48 percent. Further studies indicated an exponential relationship between cellular damage and reduction in the humidity of inhaled gases.[77]

Testing the humidity in the semiclosed circle system on the inhalation side near the Y-piece showed mixing of moist gases from the absorber and dry gases from the fresh gas hose. It is surmised[76] that no cellular damage is avoided when the fresh gas inflow in the circle system does not exceed 5 L/min.

A high inspired humidity in the anesthetic circuit will help maintain body heat, preserve the integrity of the mucociliary transport system, avoid the accumulation of viscid secretions, maintain mucous rheology, and perhaps reduce the incidence of postanesthesia pulmonary complications.[77,78] Relative humidity is the percent saturation at any given temperature and is expressed either as a percent, as the amount of water weight for volume held (mg H_2O/L) by the gas, or as the partial pressure exerted by the water vapor. At room temperature the minimum recommended[76] humidity for anesthesia is 60 percent or 12 mg H_2O/L, with optimum values[79] between 14 and 30 mg H_2O/L.

Dry gases (4 to 10 mg H_2O/L) at room temperature are partially warmed by the nose and then saturated by the lung water vapor at body temperature. In order to do this the lung must vaporize water at body temperature. Vaporization requires heat to provide the energy for the transformation to water vapor. Under normal conditions 12 to 15 percent of the total body heat is lost through the transformation process in the lung.[80] In addition, during anesthesia the operating room is cool, large peritoneum surfaces are exposed which function as a heat and moisture exchanger, and the nasopharynx may be bypassed by an endotracheal tube. A combination of these conditions will reduce the body temperature considerably.[77,81-83]

Dery[78] measured the relative humidity and temperature at various locations in the respiratory tract of patients with a prophylactic tracheostomy prior to radioactive therapy of the pharynx. During breathing of room air (relative humidity of 45 percent) the relative humidity and temperature of the gas in the nasopharynx were 65 percent and 32°C, respectively; the larynx was 69.5 percent and 33.2°C, the carina 95 percent and 36.8°C, and five cm below the carina the gas was 100 percent saturated at body temperature.

Warm water vapor exhaled by the patient condenses in the expiratory limb of the circle system and the large outer tube of the Bain circuit. The completely saturated exhaled gas leaves the patient at body temperature and rapidly cools to room temperature. Decreasing the temperature causes the water to "rain out" the difference in water vapor held at the original temperature versus the lower temperature.[77]

A circle absorber system has a humidity output[77,84] in the range of 5 to 18 mg H_2O/L. Factors which account for the wide range include (1) condensation of water vapor in the expiratory limb, (2) fresh gas inflow mixing with the inspired gases, (3) locating the pop-off valve on the expiratory side prior to the absorber, and (4) condensation of water vapor from the warm gases leaving the carbon dioxide absorber.[77]

A closed-circuit technique can provide essentially an ideal inspired humidity.[78,85] Heated humidifiers are not necessary in the circle system when low flows are used.[86] Once higher flows are used in the circle system the humidity rapidly decreases. High flows maximize the debt of moisture between precipitable water during expiration and moisture gain during inspiration.[78] Anesthetic gases can be humidified in the circuit by rinsing the corrugated tubes with warm water prior to use,[83] injecting water into the carbon dioxide absorber, flowing the gases through an "artificial nose" which acts as a heat and moisture exchanger,[87] and the use of a variety of ultrasonic nebulizers and humidifiers.[77,88] Humidification methods which require equipment may be cumbersome,[86] may become contaminated,[77] or may increase the risk to the patient.[41]

Humidity in the Bain circuit is higher than in the regular circle at the same flow rates.[24,41,77] The modified Mapleson D circuit has been found to provide a higher inspired humidity than a closed-circuit technique.[41] The large common outside tube of the Bain circuit acts as a heat and moisture exchanger during partial rebreathing and keeps the humidity[3,24,77] between 13 and 20 mg H_2O/L. Figure 6-16 compares the Bain and circle system at comparable flow rates during anesthesia. The Bain circuit starts with a relative humidity of 65 percent and increases to 100 percent after 80 minutes. The circle system[24] begins with a relative humidity of 30 percent but rises to only 60 percent after 90 minutes. CPRAM circuits[41] have been shown to stabilize within 30 minutes at a humidity between 24 and 26 mg H_2O/L.

Humidification of anesthetic gases is best accomplished by using a closed-circuit technique or a modified Mapleson D system. Care must be taken when introducing additional humidifying equipment into a complicated circle system just to preserve a high-flow technique.

RESERVOIR BAG

A reservoir (rebreathing) bag holds a volume of anesthetic gas that the patient can draw from during the beginning of inspiration, when the minute volume far exceeds the fresh gas inflow. The bag also serves as a "shock absorber" or pressure-limiting device and as a means to provide positive pressure during ventilation.[89-93]

The ANSI recommended standard[94] for the reservoir bag states the bag should be made of elastomeric material resistant to anesthetic vapor and pliable enough to remain elastic when the bag is inflated to its nominal capacity. Each bag with a volume greater than 1.5 L should not exceed a pressure of 35 cmH$_2$O when expanded to twice its volume, at six times its volume the pressure should not exceed 60 cmH$_2$O.

At flow rates from 15 to 50 L/min the reservoir bag demonstrates a passive rise in pressure with a rapid peak (see Fig. 6-17).[91] Close

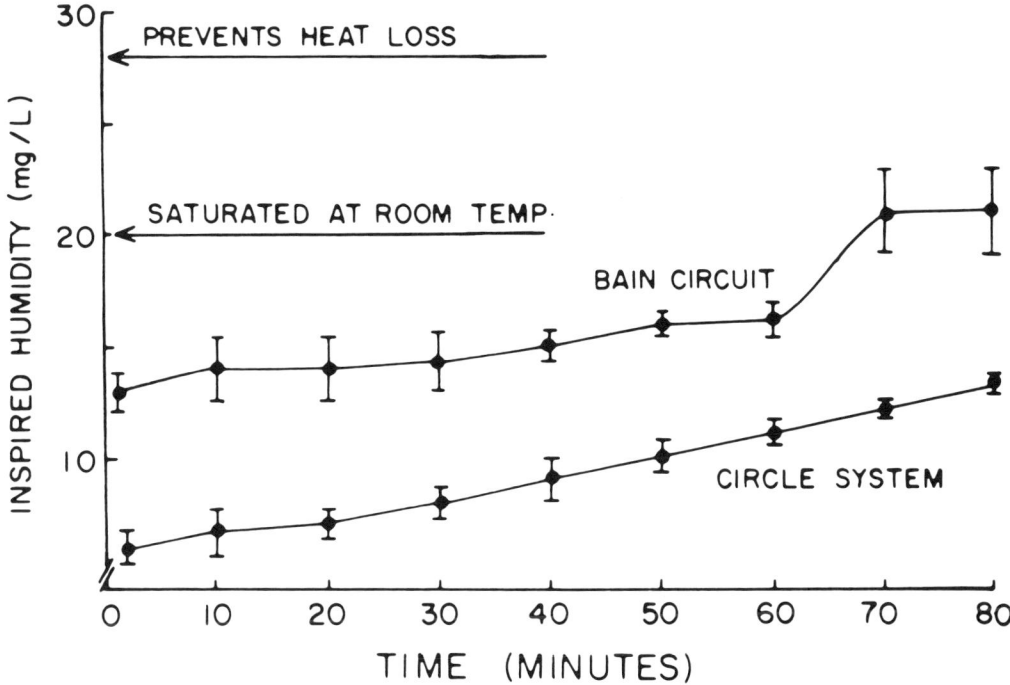

Fig. 6-16 Comparison of the humidity output of the Bain circuit and the circle absorber system: fresh gas inflow at 5 L/min, tidal volume of 700 ml, and ventilatory rate of 12 per minute. (Ramanathan S, Chalon J, Capan L et al: Rebreathing characteristics of the Bain anesthesia circuit. Anesth Analg 56:822, 1977. Reprinted with permission, The International Anesthesia Research Society.)

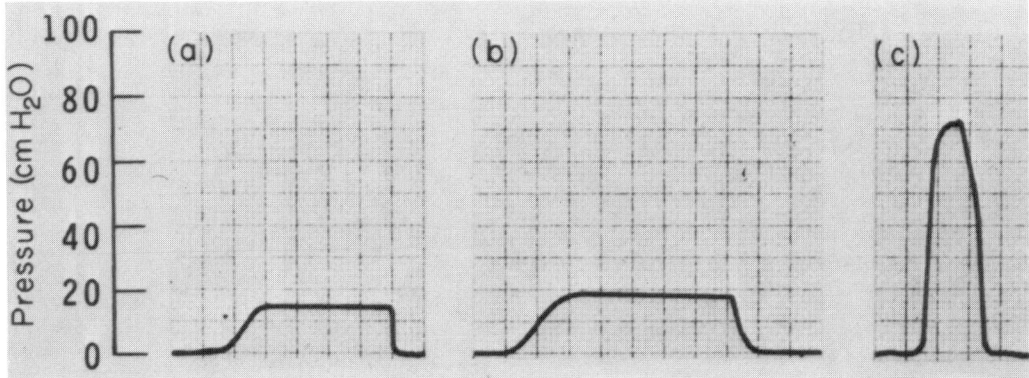

Fig. 6-17 Pressure-limiting characteristics of the reservoir bag. The fresh gas inflow is (A) 15 L/min and (B) 50 L/min. Pressure rises to a peak and remains relatively constant. The pressure will acutely increase if the reservoir bag is compressed against (C) an inflow of 15 L/min. (Newton NI, Adams AP: Excessive airway pressure during anaesthesia: hazards, effects and prevention. Anaesthesia 33:689, 1978.)

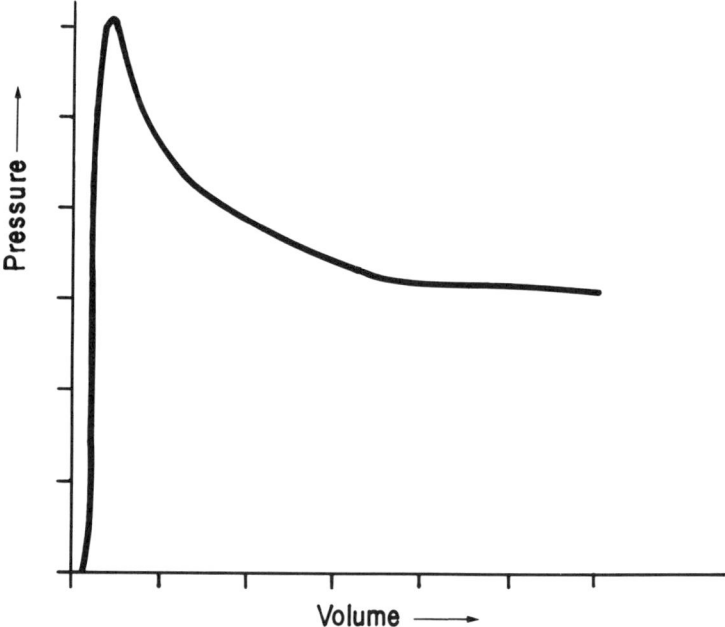

Fig. 6-18 A typical static pressure–volume curve for a rubber reservoir bag. Three phases are noted: (1) zero pressure until the bag reaches nominal volume, (2) a rapid rise to peak pressure, and (3) marked expansion of the bag with decreasing pressure. (Johnstone RE, Smith TC: Rebreathing bags as pressure-limiting devices. Anesthesiology 38:192, 1973.)

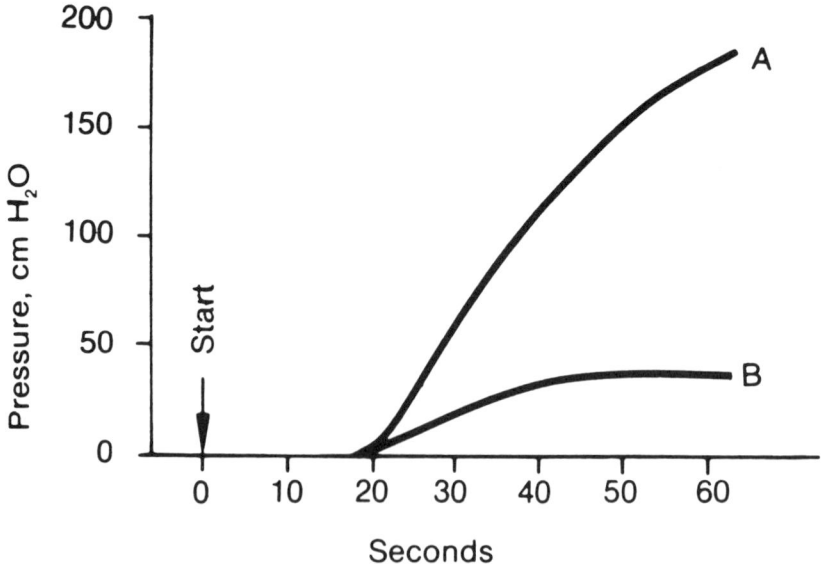

Fig. 6-19 Comparison of the peak pressures developed in a plastic reservoir bag and a rubber reservoir bag at a flow rate of 6 L/min. (Parmley JB, Tahir AH, Adriani J: Disposable plastic breathing bags and tubes. JAMA 217:1842, 1971 © 1971 American Medical Association.)

examination of the pressure–volume curve (Fig. 6-18) shows three phases: (1) negligible pressure until the nominal volume of the bag is reached, (2) a rapid rise to peak pressure, and (3) a reduction in pressure as volume increases.[90] An abrupt peak in pressure[90,91] to greater than 70 cmH_2O can occur if the bag is compressed against a fresh gas inflow of 15 L/min. Figure 6-19 illustrates the higher peak pressure and rapid rise of plastic bags when compared to rubber bags.[89] Filling the circle system with the 50 L/min oxygen flush valve can cause a 3-L rubber bag to reach a peak pressure of 50 cmH_2O within 1.5 seconds and continue to expand to 5 or 10 times its original diameter. However, some plastic bags inflate within 2 seconds, reach a peak pressure of 260 cmH_2O in 4 seconds, and then burst.[89] Newer neoprene bags compare favorably with latex bags.[95] A rapid high rise in pressure in the circle system may result in barotrauma to the lungs.[71,72,91,96,97] A slower rise in pressure which is sustained below 70 cmH_2O will avoid barotrauma but eventually lead to cardiovascular depression. Venous return to the right side of the heart is decreased by the increase in intrathoracic pressure.[91,96,97] In addition, venous return to the left side of the heart is decreased by the closing of the pulmonary capillaries secondary to the transmission of airway pressure to the alveoli.[91,97] Cardiac output will be severely limited if both sources of venous return to the heart are decreased.

CONTAMINATION OF THE BREATHING CIRCUIT

The transfer of infection from one patient to another via the breathing circuit is certainly a theoretical consideration.[15,98] Controlled studies have not been able to show a decreased incidence of postoperative pneumonia with the use of disposable circuits.[99-101] Vaporizers, nitrous oxide, and oxygen do not serve as sources of bacterial contamination.[102,103] Bacterial gas filters certainly do not decrease the incidence of postoperative pneumonia and should not be used routinely.[104,105] The use of completely disposable circle circuits or disposable Bain circuits would be useful in cases of, for example, tuberculosis and malignant hyperthermia.[106-108]

The routine use of disposable breathing tubes and bags in anesthesia in the United States certainly needs to be evaluated. In some hospitals the threat of malpractice litigation and quality assurance audits have been responsible for such policies as a mandatory change after each case. If a tonsillectomy or the placing of ear tubes lasts only 10 to 15 minutes, the entire disposable breathing tubes and bag are replaced! No one has really demonstrated a risk of infection from the reasonable repeated use of disposable anesthesia equipment. Using disposable tubes and bag for 3 to 5 hours is of less risk to the patient than the possible mistakes which could be made during the assembly of the new tubes and bag.[109] Recommended practices for the cleaning and processing of anesthesia equipment are available.[108,110-112]

MISCELLANEOUS

A multitude of unexpected and uncommon complications can occur in the circuit. Breakage of the reservoir bag mount,[113,114] a plastic partition completely obstructing the expiratory limb of a disposable circle circuit,[115] flaking of metal from the inside of components of anesthetic circuit,[116] and adhesive tape placed to ensure better circuit connection actually obstructing the circuit end[117] are just a few of those reported.

REFERENCES

1. Schreiber P: Anaesthesia equipment: Performance, classification and safety. Springer-Verlag, New York, 1972
2. Jones CS: A new look at old anesthesia circuits. Anesthesiology 56:486, 1982
3. Sykes MK: Rebreathing circuits: a review. Br J Anaesth 40:666, 1968

4. Mapleson WW: The elimination of rebreathing in various semi-closed anaesthetic systems. Anaesthesia 26:323, 1954

5. Harrison GA: Ayre's T-piece: a review of its modifications. Br J Anaesth 36:115, 1964

6. Dorsch JA, Dorsch SA (eds): Understanding Anesthesia Equipment: Construction, Care, and Complications. 2nd Ed. Williams & Wilkins, Baltimore, 1985

7. Wylie WD, Churchill-Davidson HC (eds): A Practice of Anesthesia. 3rd Ed. Lloyd-Luke, Bucks, England 1972

8. Bain JA, Spoerel WE: Why was closed circuit anesthesia abandoned? Circular 1:5, 1984

9. Cullen SC: Who is watching the patient? Anesthesiology 37:361, 1972

10. Hill DW, Lowe HJ: Comparison of concentration of halothane in closed and semiclosed circuits during controlled ventilation. Anesthesiology 23:291, 1962

11. Holaday DA: Counterpoint to the balancing opinion. Circular 1:6, 1984

12. Lin CY, Mostert JW, Benson DW: Closed circle systems: a new direction in the practice of anaesthesia. Acta Anaesthesiol Scand 24:354, 1980

13. DE Silva AJC: Normocapnic ventilation using the circle system. Can Anaesth Soc J 23:657, 1976

14. Closed and Low Flow Anesthesia Systems Society. Department of Anesthesiology. The University of Alabama in Birmingham. JT #737. University Station, Birmingham, AL

15. Jorgensen B, Jorgensen S: Carbon dioxide elimination from circle systems. Acta Anaesthesiol Scand 53:86, 1973

16. Eger EI, Epstein RM: Hazards of anesthetic equipment. Anesthesiology 25:490, 1964

17. Brown ES, Seniff AM, Elam JO: Carbon dioxide elimination in semiclosed systems. Anesthesiology 25:31, 1964

18. Eger EI, Ethans CT: The effects of inflow, overflow and valve placement on economy of the circle system: Anesthesiology 29:93, 1968

19. Purnell RJ: The position of the Wright anemometer in the circle absorber system. Br J Anaesth 40:917, 1968

20. Suwa K, Yamamura H: The effect of gas inflow on the regulation of CO_2 levels with hyperventilation during anesthesia. Anesthesiology 33:440, 1970

21. Benson DW, Graff TD, Hurt HH, Jr et al: The circle semi-closed system control of $PaCO_2$ by inflow rates of anesthetic gases and hyperventilation. Anesthesiology 29:174, 1968

22. Edsall DW: Economy is not a major benefit of closed-system anesthesia. Anesthesiology 54:258, 1981

23. Lowe HJ: Uptake and distribution: square root of time model. p. 67. In: Lowe HJ, Ernst EA (eds): The Quantitative Practice of Anesthesia: Use of the Closed Circuit. Williams & Wilkins, Baltimore, 1981

24. Ramanathan S, Chalon J, Capan L et al: Rebreathing characteristics of the Bain anesthesia circuit. Anesth Analg 56:822, 1977

25. Virtue RW: An early and safe use of low flows. Circular 1:6, 1984

26. Bushman JA, Enderby DH, Al-Abrak MH et al: Closed circuit anaesthesia: a new approach. Br J Anaesth 49:575, 1977

27. Patel A, Milliken RA: Costs of delivery of anesthetic gases re-examined. I. Anesthesiology 55:710, 1981

28. Virtue RW, Aldrete JA: Costs of delivery of anesthetic gases reexamined II. Anesthesiology 55:711, 1981

29. Spain JA: Cost of delivery of anesthetic gases reexamined. III. Anesthesiology 55:711, 1981

30. Virtue RW: Comparison of cost of high and low flows of anaesthetic agents. Can Anaesth Soc J 28:182, 1981

31. Instruction manual. Narkomed 2A: Anesthesia System. Specifications and Equipment. North American Drager, Telford, PA, 1984

32. Operation Maintenance. Modulus II: Anesthesia System. Ohmeda, Madison, WI, 1984

33. Ghani GA: Test for a leak in the anesthesia circle. Anesth Analg 62:855, 1983

34. Bain JA, Spoerel WE: A streamlined anaesthetic system. Can Anaesth Soc J 19:426, 1972

35. Rayburn RL, Graves SA: A new concept in controlled ventilation of children with the Bain anesthetic circuit. Anesthesiology 48:250, 1978

36. Dean SE, Keenan RL: Spontaneous breathing with a T-piece circuit: minimum fresh gas/minute volume ratio which prevents rebreathing. Anesthesiology 56:449, 1982

37. Rayburn R, Graves C: Homogeneous gas mixtures in the Bain circuit: a reply. Anesthesiology 50:171, 1979

38. Ayre P: The T-piece technique. Br J Anaesth 28:520, 1956

39. Brooks W, Stuart P, Gabel PV: The T-piece technique in anesthesia. Anesth Analg 37:191, 1958

40. Waters DJ, Mapleson WW: Rebreathing during controlled respiration with various semi-closed anaesthetic systems. Br J Anaesth 33:374, 1961

41. Rayburn RL, Watson RL: Humidity in children and adults using the controlled partial rebreathing anesthesia method. Anesthesiology 52:291, 1980

42. Shandro J: Resistance to gas flow in the "new" anaesthesia circuits: a comparative study. Can Anaesth Soc J 29:387, 1982

43. Bain JA, Spoerel WE: Flow requirements for a modified Mapleson D system during controlled ventilation. Can Anaesth Soc J 20:629, 1973

44. Bain JA, Spoerel WE: Prediction of arterial carbon dioxide tension during controlled ventilation with a modified Mapleson D system. Can Anaesth Soc J 22:34, 1975

45. Henville JD, Adams AP: The Bain anaesthetic system: an assessment during controlled ventilation. Anaesthesia 31:247, 1976

46. Bain JA, Spoerel WE: Carbon dioxide output in anaesthesia. Can Anaesth Soc J 23:153, 1976

47. Baraka A: PCO_2 control by fresh gas flow during controlled ventilation with a semi-open circuit. Br J Anaesth 41:527, 1969

48. Keenan RL, Boyan CP: Confusion regarding the Bain circuit. Can Anaesth Soc J 28:90, 1981

49. Spoerel WE: Bain circuit confusion? Can Anaesth Soc J 28:91, 1981

50. Stenqvist O, Sonander H: Rebreathing characteristics of the Bain circuit. Br J Anaesth 56:303, 1984

51. Ramanathan S, Gupta U, Chalon J: Homogeneous gas mixtures in the Bain circuit: to the editor. Anesthesiology 50:170, 1979

52. Nunn JF: Applied Respiratory Physiology. 2nd Ed. Butterworths, London, 1977

53. Conway CM, Seeley HF, Barnes PK: Spontaneous ventilation with the Bain anaesthetic system. Br J Anaesth 49:1245, 1977

54. Ungerer MJ: A comparison between the Bain and Magill anaesthetic system during sponta- neous breathing. Can Anaesth Soc J 25:122, 1978

55. Alexander JP: Clinical comparison of the Bain and Magill anaesthetic systems during spontaneous respiration. Br J Anaesth 54:1031, 1982

56. Bain JA, Spoerel WE: Letter to the editor. Anesth Analg 57:375, 1978

57. Byrick RJ, Janssen EG: Respiratory waveform and rebreathing in T-piece circuits: a comparison of enflurane and halothane waveforms. Anesthesiology 53:371, 1980

58. Spoerel WE, Aitken RR, Bain JA: Spontaneous respiration with the Bain breathing circuit. Can Anaesth Soc J 25:30, 1978

59. Chu YK, Rah KH, Boyan CP: Is the Bain breathing circuit the future anesthesia system? An evaluation. Anesth Analg 56:84, 1977

60. Robinson S, Fisher DM: Safety check for the CPRAM circuit: to the editor. Anesthesiology 59:488, 1983

61. Spoerel WE, Bain JA: Letter to the editor. Can Anaesth Soc J 22:626, 1975

62. Cote CJ, Petkau AJ, Ryan JF et al: Wasted ventilation measured in vitro with eight anesthetic circuits with and without inline humidification. Anesthesiology 59:442, 1983

63. Mansell WH: Bain circuit: "The hazard of the hidden tube." Can Anaesth Soc J 23:227, 1976

64. Paterson JG, Vanhooydonk V: A hazard associated with improper connection of the Bain breathing circuit. Can Anaesth Soc J 22:343, 1975

65. Hannallah R, Rosales JK: A hazard connected with the re-use of the Bain's circuit: a case report. Can Anaesth Soc J 21:511, 1974

66. Peterson WC: Bain circuit. Can Anaesth Soc J 25:532, 1978

67. Pethick SL: Letter to the editor. Can Anaesth Soc J 22:115, 1975

68. Kjnepshield WR: Safety check for the CPRAM circuit: a reply. Anesthesiology 59:489, 1983

69. Ramanathan S, Chalon J, Patel C: Letter to the editor. Anesth Analg 57:376, 1978

70. Schultz EA, Buckley JJ, Oswald AJ et al: Profound acidosis in an anesthetized human: report of a case. Anesthesiology 21:285, 1960

71. Dean HN, Parsons DE, Raphaely RC: Case report: bilateral tension pneumothorax from mechanical failure of anesthesia machine due

to misplaced expiratory valve. Anesth Analg 50:195, 1971

72. Dogu TS, Davis HS: Hazards of inadvertently opposed valves. Anesthesiology 33:122, 1970

73. Kim J, Kovac AL, Mathewson HS: A method for detection of incompetent unidirectional dome valves: a prevalent malfunction. Anesth Analg 64:745, 1985

74. Toremalm NG: Airflow pattern and ciliary activity in the trachea after tracheostomy. Acta Otolaryngol 53:442, 1961

75. Burton JDK: Effects of dry anesthetic gases on the respiratory mucous membrane. Lancet 1:235, 1962

76. Chalon J, Loew DAY, Malebranche J: Effects of dry anesthetic gases on tracheobronchial ciliated epithelium. Anesthesiology 37:338, 1972

77. Chalon J, Ali M, Ramanathan S et al: The humidification of anaesthetic gases: its importance and control. Can Anaesth Soc J 26:361, 1979

78. Dery R: The evolution of heat and moisture in the respiratory tract during anaesthesia with a non-rebreathing system. Can Anaesth Soc J 20:296, 1973

79. Weeks DB: Humidification during anesthesia. NY State J Med 75:1216, 1975

80. Clarke RE, Orkin LR, Rovenstine EA: Body temperature studies in anesthetized man: effect of environmental temperature, humidity and anesthesia system. JAMA 154:311, 1954

81. Dery R: Water balance of the respiratory tract during ventilation with a gas mixture saturated at body temperature. Can Anaesth Soc J 20:719, 1973

82. Hendricks HHL, Trahey GE, Argentier MP: Paradoxial inhibition of decreases in body temperature by use of heated and humidified gases. Anesth Analg 61:393, 1982

83. Chase HF, Trotta R, Kilmore MA: Simple methods for humidifying nonrebreathing anesthesia gas systems. Anesth Analg 41:249, 1962

84. Sare CA, Sharks CA: Estimation of inspiratory limb humidity in the circle system. Anaesth Intensive Care 3:41, 1974

85. Aldretti JA, Cubillos P, Sherrill D: Humidity and temperature changes during low flow and closed system anaesthesia. Acta Anaesthesiol Scand 25:312, 1981

86. Baumgarten RK: Humidifiers are unjustified

in adult anesthesia. Anesth Analg 64:1224, 1985

87. Weeks DB: Humidification of anesthetic gases using heat-and-moisture exchangers. Anesth Review 12:22, 1985

88. Chalon J, Patel C, Ramanathan S et al: Humidification of the circle absorber system. Anesthesiology 48:142, 1978

89. Parmley JB, Tahir AH, Adriani J: Disposable plastic breathing bags and tubes. JAMA 217:1842, 1971

90. Johnstone RE, Smith TC: Rebreathing bags as pressure-limiting devices. Anesthesiology 38:192, 1973

91. Newton NI, Adams AP: Excessive airway pressure during anaesthesia: Hazards, effects and prevention. Anaesthesia 33:689, 1978

92. Thompson PW: Prevention of the hazard of excessive airway pressure. Anaesthesia 34:593, 1979

93. Waters DJ: Use and misuse of a pressure-limiting bag. Anaesthesia 22:322

94. American National Standard for Anesthetic Equipment—Reservoir Bags. Z79.4-1983. American National Standards Institute, New York, 1983

95. Stone DR, Graves SA: Compliances of pediatric rebreathing bags. Anesthesiology 53:434, 1980

96. Sellery GR: Hazards of artificial ventilation in the operating room. Can Med J 10.421, 1972

97. Newton NI: Safety in the operating theatre: the meaning of excessive airway pressure. Br J Hosp Med 25:504, 1981

98. Neilsen H, Brinklov MM, Stokke DB et al: Cross infection from contaminated anaesthetic equipment: a reply. Anaesthesia 36:228, 1981

99. Feeley TW, Hamilton WK, Xavier B et al: Sterile anesthesia breathing circuits do not prevent postoperative pulmonary infection. Anesthesiology 54:369, 1981

100. Du Moulin GC, Hedley-Whyte J: Bacterial interactions between anesthesiologists, their patients, and equipment. Anesthesiology 57:37, 1982

101. Du Moulin GC, Hedley-Whyte J: Hospital associated viral infection and the anesthesiologist. Anesthesiology 59:51, 1983

102. Johnson BH, Eger EI: Bactericidal effects of anesthetics. Anesth Analg 56:136, 1979

103. Nielsen H, Vasegaard M, Stokke DB: Bacterial contamination of anaesthetic gases. Br J Anaesth 50:811, 1978

104. Mazze RI: Bacterial air filters. Anesthesiology 54:359, 1981

105. Garibaldi RA, Britt MR, Webster C et al: Failure of bacterial filters to reduce the incidence of pneumonia after inhalation anesthesia. Anesthesiology 54:364, 1981

106. Albrecht WH, Dryden GE: Five-year experience with the development of an individually clean anesthesia system. Anesth Analg 53:24, 1974

107. Viegas OJ, Cummins DF, Ravindran RS et al: A case for using disposable anesthesia circuitry. Anesthesiology 60:169, 1984

108. Deverill CEA, Dutt KK: Methods of decontamination of anaesthetic equipment: daily sessional exchange of circuits. J Hosp Infect 1:165, 1980

109. Drummond GB: Cross infection from contaminated anaesthetic equipment: a real hazard? Anaesthesia 36:227, 1981

110. Association of Operating Room Nurses Recommended Practices Subcommittee: Recommended practices: cleaning and processing anesthesia equipment. Assoc Oper Rm Nurses J 41:625, 1985

111. Lumley J: Decontamination of anaesthetic equipment and ventilators. Br J Anaesth 48:3, 1976

112. Enright AC, Moore RL, Parney FL: Contamination and resterilization of the Bain circuit. Can Anaesth Soc J 23:545, 1976

113. Stevenson PH, McLeskey CH: Breakage of a reservoir bag mount, an unusual anesthesia machine failure. Anesthesiology 53:270, 1980

114. Milliken RA: Bag mount detachment: a function of age? Anesthesiology 56:154, 1982

115. Register SD: Detection of defective equipment by proper preanesthetic checks. Anesthesiology 62:546, 1985

116. Austin TR: Metallic flaking: a further hazard of anaesthetic apparatus. Anaesthesia 27:92, 1972

117. Frankel DZN: Adhesive tape obstructing an anesthetic circuit. Anesthesiology 59:256, 1983

7

Scavenging and Pollution

Anesthetic gases are implicated as agents of abortion,[1] malformation,[2] cancer,[3] polyneuropathy,[4] and behavioral modification.[5,6] A plethora of studies done during recent years suggest, but do not prove, that anesthetics may be a health hazard. Critical examination of these studies reveals major pitfalls in the method of data accumulation. Numerous reviews and articles have appeared which raise reasonable doubt concerning the role of anesthetic gases as a health hazard.[7-12]

Why are we presently committed to scavenging all waste anesthetic gases? Undoubtedly the major impetus is the report of the Ad Hoc Committee on the Effect of Trace Anesthetics on the Health of Operating Room Personnel sponsored by the American Society of Anesthesiologists (ASA) in the October 1974 issue of *Anesthesiology*.[1] The initial planning meeting was attended by representatives from government, anesthesiologists, hospital associations, and other scientists. A grant proposal was written and the money for the study was furnished by the National Institute for Occupational Safety and Health (NIOSH) and the National Institutes of Health. Information was collected via questionnaires mailed to exposed and unexposed health personnel. Even though the study did "not establish a cause–effect relationship between the increases in

these diseases and exposure to the waste anesthetic gases in the operating room," a strong recommendation was issued to vent waste anesthetic gases in all anesthetizing locations. An accompanying editorial labeled the failure to use scavenging devices as "an unconscionable practice!"[3] Thus the stage was set and scavenging devices became a best seller in hospitals across the United States.

Shortly following the report of the Ad Hoc Committee on Trace Anesthetics, a government agency had to further justify its existence by overreacting to the suggestive data, and recommended strict guidelines for hospitals. In March 1977 NIOSH, an agency of the Department of Health, Education, and Welfare, issued a document outlining the criteria for a "recommended standard" for scavenging of waste anesthetic gases.[13] The recommended standards (Table 7-1) were established despite disagreeing input from the ASA Ad Hoc Committee: "All decisions and the final unrevised edition were by government edict," according to the committee chairman.[14] Permissible levels of exposure for anesthetic agents "cannot be defined as safe levels since information on adverse health effects is not completely definitive and many unknown factors still exist."[13] Control of the acceptable anesthetic level was defined. For example, a worker could not be

Table 7-1. NIOSH's Recommendations to OSHA for Occupational Exposure to Waste Anesthetic Gases and Vapors

Levels
  2 ppm of any halogenated agent
  25 ppm of nitrous oxide

Covers
  Anesthesia machine
  Nonrebreathing systems
  T-tube devices
  Nose mask

Employee requirements
  Preplacement physical exam
  Yearly physical exam
  Orientation to possible health hazards
  Keep specific records on outcome of pregnancies on employee and spouse

Anesthetic practice
  Vaporizers filled outside operating room in ventilated area
  Anesthesia machines must be taken out of service until low-pressure leak is found
  Operating room shall be closed if levels of waste anesthetic gases exceed requirement. Levels must be corrected before reopening

Monitoring
  Daily low-pressure leak test of anesthesia machine
  High-pressure leak test quarterly
  Ventilation systems–airflow measurements quarterly
  Anesthesia ventilators quarterly testing
  Sampling and analysis of operating room air
  Preventive maintenance of anesthesia machines quarterly

Records
  Must be maintained on all items above for a period of 20 years after the employee stops working

exposed to more than 2 ppm of any halogenated anesthetic agent, which was calculated from the weight of the halogenated agent collected in 45 L of air by charcoal absorption during 1 hour. Halothane at 2 ppm corresponds to the charcoal absorber collecting 16.15 mg/cm per minute. If the operating room contained 100,000 L (3,500 ft²), 2 ppm of halothane and 200 ppm of nitrous oxide would be present following 10 minutes of 50 percent nitrous oxide and 50 percent oxygen at 4 L/min with the vaporizer setting at 1 percent halothane.[15] In Sweden a level of 5 ppm for halothane was chosen as the standard. Denmark has suggested but not adapted the

levels of 1 ppm for halothane and 25 ppm for nitrous oxide.[7] All systems for anesthesia delivery in the operating room would be scavenged: the anesthesia machine, nonbreathing systems, T-tube devices, and even face masks.[13] Whitcher feels the NIOSH standards represent reasonable goals that may need to be exceeded for very specific anesthetic techniques.[16]

Procedures for the entire delivery of the anesthetic are outlined in detail. Impractical suggestions include moving the anesthesia machine from the operating room in order to fill the vaporizer in a "ventilated area" and correcting small leaks in the circle system "before use of the anesthetic delivery system."[13] Ventilation systems must have airflow measurements verified quarterly. A low-pressure leak test on the anesthesia machine must be documented quarterly and performed daily. When the low-pressure leak exceeds 100 ml/min at a pressure of 30 cmH₂O, the anesthesia machine must be removed from service until the leak is located and repaired. In fact, if the room concentration exceeds the environmental limits in Table 7-1, the leak source must be found and repaired prior to the next anesthetic!

In addition to environmental controls, each anesthesia department or hospital would have to obtain preplacement medical and occupational histories on all employees subject to potential exposure of waste anesthetic gases. Emphasis would then be given to pregnancy outcomes of the employee and spouse, as well as hepatic, renal, and hematopoietic diseases. Each employee would be advised of the potential health hazards of anesthetic exposure.[17] Yearly physical exams would be documented and all records maintained for 20 years after the employee stops working. The tremendous costs necessary to initiate and maintain such as extensive program would markedly raise the health care costs in the United States. Is the cost in money and time worth the eventual unknown outcome in an area of unproven hazard? It appears the element of overreaction has been the decisive factor in the recommended standard.

The recommended standard was submitted by NIOSH to the Department of Labor, since the Secretary of Labor enforces any standard as both legislator and prosecutor.[14] The Department of Labor assigned the Occupational Safety and Health Administration (OSHA) the task of reviewing the recommendations, and to date the recommendations have been supported in part but have not yet been enacted as law.[14] In fact, governmental intervention is probably unnecessary, since most hospitals in the United States have voluntarily instituted a waste-scavenging program.[14] A group of epidemiologist–biostatistician investigators evaluated the validity and interpretation of published reports on the efficacy of scavenging up to 1985.[18] The report noted that (1) none of the studies quantified the level of exposure, (2) the studies shared many weaknesses, and (3) there was only a small number of studies which were appropriate enough to be included in a pooled analysis. Exposure to waste gases cannot be proven to be safe or harmful. However, there is no basis, using present information, for the federal government to regulate the scavenging of waste gas anesthetics.[18,19]

The Joint Commission on Accreditation of Hospitals (JCAH) has only recommended that each anesthesia machine be provided with a gas-scavenging system.[20] In JCAH terminology, this means such action is considered desirable but not mandatory to achieve accreditation.[14] A number of studies and reviews regarding hazards to health imposed by the waste anesthetic gases have recommended the scavenging of gases despite a proven cause-and-effect relationship between inhalation of trace concentrations of anesthetics and disease.[1,8,13,14,21]

An unscavenged operating room has about 10 to 70 ppm of halothane and 400 to 3,000 ppm of nitrous oxide.[7,15,22,23] Minimal scavenging can reduce these values to 1 ppm for halothane and 60 ppm for nitrous oxide. Careful elimination of anesthesia machine leaks, utilization of low-flow techniques, and a high flow rate of fresh air in the air-conditioning system in the operating room can reduce the levels of halothane and nitrous oxide to as low as 0.005 and 1 ppm, respectively.[1,16] Ferstandig[8] calculated from long-term studies in animals the toxic level of halothane as 10 ppm and that for nitrous oxide as 850 ppm. Threshold limits for halothane or nitrous oxide can easily be reached by minimal scavenging. Anesthetic levels found in unscavenged operating rooms would be nontoxic even by conservative environmental health standards.

Reasonable changes in our habits of administrating an inhalational anesthetic could reduce the waste gas levels in the operating room. Ilsley et al.[24] assessed a number of factors affecting scavenger systems and made some reasonable suggestions for improving waste gas exposure: (1) Get a good mask fit or intubate the patient prior to turning on the nitrous oxide, (2) turn off the anesthetic and dump the anesthetic circuit reservoir bag into the scavenger system before suctioning or extubation, (3) give oxygen to the patient for as long as possible at the end of the case, (4) during mask cases make sure the mask has a tight fit, and (5) exercise reasonable care in filling the vaporizer.

Scavenging waste anesthetic gases is prudent until studies of large magnitude can rule out the slight possibility of health hazard. It has even been stated that the scavenging of waste gases is justified "if only for aesthetic reasons and to improve the morale of operating room personnel."[19] Spontaneous abortion appears to be the only health hazard which can remotely be associated with waste anesthetic gases[7,9-11, 18]; however, some authors feel the stress of the work environment may be the primary factor in the increased spontaneous abortion rate.[9-11,25] It will be years, if ever, before the following question is answered: Do waste gas anesthetics pose a threat to the health of those in the operating room environment?

SCAVENGER SYSTEMS

One of the first attempts to scavenge waste anesthetic gases used activated charcoal in a container of fixed size. The gas was ether and the reason for scavenging was to reduce the explosion hazard in the operating room.[26] A small absorber (see Fig. 7-1) with 600 g of charcoal lasted about 70 minutes, which corresponded to the delivery of 23 ml of ether. A large absorber with 1,350 g lasted about 2.5 hours, with 51 ml of ether being used for the anesthetic. Brass was used for construction to prevent corrosion by the ether. A water jacket around the absorber was recommended to reduce the heat generated by the reaction of charcoal with ether.

Gas evacuation systems[27] became commercially available around 1971. The systems were extremely variable and evacuated gases to the operating room floor, the ventilation ducts, were tied into the surgical suction of the oper-ating room, or were given a separate suction system. The site of venting became the talk of the anesthesia world. Stories were told of the scavenged gas being vented to the hospital administrators' office, the cafeteria, or the operating room lounge! In a small rural hospital in which I worked the scavenged gas was vented 6 in. from the inlet of the compressed gas system for the hospital.

A standard for scavenger systems was not defined until 1982. The American National Standards Committee on Standards for Anesthetic Equipment, Z79, submitted the proposed standard to the American National Standards Institute (ANSI), which endorsed the standard. The standard recommended by the ANSI is "intended as a guide to aid the manufacturer, the consumer, and the general public."[28] Any manufacturer can sell a scavenger system with total disregard for the standard. A schematic of scavenging systems for waste anesthetic gases is shown in Figure

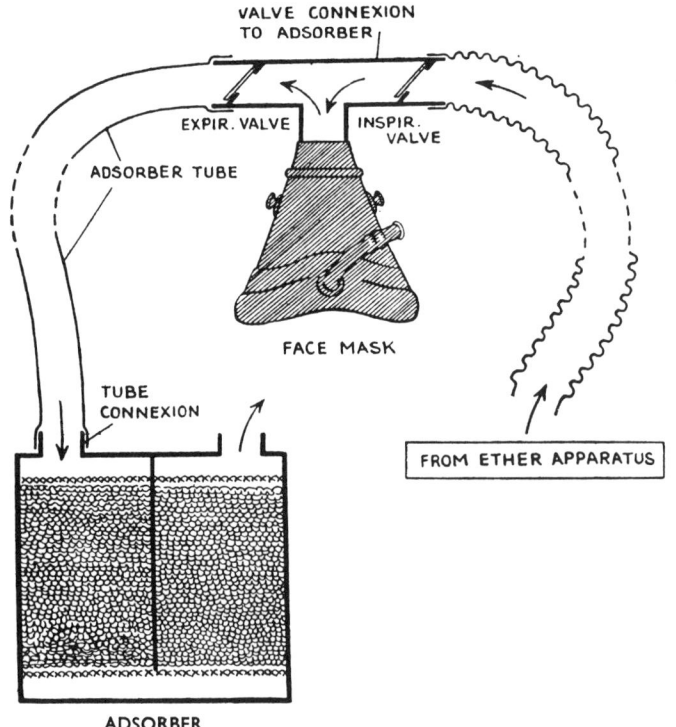

VALVE CONNEXION
TO ADSORBER

EXPIR. VALVE   INSPIR. VALVE

ADSORBER TUBE

FACE MASK

TUBE CONNEXION

FROM ETHER APPARATUS

ADSORBER

Fig. 7-1 A scavenger system for ether devised in 1944. A total of 600 g of activated charcoal could absorb about 23 ml of ether given over a period of 1 hour and 10 minutes. (Epstein HG, Berlin DP: Removal of ether vapour during anaesthesia. Lancet 1:114, 1944.)

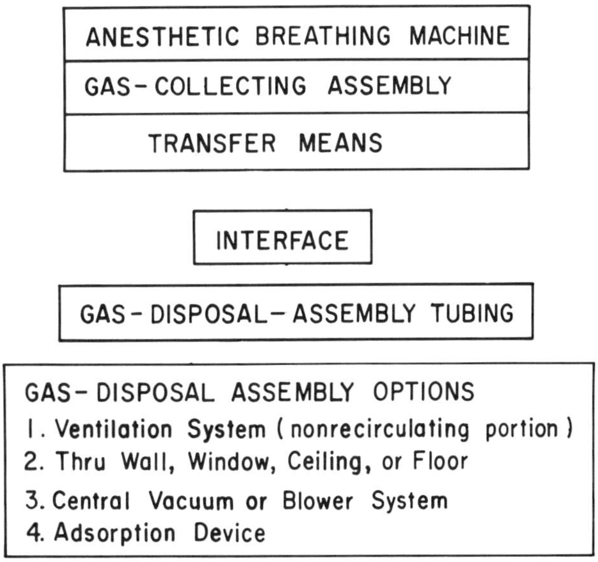

```
┌─────────────────────────────────────────┐
│  ANESTHETIC  BREATHING  MACHINE           │
├─────────────────────────────────────────┤
│  GAS – COLLECTING  ASSEMBLY               │
├─────────────────────────────────────────┤
│  TRANSFER  MEANS                          │
└─────────────────────────────────────────┘

        ┌───────────────────┐
        │   INTERFACE        │
        └───────────────────┘

   ┌─────────────────────────────────────┐
   │  GAS – DISPOSAL – ASSEMBLY  TUBING    │
   └─────────────────────────────────────┘
```

GAS– DISPOSAL ASSEMBLY OPTIONS
I. Ventilation System (nonrecirculating portion)
2. Thru Wall, Window, Ceiling, or Floor
3. Central Vacuum or Blower System
4. Adsorption Device

Fig. 7-2 Schematic of scavenging systems to remove excess anesthetic gases from the anesthesia machine. (This material is reproduced with permission from American National Standard Z79.11-1982, © 1982 The American National Standards Institute. Copies of this standard may be purchased from ANSI, 1430 Broadway, New York, NY 10018.)

7-2. The scavenging system consists of (1) an exhaust hose from the pop-off valve or ventilator, (2) an interface, (3) a gas disposal tube or hose, and (4) an exit mechanism for the gas from the operating room.

The *scavenger interface* is the most complex component of the system. Figures 7-3 to 7-5 show interface valves which are integral parts of the anesthesia machine. An interface directs the flow of waste anesthetic gas from the breathing circuit and ventilator to the hospital disposal system. Each interface should have two relief valves to minimize the effects of excessive resistance or excessive suction on the breathing circuit. The *subatmospheric intake valve* (see Fig. 7-4) opens automatically at -0.5 cmH$_2$O on the North American Drager (NAD) interface when the waste gas flow is less than the vacuum capacity. Thus the vacuum will suck in room air instead of withdrawing anesthetic gas from the breathing circuit. An additional *subatmospheric safety valve* (which opens at -1.8 cmH$_2$O) is present and opens if the primary subatmospheric valve malfunctions. Increased pressure in the scavenging system can occur when the flow of the waste gas exceeds the capacity of the

vacuum and reservoir bag. A *positive-pressure relief valve* (see Fig. 7-4) vents the gas at 5.0 cmH$_2$O and prevents pressure buildup in the breathing circuit. The *needle valve* adjusts the rate of the vacuum and thus controls the volume of the reservoir bag. Repeated adjustment is required, since the fresh gas flow to the breathing circuit is frequently changed. Once the fresh gas flow is stabilized, a lock nut, if present, can be tightened to maintain the needle valve setting. A 3- to 5-L *reservoir bag* is necessary to absorb short bursts of increased volume from the breathing circuit and contain it until the evacuation system can eliminate the excess volume. The ANSI recommends that the reservoir bag be distinguished by a different color from the reservoir bag of the anesthesia machine.[28]

A commercial scavenger–vacuum interface unit for mounting on the anesthesia machine is also available (see Fig. 7-6). A long, hollow tube with a capacity of 2,000 cc accepts the exhaust gases. No reservoir bag, valves, or adjustments (except a suction rate near 30 L/min) are necessary. Ventilator and anesthetic circuit gases interface at a T-connection prior to entering the scavenger interface.[21]

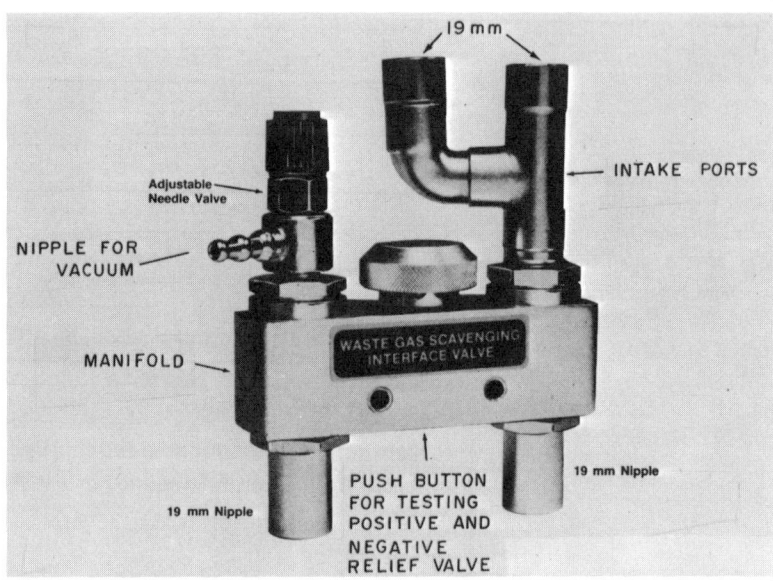

Fig. 7-3 A waste gas scavenger interface valve. The intake port(s) accepts the evacuation hose from the ventilator and the APL ("pop-off") valve. An adjustable needle valve allows the anesthesiologist to balance the rate of vacuum with the fresh gas flow rate. A nipple on the adjustable needle valve assembly allows a hose from the central vacuum system to be attached to the waste gas assembly. The reservoir bag attaches to one of the 19-mm nipples. The other 19-mm nipple may be used to evacuate waste gas to the exhaust grille of the operating room nonrecirculating exhaust system. (Courtesy of Ohmeda, The BOC Group, Inc.)

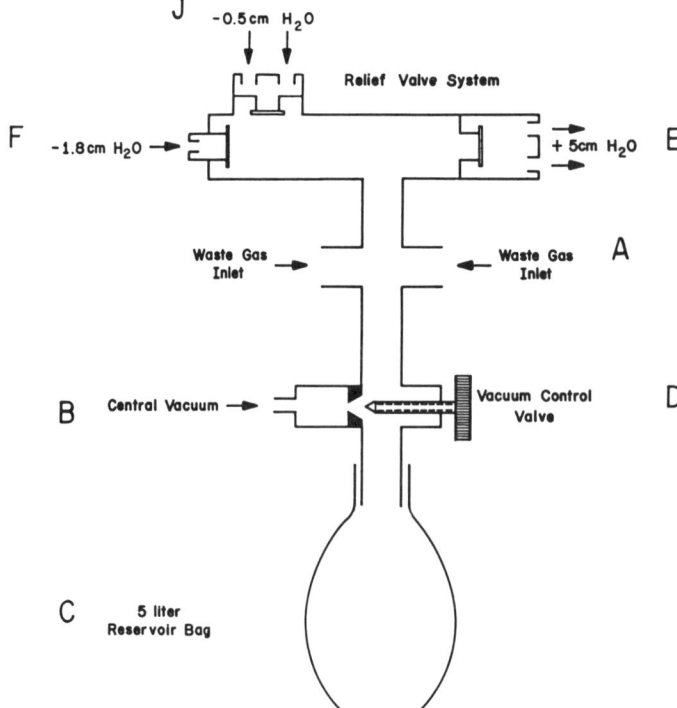

Fig. 7-4 Diagram illustrating the principles of the scavenger interface. Two inlets are available for waste anesthesia gas. Two low-pressure valves (−1.8 and −0.5 cmH_2O) admit room air when subatmospheric pressure occurs in the scavenger system. Excess pressures in the scavenger system are exited by the +5.0 cmH_2O valve. (Courtesy of North American Drager, Telford, PA.)

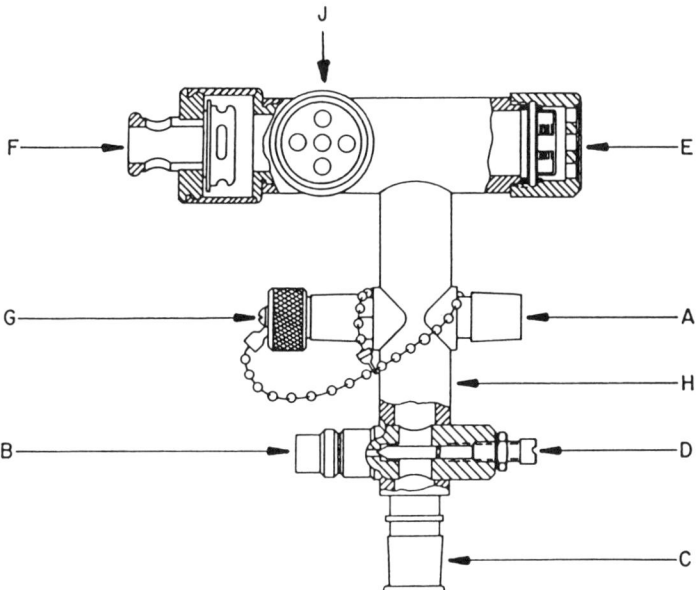

Fig. 7-5 Features of a scavenger interface valve. (A) The input port for attachment of the hose from the pop-off valve and ventilator relief valve. (B) Connection for a vacuum exhaust source. (C) Attachment port for the reservoir bag. (D) Needle valve to adjust the vacuum flow. (E) Positive-pressure relief port. (F) Subatmospheric safety relief valve. (G) Additional input port from the ventilator relief valve. (H) Body of the interface valve. (J) Subatmospheric relief valve. (Courtesy of North American Drager, Telford, PA.)

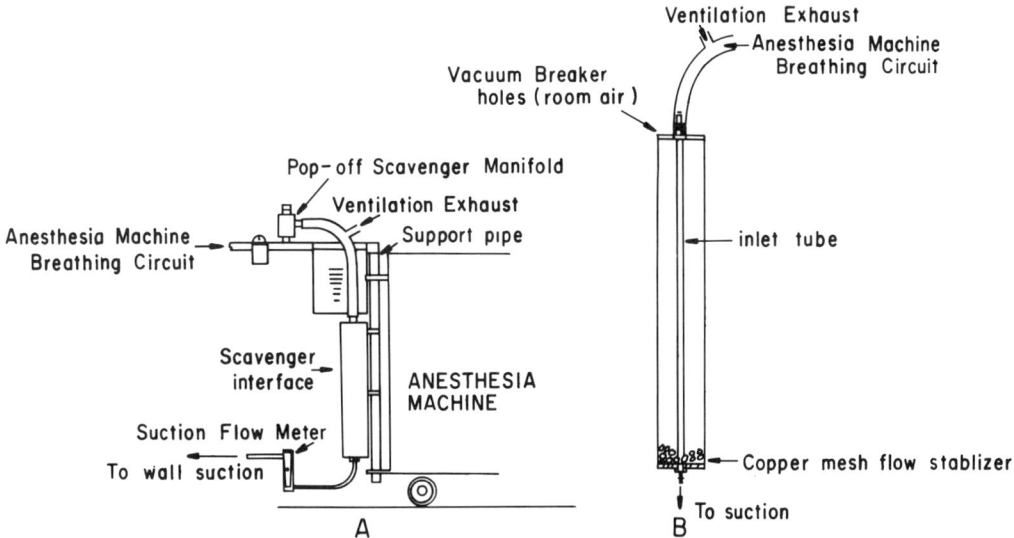

Fig. 7-6 Scavenger system that can be added to an existing anesthesia machine. (A) Connection of the scavenger interface to the anesthesia machine. Exhausted gases are exited by a separate hospital suction. (B) The add-on 2000-cc scavenger interface does not require valves or a reservoir bag. A T-connector accepts exhaust from the ventilator and anesthetic circuit. (Courtesy of Boehringer Laboratories, Wynnewood, PA.)

Table 7-2. Scavenger System Maximum Positive-Pressure Limits

Subsection	Pressure Just Downstream of the Gas-Collecting Assembly
Normal operation (10 L/min flow)	Approximately ambient pressure
Normal operation (75 L/min O_2 flush for 5 seconds)	10 cmH$_2$O
Occluded system (10 L/min flow)	10 cmH$_2$O
Occluded system (75 L/min O_2 flush for 5 seconds)	15 cmH$_2$O

(Reproduced with permission from American National Standard, ANSI Z79.11-1982, © 1982 The American National Standards Institute, 1430 Broadway, NY, NY 10018.)

Table 7-2 lists the maximum positive-pressure limits allowed for various anesthesia gas flows in the ANSI standard. A *leak rate* for the gas-scavenging system should be less than 100 ml/min, resulting in less than a 3.7 ppm ambient concentration of nitrous oxide (70 percent concentration being given).[28] Hoses that transfer waste gases to and from the scavenger interface must be rigid enough not to kink under the following conditions: A 1-m-long length of tubing is hung over a metal cylinder with a 2.5-cm diameter. A 1-kg weight is hung on each end of the tubing and an airflow of 75 L/min is passed into one end of the tubing. Only a driving pressure for the air of less than 10 cmH$_2$O above atmospheric pressure is acceptable.

The transfer tubing that runs along the floor must meet rigid ANSI occlusion requirements. A 50-kg weight is placed on a 5-cm segment of the transfer tubing and airflow at a rate of 75 L/min is started. If the pressure to drive the flow through the tube is more than 10 cmH$_2$O above atmospheric pressure, the tube is unacceptable.[28]

Scavenger systems are usually thought of as an add-on by the majority of anesthesiologists. Little attention is given to the daily checkout, maintenance, or intracase adjustments of the scavenger needle valve. Unfortunately the reality of the situation dictates the importance of buying a scavenger system that meets ANSI standards and which can be depended on for maximal safe service with minimal maintenance care.

The effective control of waste anesthetic gases depends on a combination of active scavenging, a functional circuit, a good operating room air-conditioning system, proper monitoring of the operating room air, and attention to the delivery of the anesthetic gases to the patient.

COMPLICATIONS

Serious failures of the scavenger systems have been reported, which makes one wonder if the threat to the anesthetized patient is more serious than the diseases the devices are purported to eliminate. Failure of the pop-off valve due to incorrect attachment of the exhaust hose and obstruction of the scavenging hose has resulted in an increase in the anesthesia circuit pressure.[29-32] Clinical observation by the anesthesiologists involved avoided potential pulmonary barotrauma. One study, prior to the setting of ANSI standards, warned that scavenger valves fail to function safely if the wall suction is applied directly to the exhaust port and could cause pulmonary barotrauma.[33] Ventilators have malfunctioned owing to negative or positive pressure being applied to the circuit through the venting port to the scavenger system.[34,35] Oxygen concentration in the anesthesia circuit has been reduced owing to failure of the negative-pressure safety valve and occlusion of the air intake valve.[36,37] A disconnected endotracheal tube failed to trigger the ventilator alarm because of an inappropriate Y-connection between the scavenger exhausts of the ventilator and the anesthesia circuit.[38] Scavenger systems have even been blamed for doing a good job: An anesthesia overdose went undetected owing to the absence of smell of the anesthetic agent.[35,39]

Every advance in anesthesia must be examined for the benefits and risks to the patient. Perhaps Miller and Cullen[40] are correct in assuming that the risks to the patient are less than the health hazards of exposure to waste gases for the operating room personnel. Whitcher[16] feels that scavenger systems do not interfere with safe, standard anesthetic techniques. He also feels that, until future research demonstrates nitrous oxide to be innocuous, we should scavenge routinely, as "injury caused by unnecessarily high anesthetic exposure may not be rectifiable."

MONITORING WASTE GAS LEVELS

A number of means are available for monitoring waste gas levels in the operating room. Monitoring is inaccurate if attention is not paid to when the sample is taken during administration of the anesthetic, where in the room the sample is obtained, the frequency of the sampling, and adherence to the exact methodology of the measuring device. Levels of waste gases in the operating room can be sampled continuously or spot-checked. Individual exposure can be measured by a device similar to the radiation exposure badge.

Continuous monitoring of the operating room is best achieved by using an infrared device to measure nitrous oxide. Polyatomic asymmetric molecules, which exist as vapors at room temperature, are particularly suitable for quantification and analysis by infrared techniques. Absorption of radiation (infrared light) in the infrared spectrum is related to the gas concentration and the path length in which the absorption is measured.[41] Each anesthetic gas, that is, halothane and nitrous oxide, in Figures 7-7 and 7-8 is characterized by a different absorption spectrum.[42] Figure 7-9 illustrates the narrow tall absorption peak at 4.4 μm chosen for nitrous oxide. This peak is outside the water vapor peak and decreases interference from water condensation in the sample cell. Infrared measurements are made by placing the anesthetic gas in the infrared source and the detector. An electrically heated element serves as a broad-band source of infrared energy. A spherical mirror within the source housing collimates a portion of the radiated energy and directs it down the reference and sample cells. A selective absorption filter limits the spectral range of the infrared source, allowing the gas analyzer to be made sensitive to one particular gas and insensitive to others. The analysis of very low concentrations of a gas can be enhanced by increasing the distance

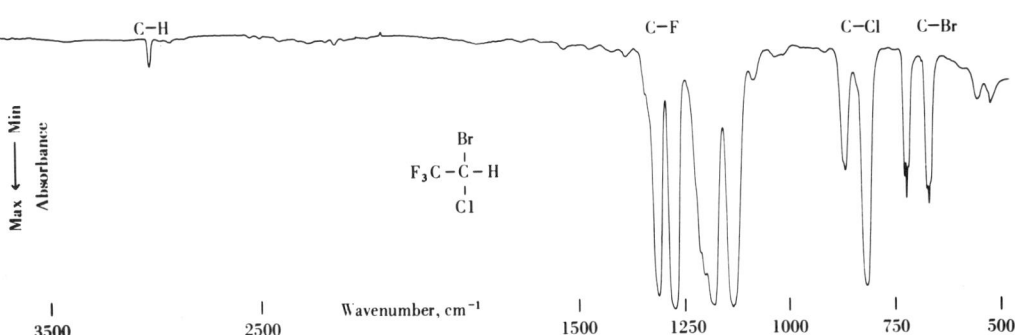

Fig. 7-7 Infrared spectra of halothane. Infrared absorption spectra are like fingerprints, characteristic of only one compound; they serve as an important tool for compound identification and analysis. Halothane was measured in a gaseous phase at a pressure of 20 mmHg in a 5-cm-path gas cell. (Chenoweth MB: Spectrophotometric fluorometric techniques. p. 279. In: Bellville JW, Weaver CS (eds.): Techniques in Clinical Physiology. © 1969 by J. Weldon Bellville and Charles S. Weaver. Reprinted with permission of Macmillan Publishing Co., New York.)

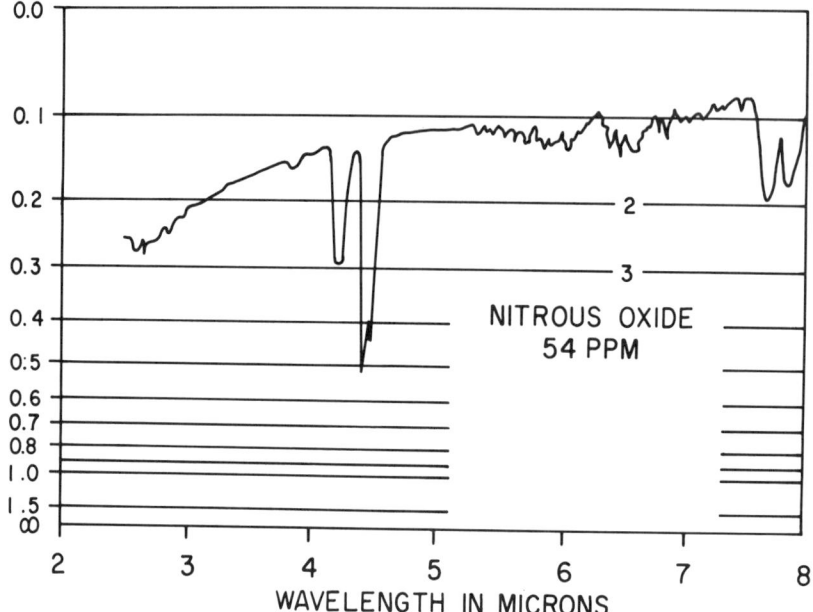

Fig. 7-8 Infrared spectra for nitrous oxide generated from a concentration of 54 ppm.

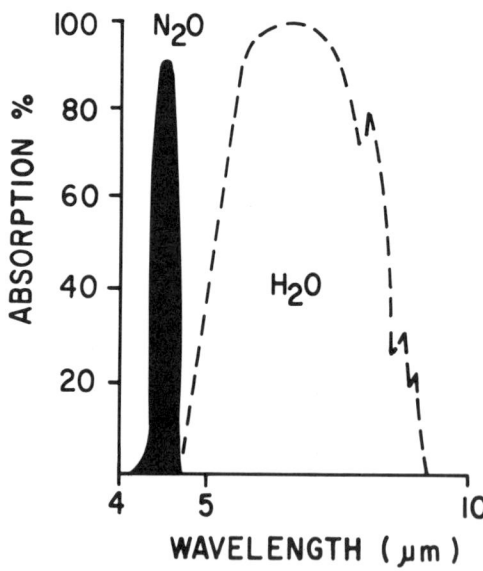

Fig. 7-9 A tall, narrow infrared spectrum peak commonly used for measuring nitrous oxide. Note the comparison to the tall but broad spectral peak for water vapor. (Courtesy of Hewlett-Packard Co., Waltham, MA. Reproduced with permission.)

the infrared beam traverses through the gas sample, as shown in Figure 7-10. Once the infrared beam passes through the gas sample, the light unabsorbed by the sample gas activates the detector cell. The electrical output voltage from the detector cell is essentially proportional to the infrared light falling upon it. An electronic signal processor compares the signal to a zero absorption level for the gas and displays the reading.

Fluorocarbon anesthetics can also be analyzed by using ultraviolet absorption spectra. Absorbance in the ultraviolet range is a convenient method to analyze a specific anesthetic gas in a gas mixture.[43,44] Limitations of the method include loss of the volatile anesthetic in specimen preparation and difficulty in the analysis of specimens which have the anesthetic gas in a solution containing substantial amounts of protein.

A continuous sampling of nitrous oxide is an excellent method to detect leaks in the anesthesia machine or eliminate poor anesthetic techniques which raise the level of waste anesthetic gases. Infrared instruments are usually stable, rugged, and can be moved to various places in the operating room for varied sampling analysis.[45] However, infrared nitrous oxide instruments are not cost effective when measuring waste anesthetic gases in a small operating suite.

Intermittent sampling of the operating room waste anesthetic gases can be done utilizing a commercial apparatus similar to the one pictured in Figure 7-11. A hermetically sealed metal "grab sample" container is used to collect air samples from the operating room for the analysis of nitrous oxide and halogenated agents by gas chromatography. Cartridges are available for spot checks or for time-weighted average sampling.[44] Analysis systems can be utilized by hospitals with less than 8 to 10 operating rooms. Initial multiple samples will establish baseline levels from various sites in each operating room and then quarterly samples can be obtained.

Individual dosimeters have recently been developed for nitrous oxide. The dosimetry system is contained within a device (Fig. 7-12) the size of a pen, worn by each member of the operating room team. Material within the device selectively absorbs nitrous oxide. After a specified time period the dosimeter device is sent to the manufacturer for nitrous oxide analysis. Results are reported as a dose-related measure of the individual's exposure.[46] Time-weighted sampling near the anesthesiologists' breathing zone have been recommended.[16] Costs for each individual will be determined by the specific monitoring strategy adopted.

Risk management factors are not yet established for the scavenging or monitoring of waste anesthetic gases. From the legal perspective it has been recommended that the ideal air-monitoring system should include an infrared analyzer and a personal dosimetry program.[47]

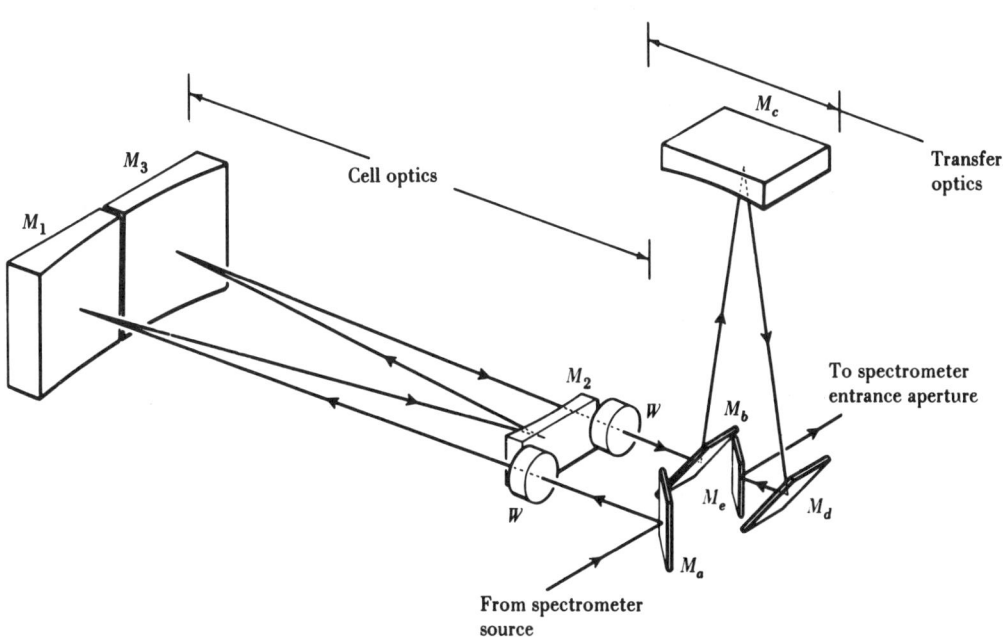

Fig. 7-10 The mirror system for infrared analysis. A 10-m path can be confined to a small space by the use of mirrors, thus allowing the infrared instrument to be smaller. (Courtesy of Perkin-Elmer Corp., Norwalk, CN.)

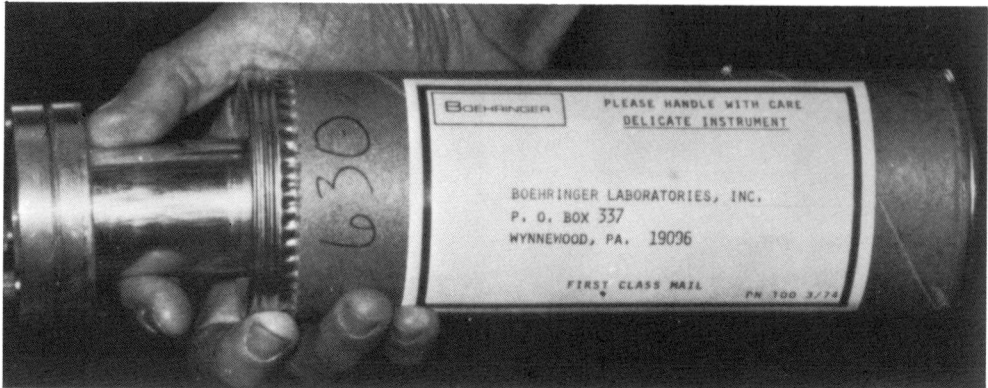

Fig. 7-11 "Grab sample" hermetically sealed metal cartridge for the sample collection of waste anesthetic gases. Each cartridge is mailed to a central laboratory for analysis by gas chromatography. (Courtesy of Boehringer Laboratories, Wynnewood, PA.)

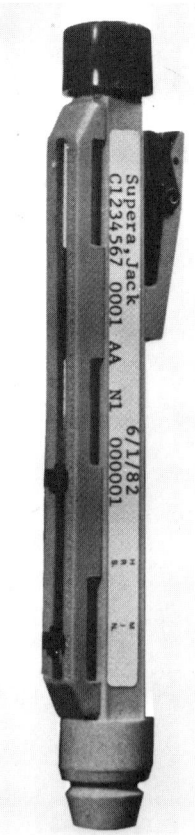

Fig. 7-12 A nitrous oxide personal dosimetry system. The device contains material which selectively absorbs nitrous oxide. Each individual wears the device for a predetermined time period prior to analysis. (Courtesy of RS Landauer, Jr. & Co., Glenwood, IL.)

REFERENCES

1. Cohen EN, Brown BW, Bruce DL et al: Occupational disease among operating room personnel: a national study. Anesthesiology 41:321, 1974
2. Corbett TH, Cornell RG, Endres JL et al: Birth defects among children of nurse anesthetists. Anesthesiology 41:341, 1974
3. Green NM: Traces of anesthetics. Anesthesiology 41:317, 1974
4. Brodsky JB: Exposure to anesthetic gases: A controversy. As Op Rm Nurs J 38:132, 1983
5. Bruce DL, Bach MJ: Psychological studies of human performance as affected by traces of enflurane and nitrous oxide. Anesthesiology 42:194, 1975
6. Bruce DL, Bach MJ, Arbit J: Trace anesthetic effects on perceptual, cognitive, and motor skills. Anesthesiology 40:453, 1974
7. Edling C: Anesthetic gases as an occupational hazard—a review. Scand J Work Environ Health 6:85, 1980
8. Ferstandig LL: Trace concentrations of anesthetic gases: a critical review of their disease potential. Anesth Analg 57:328, 1978
9. Spence AA, Knill-Jones RP: Is there a health hazard in anaesthetic practice? Br J Anaesth 50:713, 1978
10. Vessey MP: Epidemiological studies of the occupational hazards of anaesthesia—a review. Anaesthesia 33:430, 1978
11. Walts LF: Trace anesthetic gases: an unproven health hazard. As Op Rm Nurs J 37:728, 1983
12. Husum B, Wulf HC, Niebuhr E: Monitoring of sister chromatid exchanges in lymphocytes

of nurse–anesthetists. Anesthesiology 62:475, 1985

13. Institute for Occupational Safety and Health. Criteria for a recommended standard—occupational exposure to waste anesthetic gases and vapors. Publication 77-140. U.S. Dept. of Health, Education, and Welfare, Cincinnati, March 1977

14. Mazze RI: Waste anesthetic gases and the regulatory agencies. Anesthesiology 52:248, 1980

15. Linde HW, Bruce DL: Occupational exposure of anesthesiologists to halothane, N_2O, and radiation. Anesthesiology 30:363, 1969

16. Whitcher C: Controlling occupational exposure to nitrous oxide. p. 3313. In Eger EI: Nitrous Oxide/N_2O. Elsevier Science, New York, 1985

17. Lecky JH: Anesthetic pollution in the operating room: a notice to operating room personnel. Anesthesiology 52:157, 1980

18. Buring JE, Hennekens CH, Mayrent SL et al: Health experiences of operating room personnel. Anesthesiology 62:325, 1985

19. Mazze RI, Lecky JH: The health of operating room personnel. Anesthesiology 62:226, 1985

20. Joint Commission on Accreditation of Hospitals. Accreditation manual for hospitals. JCAH, Chicago, 1985

21. Boehringer Catalog. Scavenger–vacuum safety interface, Central testing service—mailable cartridge and analysis, Flow test indicator. Boehringer Laboratories, Wynnewood, PA, 1984

22. DeZotti R, Negro C, Gobbato F: Results of hepatic and hemopoietic controls in hospital personnel exposed to waste anesthetic gases. Int Arch Occup Environ Health 52:33, 1983

23. Whitcher CE, Cohen EN, Trudell JR: Chronic exposure to anesthetic gases in the operating room. Anesthesiology 35:348, 1971

24. Ilsley AH, Crea J, Cousins MJ: Assessment of waste anaesthetic gas scavenging systems under simulated conditions of operation. Anaesth Intensive Care 8:52, 1980

25. Rosenberg P, Kirves A: Miscarriages among operating room theatre staff. Acta Anaesthesiol Scand, suppl., 53:37, 1973

26. Epstein HG, Berlin DP: Removal of ether vapour during anaesthesia. Lancet 1:114, 1944

27. McInnes IC, Goldwater HL: Gas removal systems for commonly used circuits. Anaesthesia 27:340, 1972

28. American National Standard for anesthetic equipment—scavenging systems for excess anesthetic gases. Z79.11-1982. American National Standards Institute, New York, 1982

29. Flowerdew RM: A hazard of scavenger port design. Can Anaesth Soc J 28:481, 1981

30. Manti AM: Gas scavenging systems. Anesth Analg 61:162, 1982

31. Rendell-Baker L: Hazard of blocked scavenge valve. Can Anaesth Soc J 29:182, 1982

32. Tavakoli M, Havbeeb A: Two hazards of gas scavenging. Anesth Analg 57:286, 1978

33. Sharrock N, Eileith D: Potential pulmonary barotrauma when venting anesthetic gases to suction. Anesthesiology 46:152, 1977

34. Malloy WF, Wightman AE, O'Sullivan D et al: Bilateral pneumothorax from suction applied to a ventilator exhaust valve. Anesth Analg 58:147, 1979

35. O'Connor DE, Daniels BW, Pfitzner J: Hazards of anaesthetic scavenging: case reports and brief review. Anaesth Intensive Care 10:15, 1982

36. McIntyre JWR: Anesthesia equipment malfunction: origins and clinical recognition. Can Med J 120:931, 1979

37. Patel KD, Dalal FY: A potential hazard of the Drager scavenging interface system for wall suction. Anesth Analg 58:327, 1979

38. Heard SO, Munson ES: Ventilator alarm nonfunction associated with a scavenging system for waste gases. Anesth Analg 62:230, 1983

39. Sharrock NE, Gabel RA: Inadvertent anesthetic overdose obscured by scavenging. Anesthesiology 49:137, 1978

40. Miller MG, Cullen BF: The cost of scavenging—is it worth it? Anesth Analg 58:265, 1979

41. Cross AD: An Introduction to Practical Infra-Red Spectroscopy. 2nd Ed. Butterworths, London, 1964

42. Zeller MV: Infrared analysis of anesthetic chemicals. Am Lab 10:69, 1979

43. Barrett AM, Nunn JF: Absorption spectra of the common anaesthetic agents in the far ultraviolet. Br J Anaesth 44:306, 1972

44. Dumas JM, Dupuis P, Pfister-Guillouzo G et al: Ionization potentials and ultraviolet absorption spectra of flurocarbon anesthetics. Can J Spectr 26:102, 1981

45. Ilsley AH, Crea J, Cousins MJ: Evaluating of infrared analyzers used for monitoring waste anaesthetic gas levels in operating theatres. Anaesth Intens Care 8:436, 1980

46. Landauer, RS, Jr: Nitrous Oxide: Recognizing and reducing the risks. Glenwood, IL ca. 1984

47. Troyer GT: Managing the nitrous oxide risk is no laughing matter. Risk Management, 1984

8

Compressed Gases and Pressure Regulators

Anesthesiologists require anesthesia gases to be at room temperature in the operating room. Ideally the gases should be easily accessible and allow practical handling. Gases in the compressed state have evolved as the present method of choice. The physical characteristics of a gas determine exactly how the gas will be containerized and delivered. For instance, oxygen can be stored only in the gaseous state at room temperature because it has a critical temperature of $-118°C$. Oxygen or any other gas cannot exist as a liquid above its critical temperature, regardless of how much pressure is applied.[1] Nitrous oxide can exist in the liquid state in a compressed gas tank at room temperature because its critical temperature is only $36.5°C$ and a pressure of 750 psig is sufficient to convert the gas to a liquid.[1] Compressing a gas requires high pressures, which present a danger to individuals who fill, ship, store, or handle the cylinders. In 1913 the Compressed Gas Association (CGA) was created, their primary objective being[2]

to promote, develop, represent and coordinate technical and standardization activities in the compressed gas industries, including end uses of products, in the interest of safety and efficiency, and to the end that they may serve to the fullest extent the best interest of the public.

The CGA is a nonprofit service organization with a membership consisting of over 300 companies engaged in the chemical industry; firms producing and distributing compressed, liquefied, and cryogenic gases; and manufacturers of portable containers, cargo tanks, tank cars, and medical equipment.[2] Other regulatory agencies also play a role in establishing standards related to compressed gases, for example, the U.S. Department of Transportation (DOT) and the American Society of Mechanical Engineers (ASME).[3] The quality, standardization, and safety of compressed gases did not just happen but have been the result of a successful cooperation between many individuals representing a wide field of interest.

COMPRESSED GAS CYLINDERS

Construction

A cylinder begins life as a short bar of steel called a billet. The process described for cylinder manufacture will be similar to the one used by the Chesterfield Cylinder Co. of Enid, OK.[4] Heating the billet to above $1,200°C$ and piercing it with a 2,000-ton forging press to form a short cylinder with a solid base begins

119

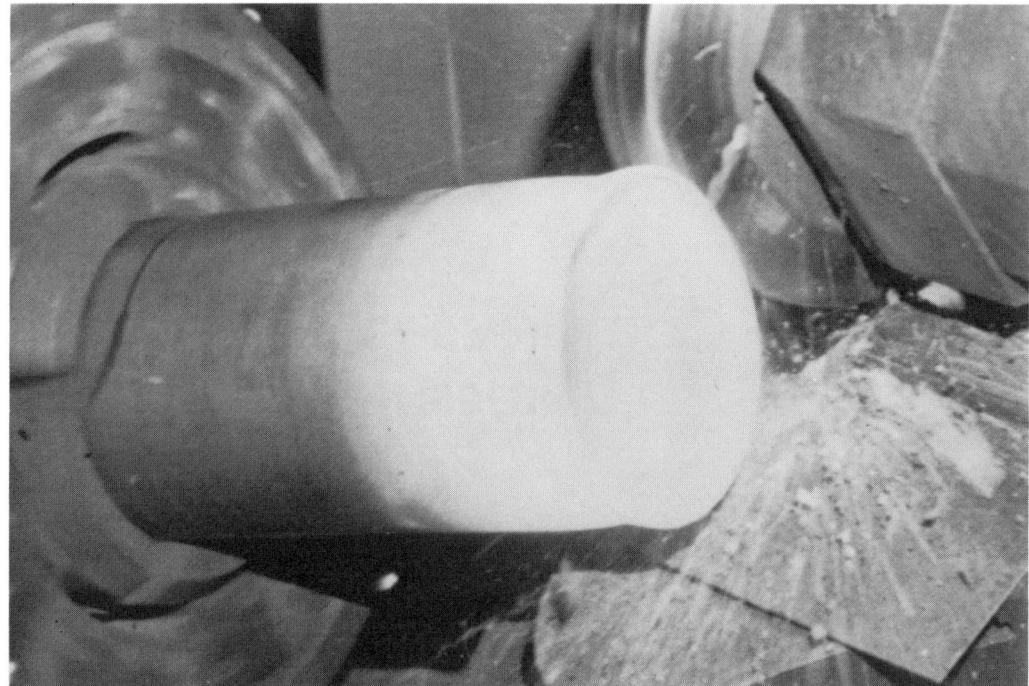

A

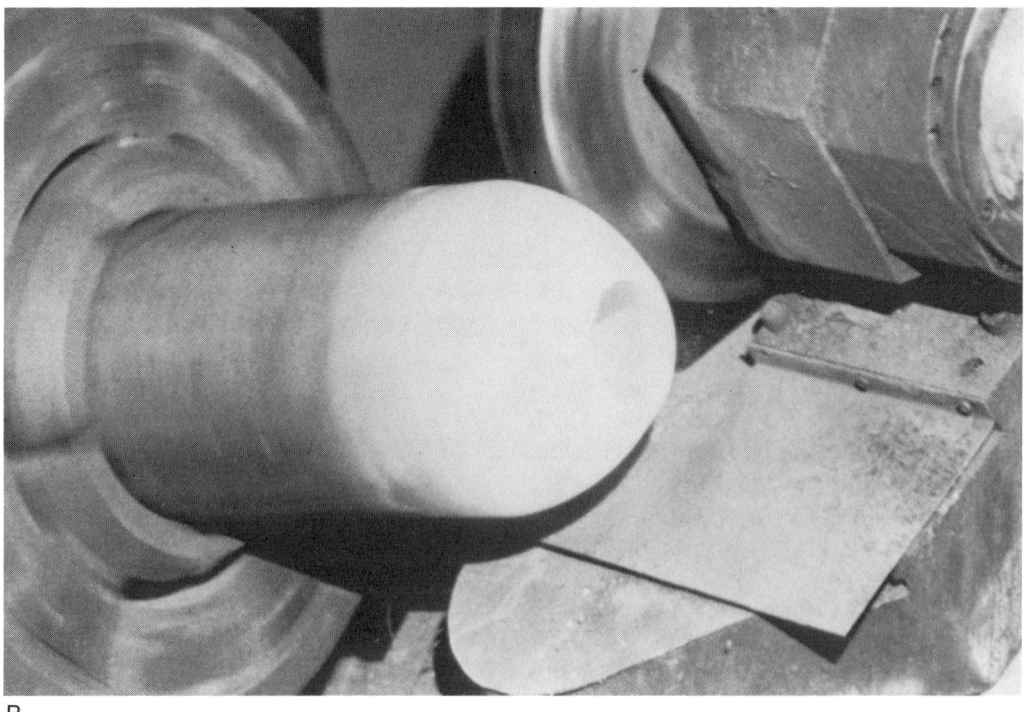

B

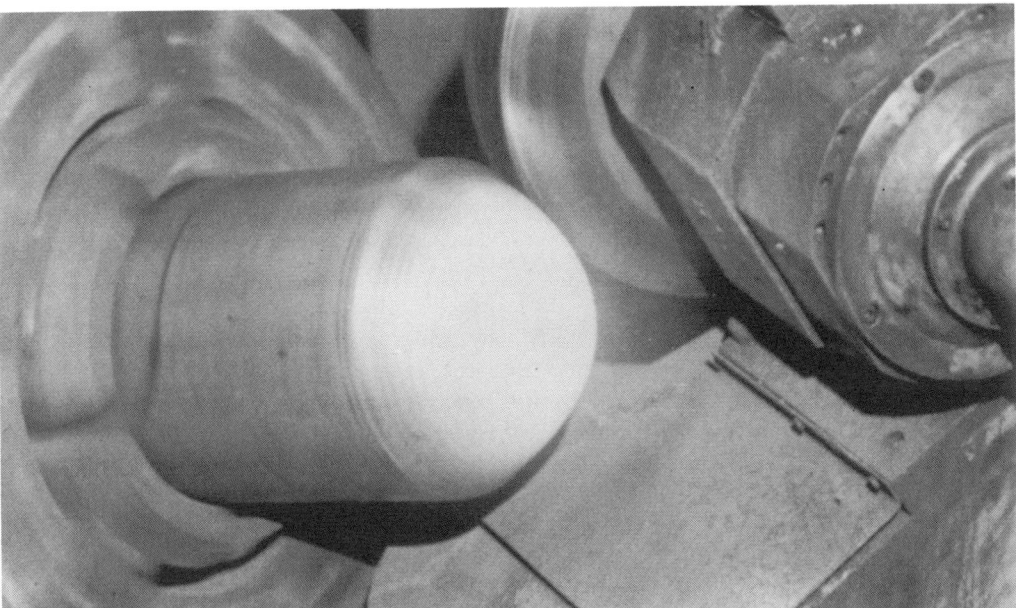

C

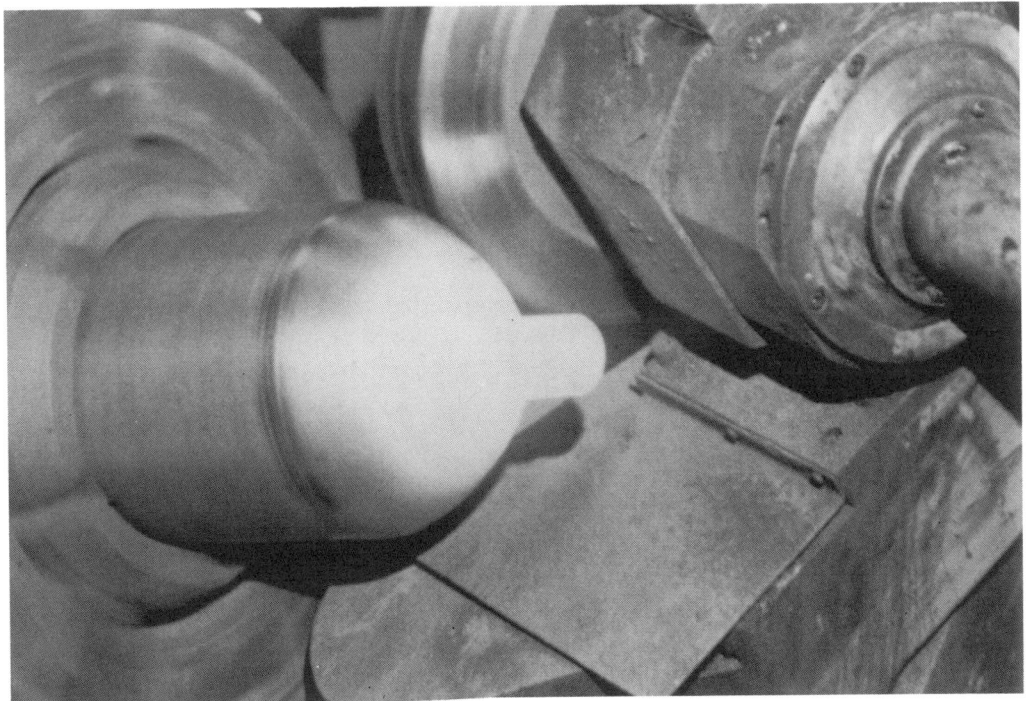

D

Fig. 8-1 Hot-spinning the anesthesia gas cylinder by a rotating wheel to form the neck. The four views (A–D) show the process from the open-ended cylinder to the making of the teatlike protrusion on the neck. (Chesterfield Seamless Steel Gas Cylinders. Chesterfield Cylinder Co., Enid, OK, 1985.)

the process. While the cylinder is still hot a mandrel is inserted into the forged blank and a series of roller dies draw out the walls to the required length and thickness. The base is then made concave and hot-stamped for cast identity. After ejection the cylinder is trimmed to length. Ultrasonic instruments test the cylinder for surface defects and ensure that the wall thickness is uniform over the entire length of the cylinder.

A programmed hot-spinning process closes the cylinder neck, leaving a teatlike protusion on the end as though a potter shaped it on a wheel (see Fig. 8-1). Heat treatment at 900°C (austenitizing temperture) polymerizes the cylinder, making it very hard and structurally sound. Next the cylinder is tempered at 580° to 680°C and air-cooled. Hardness, testing is carried out on every cylinder, followed by physical testing (i.e., tensile and flattening tests) according to DOT and CGA regulations on sample cylinders selected by the independent inspection authority.[2, 5]

A thread is machined into the cylinder neck for the appropriate valve fitting.[6] Hydrostatic testing at 167 percent of working pressure is done on every cylinder. Cylinder volume is calculated by filling with water and measuring empty and full weight values. Each cylinder is then burned out at 300°C; this effectively cleans and dries the internal surfaces. Internal shot blasting is done for scale removal, followed by inspection and cylinder stamping. A collar is riveted to the cylinder neck with threads for the valve protective cap. After the correct valve is inserted and torqued in place, a protective cap is added. External shot blasting of the cylinder is followed by the final electrostatic painting. Records of manufacture and testing for each cylinder have been kept on file by the Chesterfield Cylinder Co. for over 75 years.

Wall thickness is specified according to the pressure the tank must withstand.[3] A cylinder of nitrous oxide filled at room temperature might be shipped in the back of a hot semi-trailer, with the cylinder pressure increasing as the temperature rises. The cylinder must be constructed to withstand such expected changes in temperature. The overfilling of oxy-gen cylinders to 4,000 psig and nitrous oxide cylinders to 1,500 psig has been reported.[7] Most cylinders are able to contain twice their usual working pressure before bursting.[2]

Prior to hydrostatic testing of a used cylinder a visual inspection should be made.[5, 8] The cylinder must be condemned if it leaks, shows signs of internal or external corrosion, has dents or bulges, or shows evidence of rough usage. Visual inspection can be supplemented by using depth gauges, scales, ultrasonic devices, magnetic particle inspectors, and dye penetrant materials. In addition, high-pressure cylinders are tapped with a ½-lb metallic object (hammer test)[8]: If the cylinder has a dull or dead ring, it must be cleaned; however, if the dull or dead ring persists after cleaning, the cylinder must be condemned. Hydrostatic testing is done by (1) the water jacket volumetric expansion method, (2) the direct expansion method, (3) the pressure recession method, or (4) the proof pressure method.

Water jacket volumetric expansion method. The cylinder is enclosed in a water-filled vessel. Measurements of the volume of water displaced before and after the cylinder is pressurized are done.

Direct expansion method. A cylinder is filled with a known weight of water at a known temperature. A measurable volume of water is then forced into the cylinder and the volume of water which is expelled during pressure release is measured.

Pressure recession method. The hydrostatic test pressure is rapidly raised in the cylinder. Recession of pressure in the cylinder is observed immediately after cutting off the pressure supply.

Proof pressure method. Examination for leaks and defects is done while the cylinder is at test pressure.

Size

Compressed gas cylinders come in a variety of shapes and sizes. For some reason the nomenclature for medical gas cylinders evolved around alphabetical designations.[9] Cylinders on the anesthesia machine are referred to as

Table 8-1. Typical Anesthesia Gas Cylinders

Cylinder Style	Dimensions (cm)	Nominal Volume (L)*	Contents	Gas Oxygen	Nitrous Oxide	Air
D	10.8 × 43	2.88	psig Liters U.S. color	1,900 400 Green	745 940 Blue	1,900 375 Yellow
E	10.8 × 66	4.80	psig Liters U.S. color	1,900 660 Green	745 1,590 Blue	1,900 625 Yellow
H	23.5 × 130	43.6	psig Liters U.S. color	2,200 6,900 Green	745 15,800 Blue	2,200 6,550 Yellow

* All volumes at 21.1°C (70°F).
(Data from Compressed Gas Association pamphlet P-2, Characteristics and Safe Handling of Medical Gases, and pamphlet C-9, Standard Color-marking of Compressed Gas Cylinders Intended for Medical Use. Compressed Gas Association, Inc., 1235 Jefferson Davis Hwy., Arlington, VA)

"tanks" and are size D or E. The cylinder-manufacturing process described earlier relates to H-type cylinders; D- and E-types may be made by a similar billet route, but also from tubing or plate. Nitrous oxide banks and operating rooms without hospital pipelines usually use H cylinders. Table 8-1 lists the physical characteristics of D, E, and H cylinders and the capacity of the cylinder when filled with either oxygen, nitrous oxide, or air.

Markings

Cylinders are marked with a permanent stencil, stamp, or label and precautionary warnings indicating hazards for specific gases.[2, 5, 9, 10] Medical gas cylinders require, in addition, a color code system (see Table 8-1) adopted by the medical gas industry.[2, 9, 11]

The permanent label on cylinders of medical gases is placed on the sloping portion of the cylinder valve end. Usually the required information is stamped with letters at least 0.476 cm high.[2, 10] Information which should be stamped on every cylinder is depicted in Figure 8-2. Seven areas of importance are identified for the user: (1) the cylinder specifications, that is, the regulatory body which governs the use of the cylinder, the type and material of the cylinder, and the service pressure (in psig), (2) the cylinder serial number, (3) the identifying symbol of purchaser, user,

or manufacturer, (4) the manufacturing data, that is, date of manufacture, original test date, inspector's mark, and qualification for 110 percent filling, (5) the manufacturer's identifying symbol, (6) retest markings, and (7) the owner's identification.[5]

The CGA system of basic marking for cylinders was designed to provide immediate identification of cylinder contents, especially when special precautions must be observed for a hazardous gas.[2] A white panel contains the proper shipping name of the gas and a diamond indicates the hazard class of the gas (see Fig. 8-3). A second diamond is placed if a secondary hazard must be identified; for example, chlorine is labeled Nonflammable, Poison. If the label for the anesthesia gas does not correspond to the color code of the cylinder, the contents should be analyzed before the cylinder is used.[12]

Medical gas cylinders are color-coded with a nonfading, durable, water-insoluble paint.[2, 9, 11] At least the shoulder of the cylinder must be painted in order to identify the gas for the individual connecting the cylinder to the utilization equipment. Each country in the world seems to have its own color code system. During World War II several deaths occurred on the wards of American hospitals in England because of the differences in the color coding of oxygen cylinders. A film, *Green for Danger,* was produced to alert personnel to the hazard of substituting a British

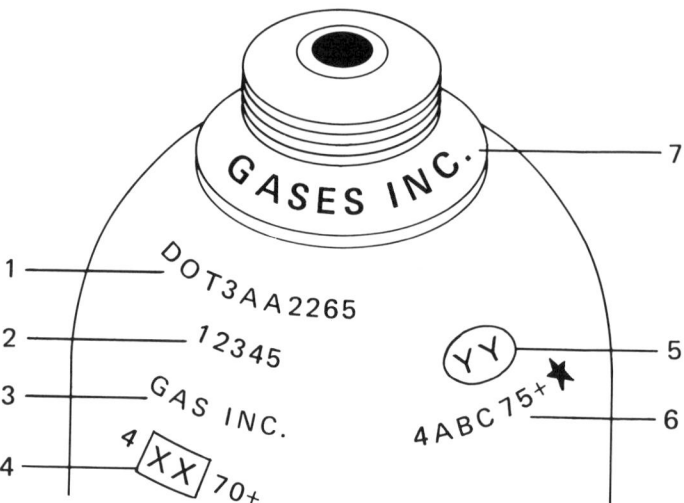

Fig. 8-2 Typical cylinder markings. (1) Cylinder specifications: DOT (Department of Transportation) is the regulatory body which governs use of the cylinder, 3AA specifies the type and material of the cylinder, and 2265 is the service pressure of the cylinder (in psig). (2) 12345 is the cylinder serial number. (3) Gas Inc. is an identifying symbol of either the purchaser, user, or manufacturer. (4) Manufacturing data: 4-70 is the date of manufacture and original test date, Boxed XX is the inspector's offical mark, + means the cylinder qualified for 110 percent filling. (5) Boxed YY is the manufacturer's identifying symbol. (6) Retest markings: 4-75 is the date of the first hydrostatic retest, ABC is the retester's identifying symbol, + means the cylinder requalifies for 110 percent filling, and the star indicates the cylinder qualifies for a 10-year retest interval. (7) Gases Inc. is the neck ring owner's identification. (CGA Pamphlet C-1: Methods for Hydrostatic Testing of Compressed Gas Cylinders. By permission of Compressed Gas Association, 1235 Jefferson Davis Hwy, Arlington, VA 22202, 1975).

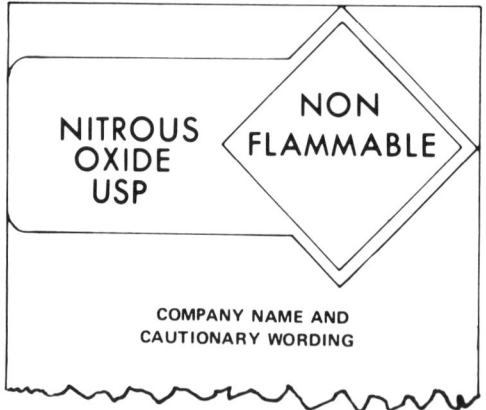

Fig. 8-3 Labels required to provide immediate identification of cylinder contents and to warn the user of any hazards inherent in the cylinder contents. Nitrous oxide is labeled as a hazard class Nonflammable. (Handbook of Compressed Gases. Compressed Gas Association. 2nd Ed. Van Nostrand Reinhold, New York, 1981.)

cylinder for an American cylinder.[13] Carbon dioxide was apparently stored in green cylinders. Prior to 1948 all anesthesia gas cylinders were painted black in Britain and were identified by a stick-on paper label and by painting the oxygen nozzles white and the nitrous oxide nozzles black.[14] Presently in the United States green is the color code for oxygen, blue is for nitrous oxide, and yellow is for air.

Cylinder Valve

The cylinder valve designed for attachment to the anesthesia machine is pictured in Figure 8-4. Two holes are drilled for the specific gas which the cylinder will hold in conformance with the pin index safety system (PISS).[6] The outlet for the gas exits in the midline on the same side as the PISS. A screw-down valve seating mechanism controls the on/off flow. Excessive pressure buildup inside the cylinder exits through the safety relief device on the cylinder yoke. A conical depression serves as a seat for the holding screw of the yoke handle. The pointed end of the yoke handle holding screw cannot be sharper than a 100° included angle.[6]

Cylinder valves are not reducing valves but serve as the mechanism to turn the cylinder on or off. Breaking off one of these valves or removing one inadvertently when the cylinder is filled with a compressed gas can result in a cylindrical flying object capable of great harm.[7, 15, 16] Even opening the oxygen cylinder can create marked commotion due to noise and turbulent air flow.

Connections of the valve to the anesthesia machine must be kept meticulously clean of oil, dirt, dust, grease, or any combustible material. Oxygen is a potent oxidizer and nitrous oxide can support combustion at elevated temperatures.[17] Opening the cylinder valve rapidly has been associated with violent combustions and explosions.[1, 18] The postulated mechanism is thought to be a rapid rise in temperature resulting from the sudden release and instantaneous compression of the gas in the cylinder. Adiabatic compression takes place, which means the generated heat does not dissipate to the outside.[1] A shock wave may also be formed, which sends powerful pressure waves from the cylinder to the low-pressure portion of the reducing valve. Shock waves from the cylinder valve produce a pressure rise when they meet the resting gas in the reducing valve and produce a higher temperature than the slower phenomenon of adiabatic change. Compressing a volume of air to one-sixth its original volume via shock waves will cause a rise in temperature of 2,000°C, whereas under adiabatic conditions the rise would be only 500°C. Either temperature would be enough to set the stage for a disaster in the presence of oxygen and a combustible material.

Pin Index Safety System

As early as 1940, medical societies and medical gas manufacturers recognized the need for a system to prevent the interchangeability of medical gas cylinders on anesthesia machines.[2, 6] Even though Dr. Philip Woodbridge[19] presented the idea for the present PISS to the Ohio Chemical Company in

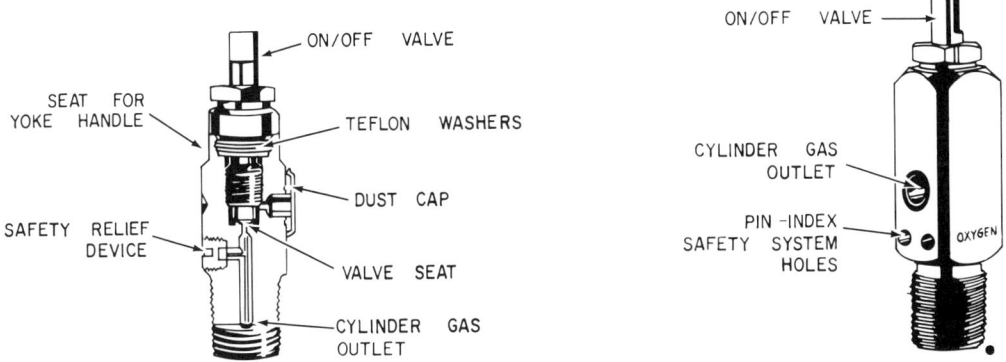

Fig. 8-4 Diagram of a cylinder valve with its Pin Index Safety System. The right view shows the two holes for the pin-indexing and the larger central hole for exit of the cylinder gas. The left view illustrates the working mechanisms of the valve. A protective plastic dust cap is placed over the gas outlet to keep out combustible materials. (Redrawn from Handbook of Compressed Gases. Compressed Gas Association. 2nd Ed. New York, Van Nostrand Reinhold, 1981; and from illustration courtesy of Ohmeda, The BOC Group, Inc.)

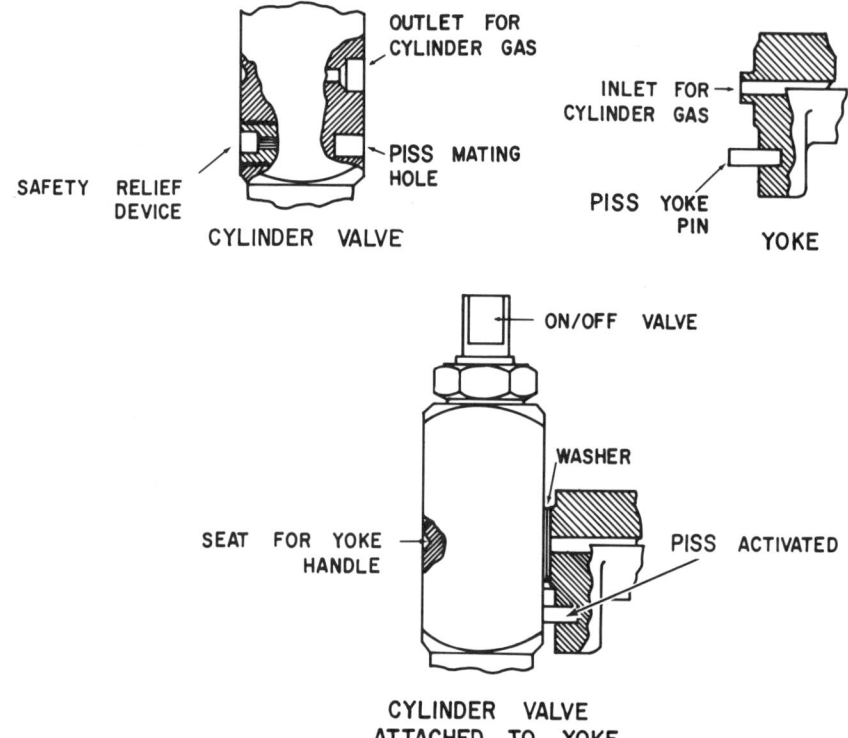

Fig. 8-5 Schematic cutaway views of the pin index safety system (PISS). Holes for the PISS can be seen in the top left view of the cylinder valve. A safety relief device is also in place in the valve. The side view of the yoke shows one of the PISS yoke pins sticking out from the body. Connecting the yoke and valve in the lower figure requires the presence of one washer. Note the position of the PISS pins and engagement into the corresponding matched holes. (Redrawn from CGA Standard V.1, ANSI B57.1, CSA B96: Compressed Gas Cylinder Valve Outlet and Inlet Connections. © 1977. By permission of the Compressed Gas Association, 1235 Jefferson Davis Hwy, Arlington, VA 22202.)

1939, it was not adopted as the standard[19, 20] until 1953. Further improvement has led to the present PISS defined by the CGA and the ANSI.[6]

Noninterchangeability of anesthesia gas cylinders is achieved by assigning each gas two pins in the yoke of the anesthesia machine and two mating holes in the cylinder valve.[6] Figure 8-5 illustrates the basic features of the pin-indexed cylinder valve–anesthesia machine yoke connection. Figure 8-6 shows the crescent positioning of all six cylinder valve holes in the PISS. Oxygen is assigned pins 2 and 5 (see Fig. 8-7), nitrous oxide pins 3 and

5, and air pins 1 and 5. The PISS is also used by the gas supplier when filling the anesthesia gas cylinders.

Pins in the yoke must have a minimum tensile strength[6] of 60,000 psig. Even this tensile strength will not stop someone from cutting the pins off.[21] Only a single washer is allowed between the valve stem and the yoke. If more than one washer is used, the pins may not extrude out far enough to engage the valve mating holes, thus bypassing the PISS.[19, 21, 22] The washer ensures a gas-tight seal and must be less than 2.4 mm thick prior to compression.[6]

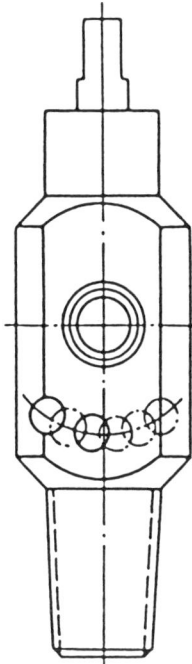

Fig. 8-6 Cylinder valve showing the placement of the six assigned holes for medical gases. Note the holes lie on an imaginary crescent. (Schreiber, P: Safety Guidelines for Anesthesia Systems. North American Drager, Telford, PA, 1984.)

The "case of the missing pin" can easily allow the wrong cylinder to be attached.[22] Some ingenious individuals[22-24] have installed hoses directly to the hospital pipeline with PISS fittings on the anesthesia machine end, then they say the anesthesia machine design is faulty as they proceed to put the PISS in the yoke upside-down! However, the most insidious and dangerous problem occurs when the PISS is bypassed by the supplier by filling the cylinder with another gas and not changing the label, the pins, or the cylinder color.[25]

Hanger yokes must have the PISS pins and be provided with a mechanism which will prevent tightening the cylinder until it is properly engaged in the yoke (Fig. 8-8). The yoke must have (1) a cylinder pressure gauge, (2) a filter to remove particulate matter, (3) a clamping device with a 100° to 120° conical point at least 7 mm in diameter, (4) a nipple at least 6.35 mm in diameter for a gas conduit, (5) a permanent identification by name or chemical symbol, and (6) a color code for the gas it accepts.[26] When a two-yoke system (Fig. 8-9) is used, there must be a means, such as a check valve (Figs. 8-8 and 8-10), provided to prevent leakage (transfilling) from a full cylinder to an empty cylinder.

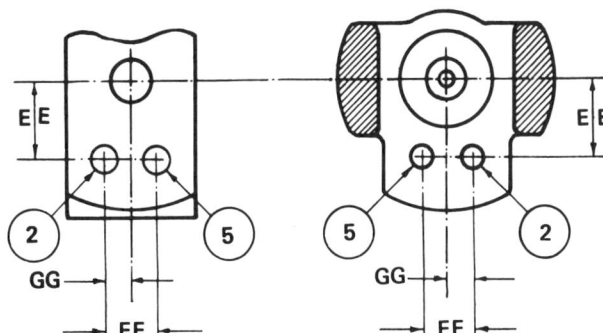

DIMEN-SIONS	INCHES	MM
EE	.535 ± .003	13.6 ± .07
GG	.174 ± .005	4.4 ± .15
FF	.348 ± .003	8.8 ± .07

Fig. 8-7 Pin index safety system (PISS) for oxygen. Each anesthesia gas is assigned two pins; those for oxygen are 2 and 5. Two holes are drilled in the cylinder valve at a distance FF just below the cylinder gas outlet (left). Two corresponding pins are placed on the yoke of the anesthesia machine (right). (CGA Standard V.1, ANSI B57.1, CSA B96: Compressed Gas Cylinder Valve Outlet and Inlet Connections. © 1977. By permission of the Compressed Gas Association, 1235 Jefferson Davis Hwy, Arlington, VA 22202.)

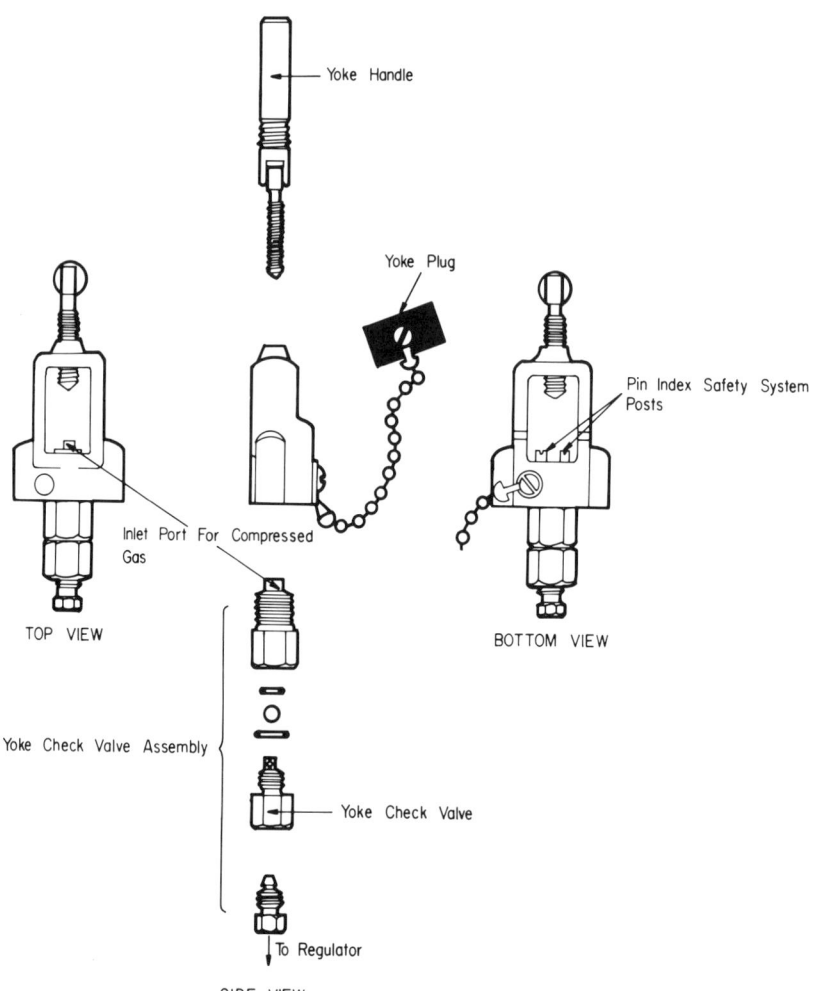

Fig. 8-8 Anesthesia machine yoke assembly. The side view shows the multiple parts that make up the yoke as seen in the top and bottom views. The PISS ports are seen in the bottom view and the inlet port for the compressed gas is shown in the top view. Note the yoke plug and yoke check valves which help prevent backflow. (Redrawn from Parts Manual. North American Drager, Telford, PA, 1984.)

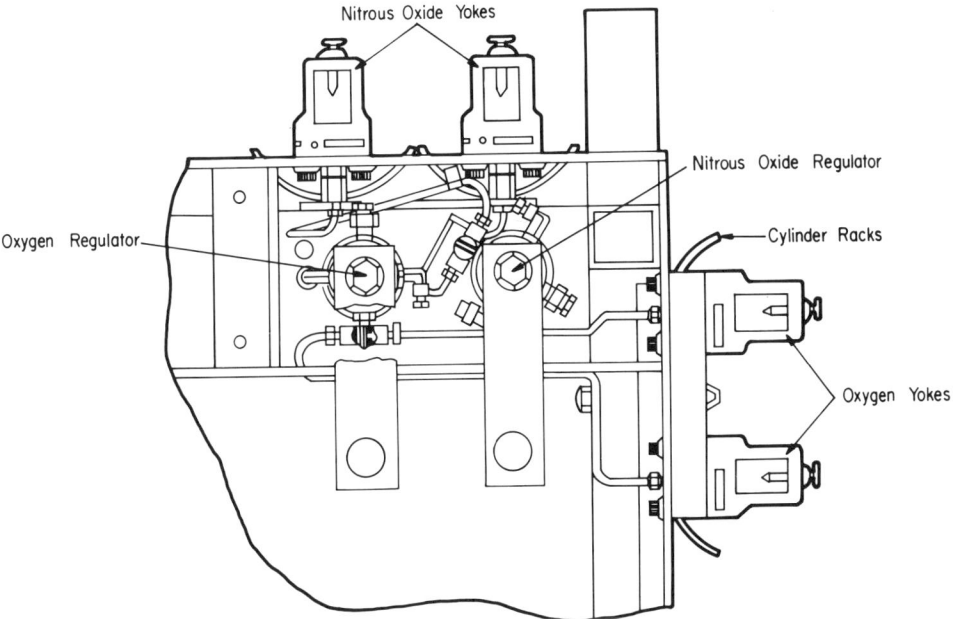

Fig. 8-9 Two-yoke arrangement for oxygen and nitrous oxide. Each regulator reduces the individual compressed cylinder pressure to an adjustable line pressure between 40 and 48 psig. (Redrawn from Parts Manual. North American Drager, Telford, PA, 1984.)

Fig. 8-10 The hanger yoke system for compressed gases. In yoke A the compressed gas cylinder is on and the check valve is forced off the valve seat allowing the gas in the cylinder to flow into the anesthesia machine piping. In yoke B the compressed gas cylinder is absent. The check valve is seated against the valve seat preventing retrograde flow of gas from yoke A out through yoke B. The yoke plug prevents gas from escaping to the atmosphere and keeps the gas inlet clean and safe from accidental damage to the pin index configuration or the structural housing. (Reproduced with permission from Bowie E, Huffman LM: The Anesthesia Machine: Essentials for Understanding. Ohmeda, The BOC Group, Inc., 1985)

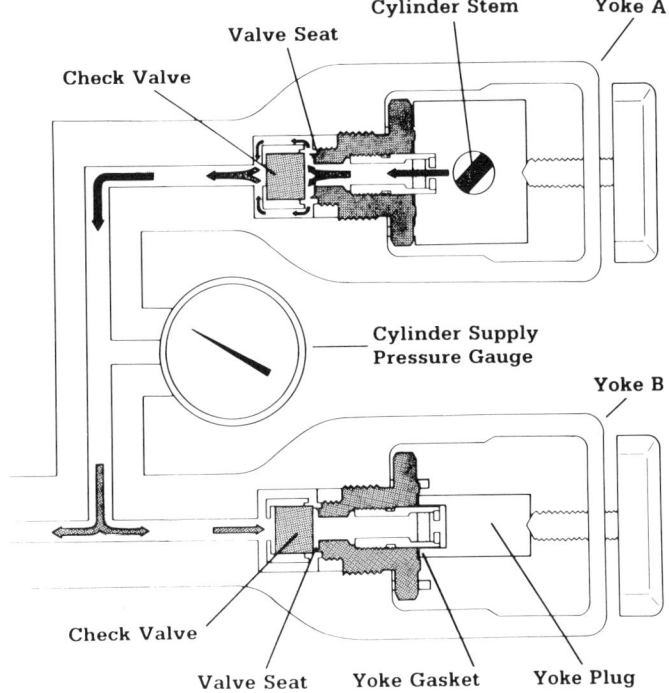

Pressure Relief Devices

A pressure relief device designed to prevent rupture of a compressed gas cylinder placed in a fire is required[27] by DOT Section 173.34. Additional city and state pressure vessel laws and regulations must be adhered to on an individual basis. Seven types of pressure relief devices are defined by the CGA.[27] Each gas is assigned a device on the basis of the intended pressure and the risk of rupture.

Oxygen, nitrous oxide, and air cylinders require the same CGA types of pressure relief devices. Each cylinder must have two devices: a CG-1 rupture disk and a CG-4 rupture disk with a 74°C fusible alloy backing.[27] A rupture disc is a nonreclosing device which bursts when actuated by inlet static pressure.[2] Fusible plug devices are also nonreclosing but function by either "yielding" or melting at a temperature dependent on the alloy in the plug. The yield temperature is reached when the fusible plug extrudes from its holder and allows the contents of the cylinder to exit. A rupture disk and a low-temperature fusible plug combination device prevent the cylinder from bursting when it reaches the preset bursting pressure of the rupture disk unless the temperature is high enough to cause the fusible plug to yield or melt.[27]

Storage and Handling

Years of experience with compressed gas cylinders have led to the evolution of handling and storage techniques which, if employed, will result in complete safety.

Gas suppliers are given a long list of standards regarding the filling, painting, maintenance, retesting, moving and lifting, storage, and connection of the gas cylinder or container at the user's site.[2, 9, 28] In the hospital, gas cylinders should be attached to the anesthesia machine, chained to a secure gas hand truck or to a wall or some other secure fixture. Cylinders should never be left standing free. The weight of a cylinder—an empty H cylinder weighs 59 kg—can cause personal injury.[16] A cylinder that falls may break off the valve, which can result in either the valve, the cylinder, or both becoming a projectile.[7, 15, 16] Falling increases the likelihood of contamination of the cylinder gas outlet with dust, dirt, or other combustibles. Regulations do not preclude the user from storing the cylinders horizontally but merely indicate the need for proper securement, no matter what the position may be. Protective caps should be placed on the cylinders except when in use. During storage, cylinders should be placed in a well-ventilated, dry, cool, and, if possible, fire-resistive room of the hospital, and never in the operating room.[15] Cylinders should obviously be kept away from sparks, flames, combustible material, or exposure to high temperatures. Local and state governmental agencies have regulations pertaining to anesthesia gas storage. Anesthesiologists or designated hospital personnel responsible for the storage of anesthesia gases should be familiar with local and state, as well as federal, government regulations regarding gas storage.

Cylinder valves should be opened slowly.[15] The process of "cracking the cylinder" prior to mounting on the yoke will serve to blow out any dirt or dust in the stem valve. Only two turns of the valve tap are required to completely open the cylinder. Damage to the valve may occur if the tap is opened excessively.[16] Opening the valve on a large cylinder when only the cylinder end of the anesthesia machine connecting hose is attached can result in significant damage, as the unattached yoke end acts as an air hammer.[29] A cylinder connection which does not fit easily should never be forced. All cylinders connected to the anesthesia machine should have a check valve to prevent feedback, a pressure regulator, and a system pressure relief device.[15, 26] Specific details regarding standards for handling and storage are available.[2, 9, 15, 26]

Anesthesiologists should be especially alert to the potential abuse of nitrous oxide.[16, 30-33] Theft of nitrous oxide cylinders from suppliers, dental offices, and hospitals is increasing.

Strangers have been discovered in operating room lounges in the middle of the night inhaling nitrous oxide from anesthesia machines.[16] Some of the steps recommended by the Compressed Gas Association to limit access to nitrous oxide cylinders include the following: (1) Lock the cylinder storage area, (2) allow only authorized personnel in the cylinder storage area, (3) return "empty" cylinders to the storage room promptly, (4) establish a cylinder inventory accounting system, and (5) report thefts immediately.[30]

Compressed Anesthesia Gases

OXYGEN

Oxygen is manufactured by (1) fractional distillation of liquefied air,[2, 17, 34] (2) electrolysis of water,[2, 17] or (3) chemical reaction,[35] that is, thermal decomposition of sodium chlorates. Fractional distillation of air is by far the most important manufacturing method. The steel and chemical industries use over 80 percent of the oxygen produced.[17] Rigid standards control the purity and product qualification testing,[2, 17, 35, 36] as well as the valves[6] and cylinders.[3, 5, 10] Physical constants for oxygen are listed in Table 8-2.

High-purity oxygen is readily available at a reasonable cost because of the high nationwide demand for the gas. Oxygen is used to power the anesthesia ventilator because it is inexpensive, contains little or no water, and is readily available in the operating room.

Medical-grade gaseous and liquefied oxygen is given the CGA classification of A and B. Both grades are classified as drugs by the USP and must meet the requirements of the Federal Food, Drug, and Cosmetics Act.[36-38] Grade A requires a minimum of 99 percent oxygen and grade B requires a minimum of 99.5 percent oxygen. Research-grade oxygen is also available[17] with a minimum purity of 99.995 percent.

An H cylinder of oxygen contains 6,900 L at a pressure of 2,200 psig (see Table 8-1). H-type cylinders of oxygen are assigned CGA valve no. 540, while smaller D or E cylinders use the PISS 2–5 valve.[6] Oxygen is above its critical temperature ($-118.6°C$) at room temperature, so the volume of oxygen remaining in the cylinder is directly proportional to the cylinder pressure. Cylinders of oxygen have a safety device which is either the frangible disk type or the frangible disk type backed up with fusible metal,[17] melting at approximately 100°C. Either a single-stage or two-stage regulator can be used to reduce the pressure from 2,200 psig to the required 40 to 55 psig of the anesthesia pipeline.

NITROUS OXIDE

Nitrous oxide is commercially manufactured by the thermal decomposition of ammonium nitrate. Nitrous oxide, water, and a host of toxic impurities are present in the initial reaction. Further purification is achieved by removing water by condensation, passing the gas through a series of scrubbing towers, and, after compressing it, passing it through a bed

Table 8-2. Physical Constants of Oxygen, Nitrous Oxide, and Air

	Oxygen	Nitrous Oxide	Air
International symbol	O_2	N_2O	Air
Molecular weight	31.999	44.013	28.97
Boiling point (°C)	-183.0	-88.5	-194.35
Critical temperature (°C)	-118.6	36.4	-140.6
Weight of 1 mole (kg)	0.0319988	0.044013	0.02896

(Data from Braker W, Mossman AL: Matheson Gas Data Book. 6th Ed. Matheson Gas Products, Secaucus, NJ 07094; and CGA pamphlets G-7, Compressed Air for Human Respiration, and G-4, Oxygen. Compressed Gas Association, Inc., 1235 Jefferson Davis Highway, Arlington, VA, 1980.)

of desiccant in the final drying process.[2] Nitrous oxide may also be obtained by a controlled reduction of nitrites, a slow decomposition of hyponitrites, and thermal decomposition of hydroxylamine.[17, 39] Regulations and standards control the cylinders,[4, 5, 10] cylinder valves,[6] and purity[40, 41] of nitrous oxide. Physical constants for nitrous oxide are listed in Table 8-2. Nitrous oxide is also classified as a drug by the USP and must meet the regulations of the Federal Food, Drug, and Cosmetic Act.[38, 40]

Nitrous oxide cylinders must contain a minimum of 99.0 percent nitrous oxide by volume.[33, 41] Maximum allowable parts per million (ppm) in the vapor phase include[41] carbon monoxide, 10 ppm; nitric oxide, 1 ppm; nitrogen dioxide, 1 ppm; carbon dioxide, 300 ppm; ammonia, 25 ppm; and water, 198 ppm.

Nitrous oxide H cylinders contain 15,800 L at a pressure of 745 psig. Nitrous oxide at room temperature is below its critical temperature (36.4°C); therefore the volume of nitrous oxide in a cylinder is *not* proportional to the cylinder pressure. The only reliable practical method to find the remaining volume in a nitrous oxide cylinder is to weigh the cylinder and compare the weight to the full cylinder value.[9, 42] Since the cylinder pressure gauge does not indicate content, why do we need the gauge at all? Two reasons are suggested to support the need of a cylinder gauge: to detect pressures below the limit necessary to maintain adequate pressures at the flowmeter needle valve and to indicate when the cylinder is completely empty.[42]

Rapid removal of nitrous oxide may cause the liquid to cool very quickly, thus creating a drop in pressure and flow below the required level (see Fig. 8-11).[42] When nitrous oxide flows from a cylinder at rates greater than 4 L/min, frost will begin to develop. If flow continues, a frost demarcation line will form approximately halfway down the cylinder[42] as the cylinder pressure drops to 300 psig. The frost develops because of cooling of the liquid

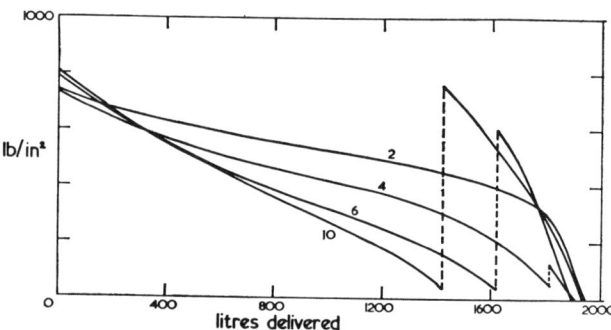

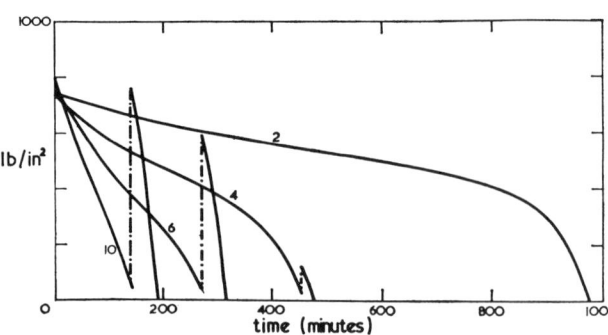

Fig. 8-11 Pressure changes in 1,800-L nitrous oxide cylinders emptying at continuous flow rates between 2 and 10 L/min. Note in the bottom diagram the rapidity with which a 10-L flow decreases the pressure in the cylinder. Each broken line indicates rewarming of the cylinder to room temperature. (Jones PL: Some observations on nitrous oxide cylinders during emptying. Br J Anaesth 46:534, 1974.)

nitrous oxide from vaporization. Heat is necessary to convert liquid nitrous oxide to a vapor (latent heat of vaporization). Initially the cooling effect is minimal, since the latent heat of vaporization is less as the gas approaches its critical temperature.[1] Near the critical temperature it takes very few calories to convert a liquid to a gas (see Fig. 8-12). Rapid condensation and freezing of water vapor (frost) in the ambient air begin to occur when the liquid nitrous oxide has cooled to less than 5 to 10°C. As the liquid cools, the vapor pressure decreases (see Fig. 8-13) in a predictable fashion.[1, 42, 43] Closing the cylinder and allowing equilibration to room temperature will restore the original cylinder pressure.

High flow rates from the nitrous oxide cylinder not only cool the nitrous oxide liquid but can also freeze up the nitrous oxide pressure regulator. Sometimes the first indication of freezing problems in the regulator will be fluctuation of the flowmeter float.[44] A commercial nitrous oxide heater is available which is placed between the cylinder and the regulator.[17] Most anesthesiologists are not familiar with the problems of decreasing vapor pressure in the nitrous oxide cylinders or freezing pressure regulators because of the widespread use of hospital pipelines.

Nitrous oxide is classified as a nonflammable gas but will support combustion. Each cylinder is provided with a frangible disk in the valve as a safety device: H-type cylinders use the CGA valve outlet connection no. 326 and D and E cylinders use the PISS 3–5 valve.[6] Either a single-stage or two-stage regulator is sufficient to reduce the 745-psig cylinder to the working pressure of 50 psig.

AIR

Air is a mixture of gases (see Table 8-3). Sample composition will vary with the altitude and place of sampling; for example, air over Los Angeles will differ from that over Denver. Air has four major components: nitrogen, oxygen, argon, and carbon dioxide. The remaining portion is comprised of rare gases and other highly variable components. Since air can be easily liquefied, the components can be separated by fractionation and rectification.[17] The average adult man will consume approximately 26 ft³ of oxygen in 24 hours. It is interesting to note that the weight of the oxygen consumed (2.5 lb) is equal to the weight of food consumed during the same time period. Over 500 ft³ of air must be respired in order to obtain the required oxygen.[45]

Compressed air cylinders used for human respiration must be either D,E,F,G,H, or J CGA specification.[45, 46] Water vapor in cylinders will depend on the compressor utilized. Removing water vapor to the point of "dry" air is expensive. Using compressed air with even minimal water vapor to power an anesthesia ventilator can cause damage to the ventilator.[47]

An H cylinder of air contains 6,550 L at a pressure of 2,200 psig. Air exists in the cylinder as a gas because at room temperature it is above critical temperature (−140.6°C). H-type cylinders are assigned CPG valve no. 590, with D and E cylinders using the PISS 1–5 designation. Cylinder valves either are the frangible disk type or have a frangible disk backed up with fusible metal (melting at 100°C).[17]

Table 8-3. Composition of Air

Component	Chemical Symbol	Percent by Volume
Nitrogen	N_2	78.084
Oxygen	O_2	20.9476
Argon	Ar	0.934
Carbon dioxide	CO_2	0.0314*
Neon	Ne	0.001818
Helium	He	0.000524
Methane	CH_4	0.0002*
Krypton	Kr	0.000114
Hydrogen	H_2	0.00005
Nitrous oxide	N_2O	0.00005*
Xenon	Xe	0.0000087

* Variable

(Data from CGA pamphlet G-7, Compressed Air for Human Respiration, Compressed Gas Association, Inc., 1235 Jefferson Davis Highway, Arlington, VA, 1984.)

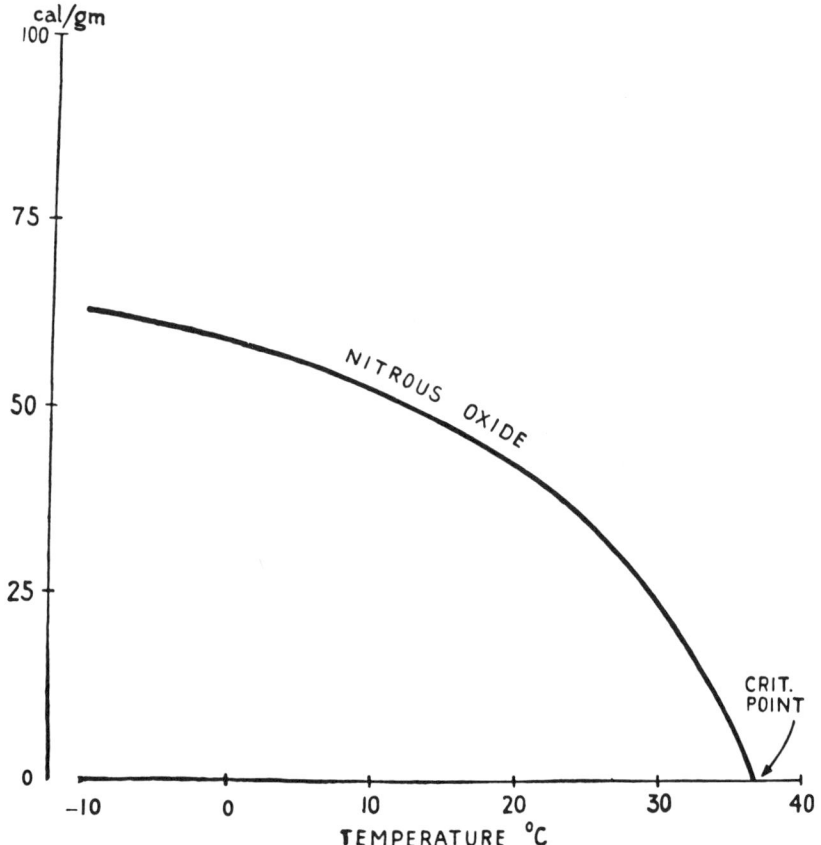

Fig. 8-12 The latent heat of evaporation of nitrous oxide. At the critical temperature the latent heat of evaporation is nil. More heat (cal/g) is required to convert nitrous oxide to a vapor as the temperature of the liquid decreases. (Redrawn from MacIntosh R, Mushin WW, Epstein HG: Physics for the Anaesthetist. 3rd Ed. Blackwell, Oxford, 1963.)

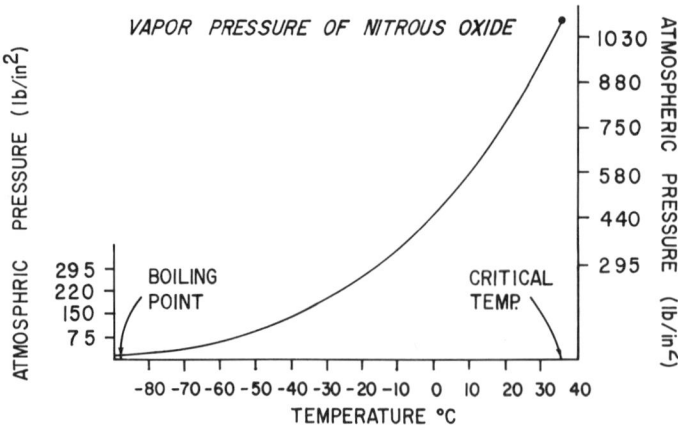

Fig. 8-13 Effect of temperature on the vapor pressure of nitrous oxide. Lowering the temperature of nitrous oxide in the cylinder via rapid vaporization will decrease the vapor pressure and eventually the rate of flow at the flowmeter needle valve. (Redrawn from MacIntosh R, Mushin WW, Epstein HG: Physics for the Anaesthetist. 3rd Ed. Blackwell, Oxford, 1963.)

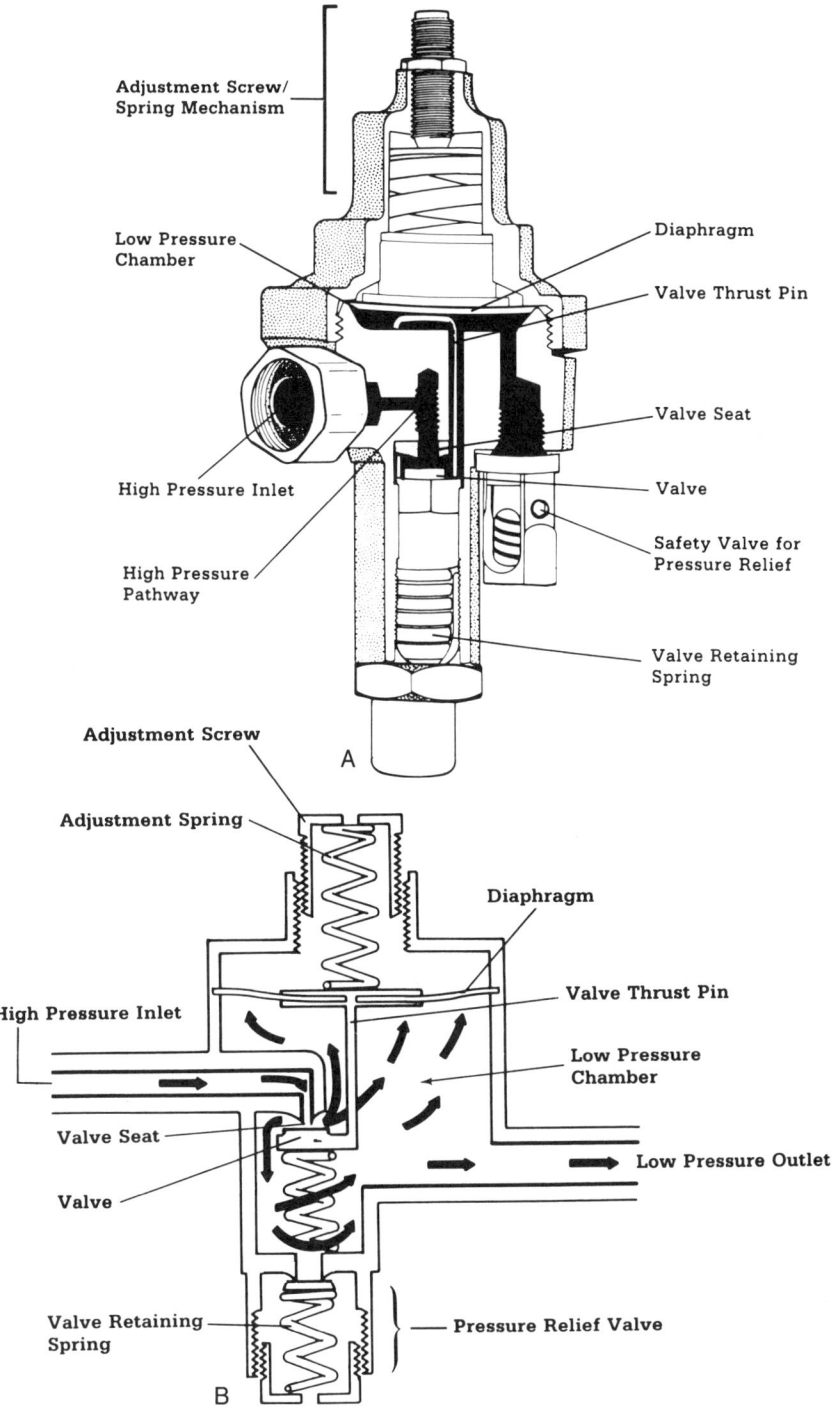

Fig. 8-14 Cylinder pressure reducing regulator. (A) Schematic of the functional parts of the regulator. (B) Cutaway view of a regulator. See text for a description of the mechanism. (Reproduced with permission from Bowie E, Huffman LM: The Anesthesia Machine: Essentials for Understanding. Ohmeda, The BOC Group, Inc., 1985.)

OTHER GASES

Other gases have found various applications in anesthesia and are found intermittently on the anesthesia machine. Cyclopropane in the United States has become of historical importance in anesthesia. The physical properties and specifications of the infrequently used gases, carbon dioxide,[2, 17, 48-50] helium,[2, 17, 51] and nitrogen,[2, 17, 52] are available. Each compressed gas is assigned a specific CGA valve number and type of pressure safety release device.

SAFETY PRECAUTIONS

Safety in the use of anesthesia compressed gases has required the cooperation of many individuals and institutions. Regulations and standards for the construction, inspection, testing, storage, and handling of compressed gas cylinders ensure dependability. Additional safety precautions consist of marking the cylinder, hazard labels, color codes, specific valve connections, the pin index safety system, the diameter index safety system, and a safety relief device, and these help to ensure excellence in performance. Not only does the cylinder have to meet rigid criteria, but also the anesthesia gas contained in the cylinder is under rigid scrutiny. All these factors come together when we turn on the compressed gas cylinder on the anesthesia machine and turn up the flowmeter to deliver the gas to the patient.

PRESSURE REGULATORS

A cylinder gas pressure-reducing regulator consists of a spring-loaded diaphragm which controls the opening and closing of a delivery orifice. Figure 8-14 is a schematic diagram and a cutaway view of a pressure regulator and illustrates the basic operating mechanism of a pressure regulator. Compressed gas from the cylinder enters at the high-pressure inlet,

forcing the valve seat to open. As the valve seat is pushed open, a spring is compressed and pulls down the large diaphragm via a valve thrust pin. Descent of the diaphragm releases tension on the adjustment spring. High-pressure gas entering the low-pressure chamber rapidly increases the pressure, which causes the diaphragm to be forced upward. The low pressure pushing against a large diaphram area overcomes the counteracting high pressure pushing against the small area of the valve.[1] The diaphragm is pushed up, closes the valve, which in turn shuts off entry of high-pressure gas. An adjustment screw controls the tension on the adjustment spring. Increasing the spring tension requires a higher buildup of low pressure in the chamber to seat the high-pressure valve. Outlet pressure from the low-pressure chamber can be controlled within a narrow range.

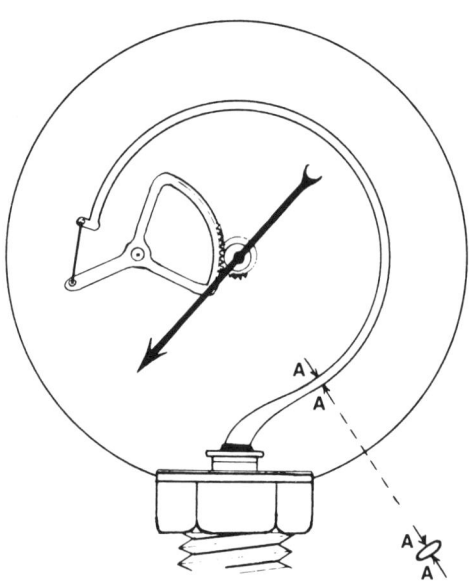

Fig. 8-15 Bourdon spring-type pressure gauge. A small metallic tube is bent in a circular fashion and soldered into place. A–A shows the flattened cross-sectional area of the tube. Pressure inside the tube straightens out the tube and causes the gear mechanism to move the pointer. (Schreiber P: Anaesthesia Equipment: Performance, Classification and Safety. Springer-Verlag, New York, 1972.)

Each anesthesia machine cylinder pressure regulator must be adjusted below the pipeline pressure to ensure the machine uses gas from the reserve source[26] only when the pipeline inlet pressure falls below 50 psig. A leak no greater than 10 ml/min can be present at an outlet pressure of 50 psig. The oxygen flush valve supplies 35 to 70 L/min and, when activated, causes a rapid reduction in anesthesia pipeline pressure. An oxygen regulator is provided to restore a flow rate of 2 L/min to its previous value (±0.1 L/min) immediately following each operation of the oxygen flush valve.[26]

The reclosing pressure relief valve is a small-area valve diaphragm held in place by the valve retaining spring (see Fig. 8-14). Should the diaphragm rupture or the valve not seat properly, the gas will exit the pressure relief valve at a preset pressure. Anesthesia machine relief valves must open at not more than four times the normal delivery pressure and not more than two-thirds of the minimum burst pressure of the diaphragm.[26]

The regulator in Figure 8-14 is a single-stage regulator which can show slight variation in delivery pressure as the flow rate is increased or the cylinder pressure decreases.[2] Some anesthesia machines have two-stage regulators (two single-stage regulators in series) for the compressed gas cylinders. Oxygen pressure might be reduced from 2,200 to 800 psig in the first regulator and then from 800 to 50 psig in the second regulator. When selecting a pressure regulator, it is important to keep in mind (1) the required range of the delivery pressure, (2) the degree of accuracy of the delivery pressure, and (3) the flow rate required.

Pressure regulators must be constructed of

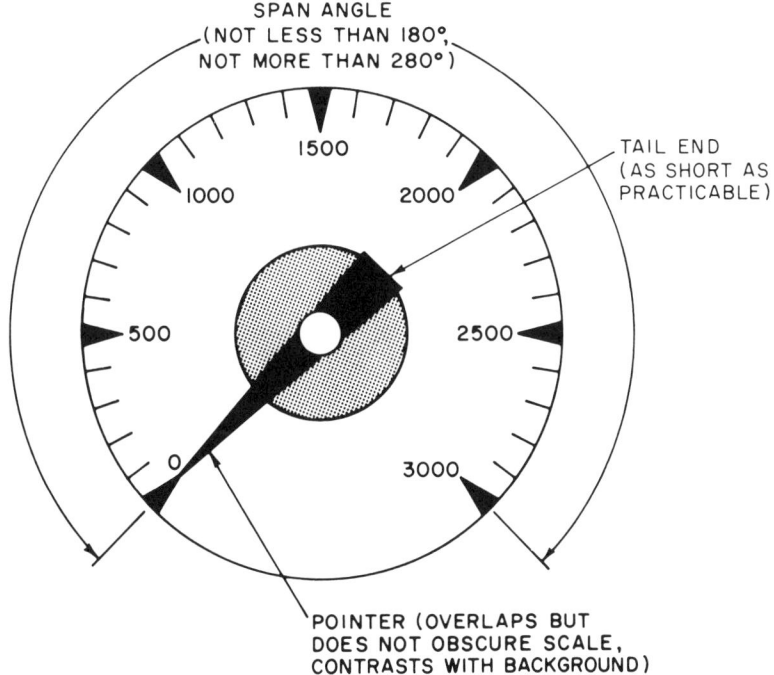

Fig. 8-16 Pressure gauge features. (This material is reproduced with permission from American National Standard: Minimum Performance and Safety Requirements for Components and Systems of Continuous-Flow Anesthesia Machines for Human Use. Z79.8-1979. © 1979, American National Standards Institute. Copies of this standard may be purchased from ANSI, 1430 Broadway, New York, NY 10018.)

materials which will not react chemically with the gas being controlled. Function must be maintained[53] over a temperature range of −18 to 50°C. Inlet connections must conform to CGA valve connection standards.[6] A corrosion-resistant filter of less than 66 μm is required upstream of the first valve seat.[53] The high-pressure portion of the regulator inlet must be capable of withstanding four times the maximum rated inlet pressure; for example, for an oxygen regulator this would be 8,800 psig. Rupture of the regulator diaphragm[53] must occur at a pressure below 400 psig but higher than 200 psig.

Cylinder pressure regulators must have a pressure-indicating gauge with a scale graduation readable by someone with 20/20 vision at a distance of 3.3 ft under 20 ft-candles of illumination.[53] Pressure gauges for anesthesia machines are usually of the Bourdon spring type (see Fig. 8-15). A small metallic tube with a flattened cross section is bent in a circular fashion and soldered into a socket. The opposite end is sealed and linked to the gear mechanism. Pressure inside the tube straightens out the tube, causing the sealed end to move slightly. Any movement on the sealed end of the fulcrum moves the gauge pointer.[44, 54] The full-scale pressure gauge indication must be 33 percent greater than the maximal cylinder pressure.[5] Markings, size, units of calibration, and cleanliness requirements are very specific.[26] Figure 8-16 illustrates some of the required pressure gauge features outlined by the ANSI.

REFERENCES

1. MacIntosh R, Mushin WW, Epstein HG: Physics for the Anaesthetist. 3rd Ed. Blackwell, Oxford, 1963
2. Handbook of Compressed Gases. Compressed Gas Association. 2nd Ed. Van Nostrand Reinhold, New York, 1981
3. Boiler and Pressure Code. American Society of Mechanical Engineers, New York, 1980
4. Douch ME, technical director. personal communication. Chesterfield Cylinder, Co, Enid, OK, 1985
5. CGA Pamphlet C-1: Methods for Hydrostatic Testing of Compressed Gas Cylinders. Compressed Gas Association, Arlington, VA, 1975
6. CGA Standard V.1, ANSI B57.1, CSA B96: Compressed Gas Cylinder Valve Outlet and Inlet Connections. Compressed Gas Association, Arlington, VA, 1977
7. Feeley TW, Bancroft ML, Brooks RA et al: Potential hazards of compressed gas cylinders: a review. Anesthesiology 48:72, 1978
8. CGA Pamphlet C-6: Standards for Visual Inspection of Compressed Gas Cylinders. Compressed Gas Association, Arlington, VA, 1975
9. CGA Pamphlet P-2: Characteristics and Safe Handling of Medical Gases. Compressed Gas Association, Arlington, VA, 1978
10. CGA Pamphlet C-4. ANSI/CGA C-4-1978: American National Standard. Method of Marking Portable Compressed Gas Containers to Identify the Material Contained. Compressed Gas Association, Arlington, VA, 1978
11. CGA Pamphlet C-9: Standard Color-Marking of Compressed Gas Cylinders Intended for Medical Use. Compressed Gas Association, Arlington, VA, 1982
12. Sawhney KK, Yoon YK: Erroneous labeling of a nitrous oxide cylinder. Anesthesiology 59:260, 1983
13. MacIntosh R: Wrongly connected gas-pipe lines. Anaesthesia 33:65, 1978
14. Editorial: Medico-legal. Identification of gas cylinders. Br Med J 1:381, 1945
15. Finch JS: A report of a possible hazard of gas cylinder tanks. Anesthesiology 33:467, 1970
16. Webb AI, Warren RG: Hazards and precautions associated with the use of compressed gases. J Am Vet Med Assoc 181:1491, 1982
17. Braker W, Mossman AL: Matheson Gas Data Book. 6th Ed. Matheson Gas Products, New Jersey, 1980
18. Garfield JM, Allen GW, Silverstein P et al: Flash fire in a reducing valve. Anesthesiology 34:578, 1971
19. Hogg CE: Pin-indexing failures. Anesthesiology 38:85, 1973
20. U.S. Department of Commerce. National Bureau of Standards. Handbook H-28, Part III, Washington, DC, 1957
21. Goebel WM: Failure of nitrous oxide and oxy-

gen pin-indexing. Anesth Prog 189, 1980
22. Steward DJ, Sloan IA: Additional pin-indexing failures. Anesthesiology 39:355, 1973
23. Wolff JDP, Lionarons HB, Mesdag MJ: A failure of the pin-index system of anesthetic gas tube connections. Arch Chir Neerl 22:243, 1970
24. Rawstron RE, McNeill TD: Pin index system. Br J Anaesth 34:591, 1962
25. Mazze RI: Therapeutic misadventures with oxygen delivery systems: the need for continuous in-line oxygen monitors. Anesth Analg 51:787, 1972
26. American National Standard: Minimum Performance and Safety Requirements for Components and Systems of Continuous-Flow Anesthesia Machines for Human Use. Z79.8-1979. American National Standards Institute, New York, 1979
27. CGA Pamphlet S-1.1: Pressure Relief Device Standards. Part I—Cylinders for Compressed Gases. Compressed Gas Association, Arlington, VA, 1979
28. CGA Pamphlet P-1: Safe Handling of Compressed Gases in Containers. Compressed Gas Association, Arlington, VA, 1974
29. Jones RJ: External vigilance. Anesthesiology 32:56, 1970
30. CGA Safety Bulletin SB-6: Nitrous Oxide Security and Control. Compressed Gas Association, Arlington, VA, 1980
31. Layzer RB: Nitrous oxide abuse. In Eger EI: Nitrous Oxide/N_2O. Elsevier Science, New York, 1985
32. Danto BL: A bag full of laughs. J Psychiatry 121:612, 1964
33. Nagle DR: Anesthetic addiction and drunkenness: a contemporary and historical survey. Int J Addict 3:25, 1968
34. CGA Pamphlet G-4: Oxygen. Compressed Gas Association, Arlington, VA, 1980
35. CGA Pamphlet G-4.5: Commodity Specification for Oxygen Produced by Chemical Reaction. Compressed Gas Association, Arlington, VA, 1983
36. CGA Pamphlet G-4.3: Commodity Specification for Oxygen. Compressed Gas Association, Arlington, VA, 1980
37. Oxygen. U.S. Pharmacopeia. 21st Ed. U.S. Pharmacopeial Convention, Rockville, MD, 1984
38. Federal Food, Drug and Cosmetic Act. Code of Federal Regulations, Title 21, Part 207.
39. Wynne JM: Physics, chemistry, and manufacture of nitrous oxide. In Eger EI: Nitrous Oxide/N_2O. Elsevier Science, New York, 1985
40. Nitrous oxide. U.S. Pharmacopeia. 21st Ed. U.S. Pharmacopeial Convention, Rockville, MD, 1984
41. CGA Specification G-8.2: Commodity Specification for Nitrous Oxide. Compressed Gas Association, Arlington, VA, 1980
42. Jones PL: Some observations on nitrous oxide cylinders during emptying. Br J Anaesth 46:534, 1974
43. Couch EJ, Kobe KA: Volumetric behavior of nitrous oxide: Pressure–volume isotherms at high pressures. J Chem Eng Data 6:229, 1961
44. Schreiber P: Anaesthesia Equipment: Performance, Classification and Safety. Springer-Verlag, New York, 1972
45. CGA Pamphlet G-7: Compressed Air for Human Respiration. Compressed Gas Association, Arlington, VA, 1976
46. CGA Pamphlet G-7.1, ANSI Z86.1-1973: Commodity Specification for Air. Compressed Gas Association, Arlington, 1973
47. Howell RSC: Piped medical gas and vacuum systems. Anaesthesia 35:676, 1980
48. Carbon dioxide. U.S. Pharmacopeia. 21st Ed. U.S. Phamacopeial Convention, Rockville, MD, 1984
49. CGA Specification G-6.2: Commodity Specification for Carbon Dioxide. Compressed Gas Association, Arlington, VA, 1973
50. CGA Pamphlet G-6: Carbon dioxide. Compressed Gas Association, Arlington, VA, 1984
51. CGA Specification G-9.1: Commodity Specification for Helium. Compressed Gas Association, Arlington, VA, 1972
52. CGA Specification G-10.1: Commodity Specification for Nitrogen. Compressed Gas Association, Arlington, VA, 1976
53. CGA Pamphlet E-7: Standard for Flowmeters, Pressure Reducing Regulators, Regulator/Flowmeter and Regulator/Flowgauge Combinations for the Administration of Medical Gases. Compressed Gas Association, Arlington, VA, 1982
54. Schreiber P: Safety Guidelines for Anesthesia Systems. North American Drager, Telford, PA, 1984

9

Piping Systems for Gases Used in Anesthesia

Anesthesia gases are manufactured, transported, and then delivered via the anesthesia machine to the patient. Oxygen and nitrous oxide after manufacture are stored in bulk liquid form or as compressed gases. Local economic considerations determine which form is used at the source. The majority of hospitals in the United States use bulk liquid oxygen storage tanks. A high consumption rate makes liquid oxygen very cost efficient. Only in a few hospitals is low-pressure bulk liquid nitrous oxide economical. Nitrous oxide banks composed of multiple tanks of high-pressure liquefied nitrous oxide are used in the majority of hospitals in the United States.

The design and construction of piping systems delivering anesthesia gases to the anesthesia machine are critical to the safety and welfare of the patient. Molecules of anesthesia gases, like water droplets, follow the path of least resistance. Any defect will direct the molecules to leave the hospital piping system or enter a wrong conduit. Small defects in pipelines, interface misconnections, gases in the wrong pipeline, and a host of other errors have resulted in significant injuries to patients. The anesthesiologist is responsible for knowing the source of the gases used in the operating room and the kind of system utilized by the hospital to deliver the gases to the operating room. Figure 9-1 is a schematic delivery flow sheet for the anesthesia gases, beginning at the source (liquid or compressed gas) and ending with delivery to the patient.

The National Fire Protection Association (NFPA) has recognized the public health problem of hospital piping systems and has developed very specific regulations applicable to all phases of the anesthesia gas system.[1] However, there does not seem to be a significant national or state inspection system to ensure hospital compliance with the regulations. A 1976 hospital survey showed a high incidence of serious hazards related to anesthesia gas supply systems.[2] The Joint Commission on Accreditation of Hospitals (JCAH) requires compliance to the NFPA regulations for hospital accreditation but is unable to make a detailed on-site inspection of the anesthesia gas supply.[2] Installation, final testing, and maintenance of any anesthesia gas system should be done only by specialists.

In discussing the delivery of gases from the source to the patient, it is convenient to divide the piping system into two divisions: external to the anesthesia machine and internal to the anesthesia machine. (See Chapter 8 for principles of compressed gases and regulators.)

141

PIPELINE SYSTEM EXTERNAL TO THE ANESTHESIA MACHINE

Nitrous Oxide Compressed Gas Banks

High-pressure tanks of compressed liquefied nitrous oxide are arranged in single or double rows connected to a single manifold control box. A manifold bank can be used for compressed gas tanks of oxygen, nitrogen, or ni-

trous oxide. Figure 9-2 shows a manifold control system for nitrogen that resembles a character from outer space. Each gas enters the high-pressure header of the manifold via coiled high-pressure copper lines attached to the regulator of the compressed gas tank. A nitrous oxide bank is divided into a left bank and a right bank, as shown in Figure 9-3. Only one of the banks is utilized at any given time, the other constituting a "reserve bank." A central manifold control box (Fig. 9-4) monitors the pressure from each bank and regulates the pressure (usually about 50 psig)

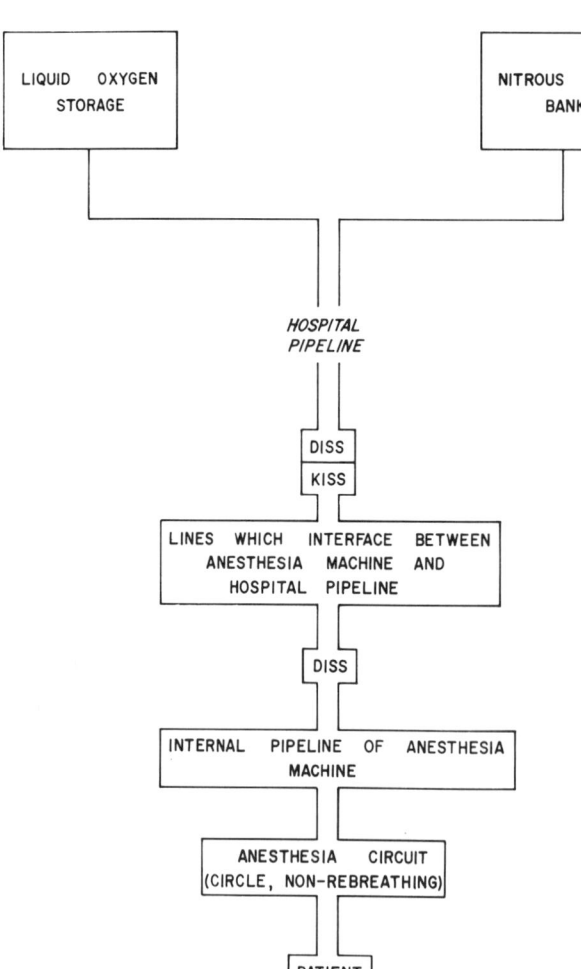

TRANSPORTATION SCHEMATIC OF ANESTHESIA GASES FROM SOURCE TO PATIENT

Fig. 9-1 Flow sheet of the delivery of gases used in anesthesia from the source to the patient.

delivered to the hospital pipeline system. Changeover from the primary bank to the reserve bank takes place automatically when the pressure in the primary bank drops below a preset level. As the changeover occurs an alarm is activated in the hospital engineer's office and other appropriate surveillance areas to notify personnel of the need to replace the empty nitrous oxide tanks in the primary bank. Hospitals should establish a procedure for changing the gas cylinders which defines who is responsible for the task and who is responsible for teaching others how to change the tanks.[3] On a rare occasion the nitrous oxide flowmeter may be turned on just as the central supply of nitrous oxide is becoming exhausted. Nitrous oxide flow from the anesthesia machine could increase as the reserve bank begins to supply gas and result in a hypoxic mixture.[4] The author practiced in a small hospital in which the daily use of nitrous oxide outgrew the original size of the nitrous oxide bank. On one occasion the hospital engineer had a delayed response to the switchover

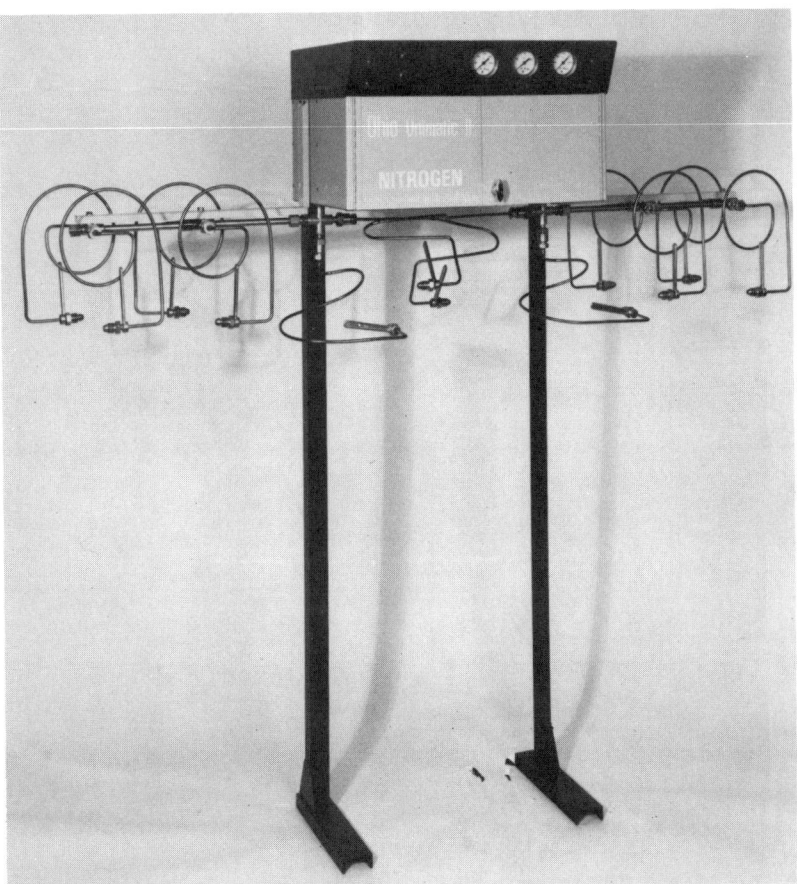

Fig. 9-2 A nitrogen bank and control box. This spacelike creature is divided into two separate banks. Each arm connects to the central manifold control box. The coiled lines attach to nitrogen cylinders. Changeover from the primary bank to the secondary bank occurs automatically when the pressure in the primary bank is less than 135 psig. (Courtesy of Ohmeda, The BOC Group, Inc.)

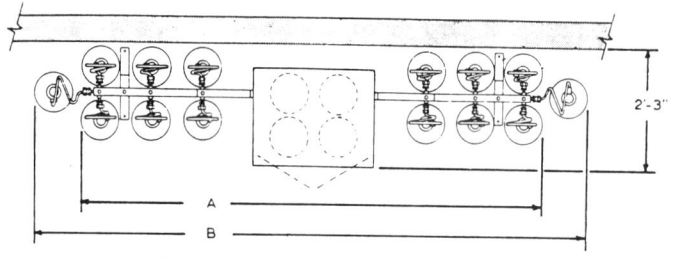

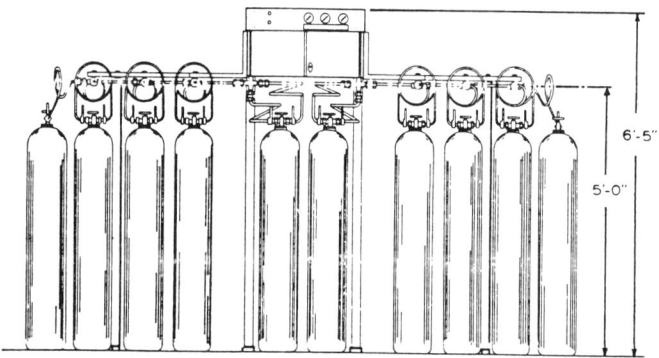

Fig. 9-3 Nitrous oxide bank. The top view illustrates a 2-row 18-cylinder bank. The front view shows the coiled lines attached to the cylinders and the manifold high-pressure header. B is the distance required when each arm of the bank has an odd number of cylinders, while A is the distance for an even number of cylinders on each bank. (Courtesy of Ohmeda, The BOC Group, Inc.)

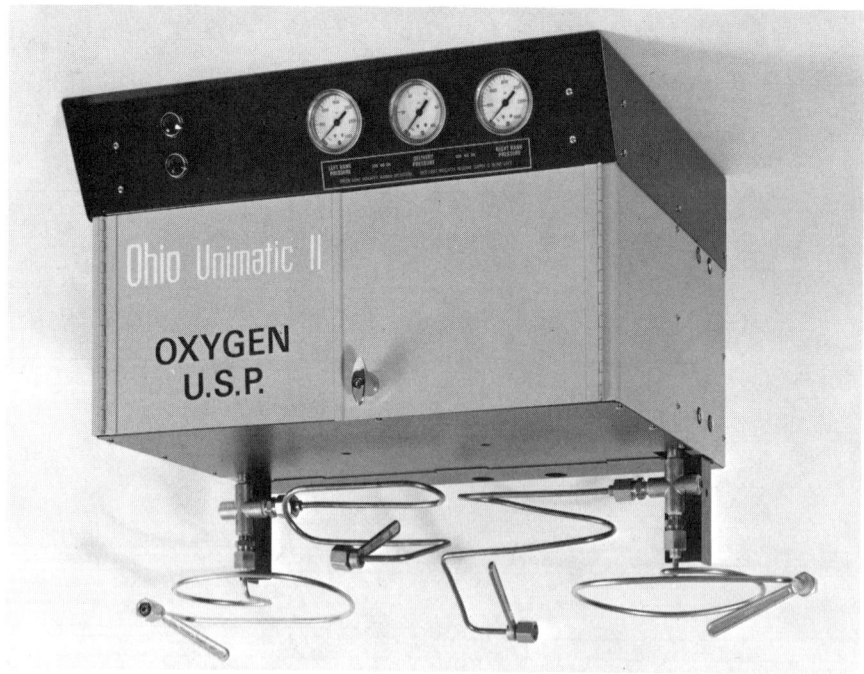

Fig. 9-4 A close-up view of a central oxygen bank manifold control box. A pressure gauge indicates the pressure in the left and right banks and the main hospital line. The manifold will deliver oxygen continuously at 50 ± 5 psig. (Courtesy of Ohmeda, The BOC Group, Inc.)

alarm and upon arrival at the nitrous oxide bank found the primary bank empty and the reserve near empty. The engineer elected to change the reserve bank first. In the operating room each anesthesiologist adjusted the nitrous oxide flow to compensate for the rapidly dropping pressure. When the pressure dropped to zero, the nitrous oxide bobbin fell to the bottom of the flowmeter and the flowmeter knob was not turned off. Upon restoration of full pressure in the nitrous oxide bank the bobbins rose to the very top of the flowmeters and a hypoxic mixture was present in the fresh gas flow tube. Fortunately the hypoxic mixture was immediately detected without patient harm. In-depth training on how to change the nitrous oxide bank and notification of the anesthesiologist prevented a repeat of the episode.

Additional safety features of nitrous oxide banks are detailed in Figure 9-5. The check valve between the gas cylinder regulator and the high-pressure manifold header prevents loss of gas if a cylinder pressure relief fails or a leak occurs in the tubing exiting the gas cylinder.[1] All pressure relief valves are set to exit gases at pressures 50 percent above normal line pressure and will close automatically once the excess pressure is exited. The pressure relief value which exits is only necessary if

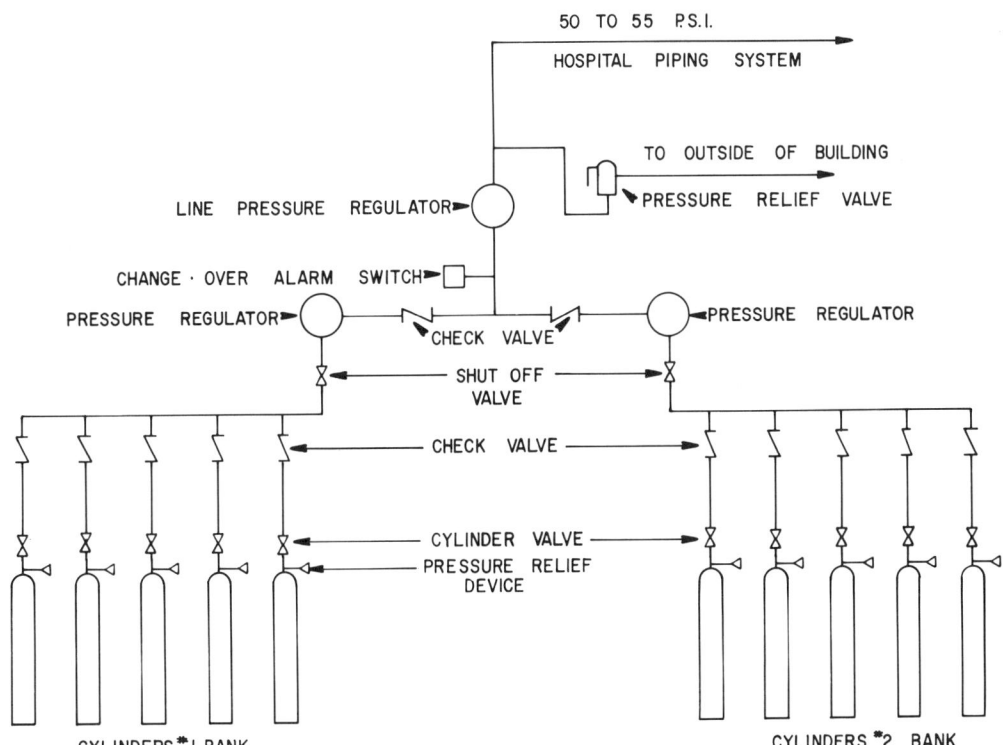

Fig. 9-5 Schematic of a typical nitrous oxide or oxygen cylinder supply system. Note the arrangement of the valves and regulators required to provide safety in the system. (Reprinted with permission from NFPA 56F-1983, Nonflammable Medical Gas Systems. © 1983, National Fire Protection Association, Quincy, MA 02269. This reprinted material is not the complete and official position of the NFPA on the referenced subject, which is represented only by the standard itself.)

the supply system is in excess of 2,000 ft³ of gas (four H tanks of nitrous oxide contain 2,228 ft³ of gas).

Nitrous oxide, nitrogen, and carbon dioxide banks are usually located near the loading dock of the hospital in order to minimize transportation of full tanks and storage of empty tanks. Anesthesia gas supply systems must be in a special room or enclosure.[1] Only containers of nonflammable gases may be stored in these areas. Provision of adequate ventilation will avoid oxygen-deficient atmosphere in the event a cylinder or manifold pressure device malfunctions.

Each anesthesiologist should know the location of the nitrous oxide bank, the person(s) responsible for changing the tanks, and the basic method of operation of the bank.

Liquid Oxygen Storage

Storing oxygen as a liquid is economical and greatly reduces the amount of space required to store large quantities of gas. Any large hospital would find the handling of compressed oxygen tanks a very impractical method of supplying oxygen to the numerous sites within the hospital. Liquid oxygen storage is considered more economical than the manifold system when the hospital uses over 100,000 L of oxygen per week.[3] When warmed to room temperature at 1 atm, 1 volume of liquid oxygen will vaporize to 860.6 volumes of oxygen.[5]

Liquid oxygen is light blue and is produced by liquefaction of atmospheric air followed by fractionation.[5] Liquid oxygen is stored between $-150°$ and $-175°C$ in a welded double-walled austenitic stainless steel container specified by the ASME Boiler and Pressure Vessel Code.[3, 6, 7] A simplified diagram of a liquid oxygen storage system is shown in Figure 9-6. One way to understand the vacuum-insulated evaporator containing liquid oxygen is to think of it as a large sealed and pressurized Dewar or vacuum flask.[3] The stainless steel container is insulated within the double

wall by silicone-based Pearlite powder.[8] Gaseous oxygen is withdrawn from the top of the container, passed through a vaporizer, and then into the hospital pipeline. During pressure drops secondary to high consumption rates, liquid oxygen is withdrawn from the bottom of the container, vaporized by the pressure-building coil, and passed through the vaporizer and into the hospital piping system. If extremely high quantities are required, liquid oxygen can be withdrawn and passed through the vaporizer and directly into the hospital piping system.

Duplicate pressure relief valves are found in liquid oxygen systems because of the potential of extremely high pressures. For instance, 1 volume of liquid helium vaporized in a closed container to room temperature has the potential of generating a pressure of over 14,500 psig. The double-walled oxygen container[8] is built to withstand a pressure of about 250 psig. In addition, a DOT 4-L oxygen cylinder must have a CGA CG-1 rupture disk set at a specified burst pressure.[9] The rupture disk is actuated by inlet static pressure, releases the gas to avoid excess pressure, and will not reclose automatically.[5]

Bulk oxygen systems must be located in an accessible area and meet the NFPA standards for systems at consumer sites.[6] The diagram in Figure 9-7 shows how far the system must be from such things as public sidewalks, non-ambulatory patients, parked vehicles, and other flammable gas storage. It is important to know where the main lines from the storage and reserve tanks are located in reference to the hospital. Lines can be run over by heavy trucks, disrupted by earthquakes, or inadvertently torn up by construction. When disruption occurs, an oxygen supply connection located on the loading dock of the hospital will allow the commercial supplier to immediately connect an emergency source of oxygen.[1]

The NFPA standards require hospitals to have a reserve supply of oxygen equivalent to 1 day of consumption.[1] Large hospitals (of 500 or more beds, using at least[8] 717,000 L/day) utilize a second liquid reserve system to

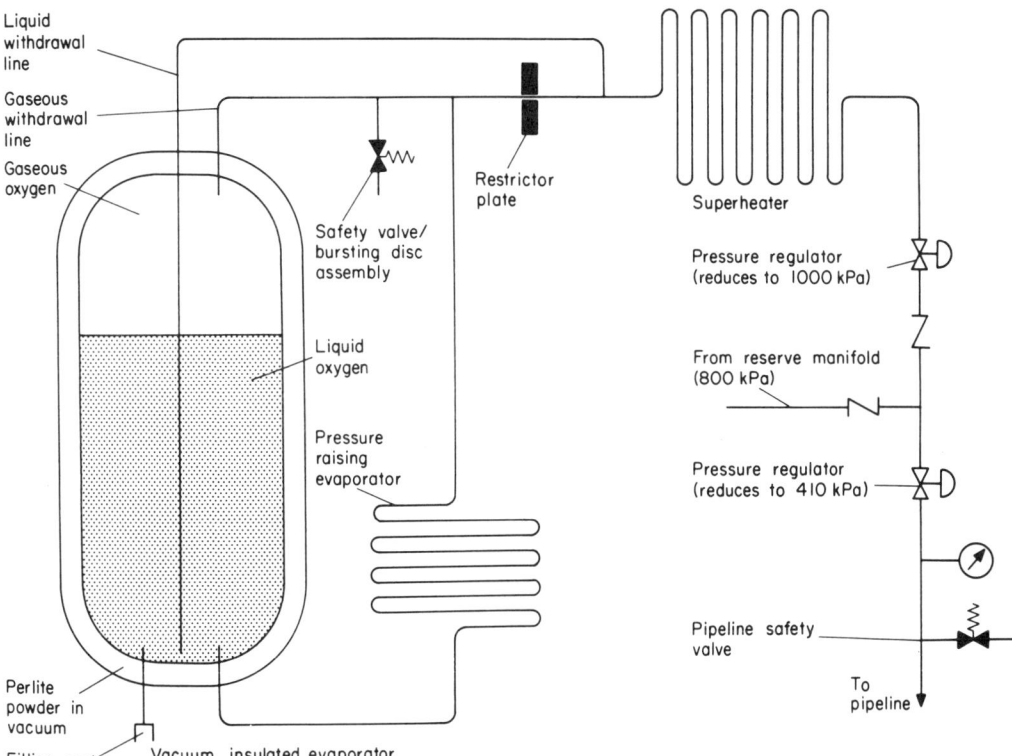

Fig. 9-6 Schematic of a liquid oxygen storage system. The liquid oxygen is surrounded by a double-walled stainless container packed with Perlite powder. Gaseous oxygen passes out the superheater and into the hospital pipeline. Consult text for a detailed description. (Howell RSC: Piped medical gas and vacuum systems. Anaesthesia 35:676, 1980.)

meet their needs, but smaller hospitals usually use a high-pressure oxygen manifold bank similar to the nitrous oxide bank. A schematic of a complete liquid oxygen bulk system, including a liquid storage tank and cylinder reserve supply, is shown in Figure 9-8.

A master alarm system must monitor the conditions and operation of the oxygen supply source.[1] Monitor alarms for the source can be low-liquid-level detectors, low-supply-pressure detectors, and/or detectors that sense a variation of 20 percent above or below the line pressure in the main supply line.

Oxygen is an oxidizer and will vigorously support and accelerate the combustion of other materials. Oxygen valves are turned on and off slowly to avoid the possibility of igniting contaminants in the system. Smoking, open flames, and the storage of combustible materials should not be permitted in the immediate vicinity of oxygen.[5]

Despite many builtin safety features, liquid storage systems have failed. In 1976 Feeley and Hedley-Whyte[2] found a serious or potentially serious accident related to bulk oxygen delivery systems in one-third of 190 hospitals surveyed. The most frequent malfunction was insufficient oxygen pressure due to damage of the pipelines during construction, obstructed pipelines, or insufficient capacity to supply a high demand for oxygen. Erroneous filling of the liquid oxygen reservoir with nitrogen[10] or argon[11] has resulted in intraoperative hypoxia and death. The majority of hazards associated

148 • *The Anesthesia Machine*

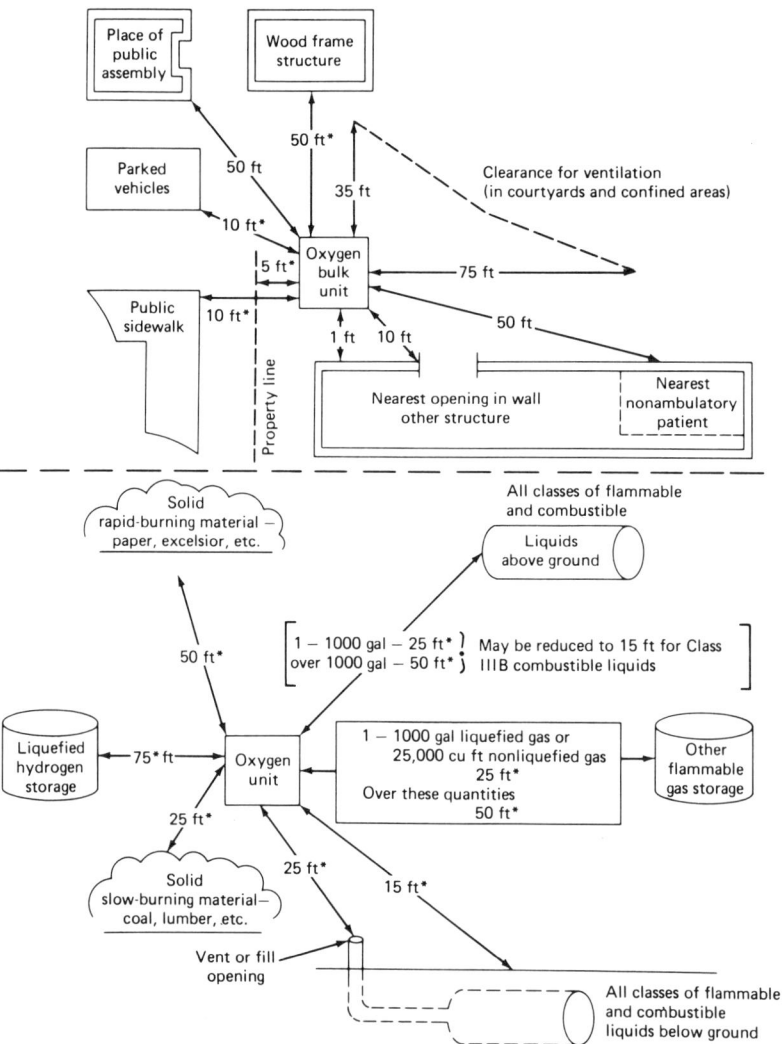

Fig. 9-7 Distances allowed between bulk oxygen storage systems for ventilation and exposure to flammables and combustibles. The top half of the figure shows the clearances for ventilation. The bottom half of the figure indicates the minimum distance separating various classes of flammables and combustibles from the oxygen unit. (Reprinted with permission from NFPA 50-1979 Bulk Oxygen Systems. © 1979, National Fire Protection Association, Quincy, MA 02269. This reprinted material is not the complete and official position of the NFPA on the referenced subject, which is represented only by the standard itself.)

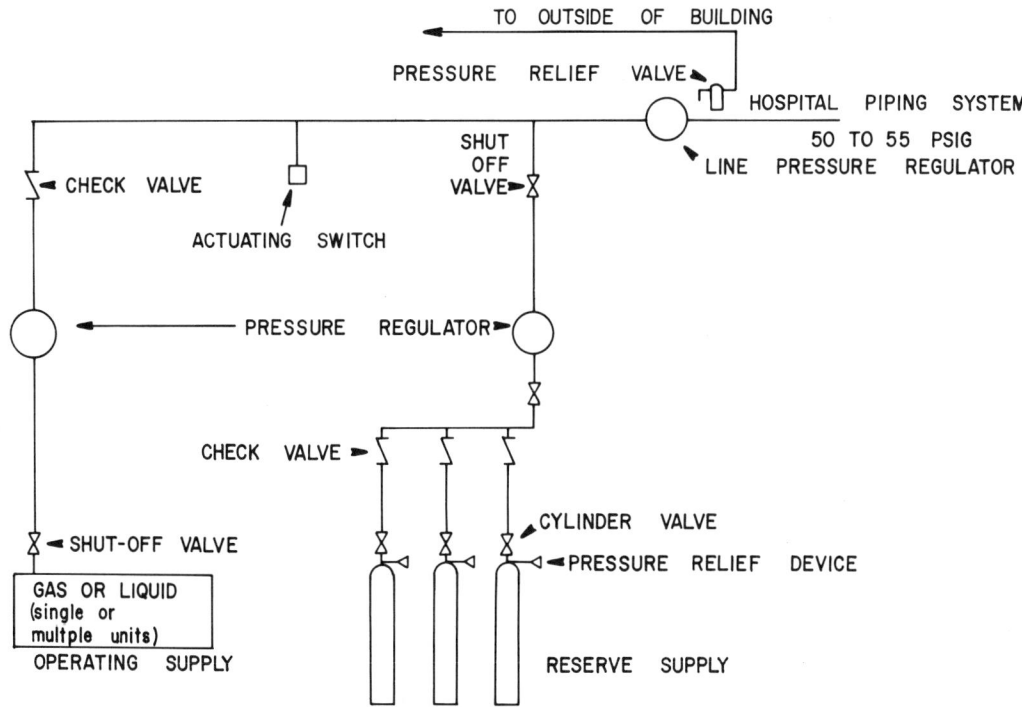

Fig. 9-8 Schematic of a typical oxygen bulk system with an oxygen cylinder reserve bank. Note the multiple valves and pressure regulators to maintain a high level of system safety and reliability. (Reprinted with permission from NFPA 56F-1983 Nonflammable Medical Gas Systems. © 1983, National Fire Protection Association, Quincy, MA 02269. This reprinted material is not the complete and official position of the NFPA on the referenced subject, which is represented only by the standard itself.)

with bulk oxygen delivery systems are due to lack of awareness of system design and function among hospital personnel.[2, 8] During 1 year at a 500-bed hospital, 18 potentially serious mishaps occurred in the liquid oxygen delivery system.[8] Included were five false alarms and five occasions of excessive depletion of the reserve oxygen supply.

Hospital Pipelines

A typical hospital oxygen pipeline installation is illustrated in Figure 9-9. Multiple outlets are required. All pressure gauges must be connected to a master alarm system. The outlets available for connection to the anesthe-sia machine can be on the wall or ceiling.

Copper is recommended as the material for the pipelines, because it is clean and rust free.[7] The NFPA standard requires either seamless copper tubing or standard-weight brass pipe.[1] All piping for medical gases must be thoroughly cleaned according to rigid standards prior to installation.[12, 13] When cleaning oxygen pipelines, the following applies:[13]

Cleaning a component or system for oxygen service involves the removal of combustible contaminants including the surface residue from manufacturing, hot work, and assembly operations, as well as the removal of all cleaning agents and the prevention of recontamination before final assembly, installation and use.

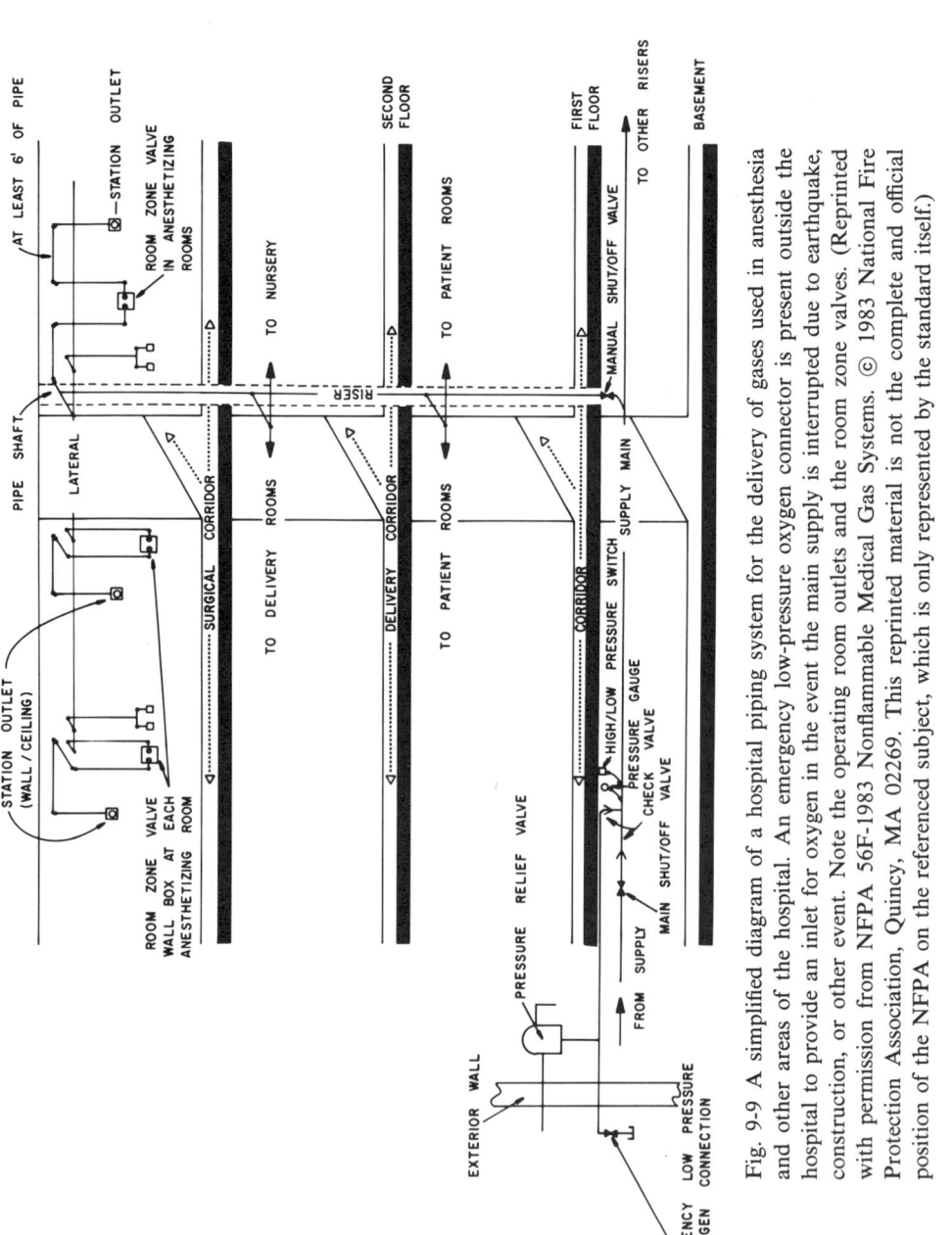

Fig. 9-9 A simplified diagram of a hospital piping system for the delivery of gases used in anesthesia and other areas of the hospital. An emergency low-pressure oxygen connector is present outside the hospital to provide an inlet for oxygen in the event the main supply is interrupted due to earthquake, construction, or other event. Note the operating room outlets and the room zone valves. (Reprinted with permission from NFPA 56F-1983 Nonflammable Medical Gas Systems. © 1983 National Fire Protection Association, Quincy, MA 02269. This reprinted material is not the complete and official position of the NFPA on the referenced subject, which is only represented by the standard itself.)

Once cleaning is completed, the ends of the pipes are capped until the actual installation. During installation, cutting or reaming tools must be kept free of oil or grease to avoid internal contamination of the pipes. Fittings used for connecting the copper tubing must be wrought copper, brass, or bronze.[1] Only silver brazing alloy (no flux) may be used in the welding process. Each anesthesia gas pipe must be clearly labeled throughout the system at a minimum of every 20 ft, in every room, on every floor and at each outlet.

Once the pipes are installed, they must be blown out with dry, oil-free air or nitrogen. The station outlets are then installed and initial testing begins. Each section of the pipeline is filled with either dry, oil-free air or nitrogen to a minimum pressure of 150 psig for the leakage test.[1, 14] This pressure is maintained while each joint is examined for leaks. Leaks are repaired and the remaining system components are installed. A standing pressure test is then accomplished by pressurizing the system with air or nitrogen at 20 percent above the normal operating line pressure. During the next 24 hours the only acceptable pressure changes are fluctuations secondary to ambient temperature changes around the piping system.[1, 14] One of two detailed procedures are used to detect cross-connections.[1] A final purging of test gases is done with the gas to be carried in each specific pipeline. Purge gas flows from each station connector onto a white cloth material at a minimum flow rate of 100 L/min; there should be no evidence of discoloration. Finally, each anesthesia gas outlet is tested with an oxygen analyzer to confirm the presence or absence of the appropriate concentration of oxygen.[1, 14] Nitrous oxide outlets can be tested with a nitrous oxide analyzer if available. Records of the testing personnel, the date, and the test results should be maintained by the hospital and other interested parties.

Commercial inspection services are available that offer certification of medical gas pipeline inspection. The service verifies that (1) the gas outlets are properly labeled, (2) the gas delivered at each outlet originated at the correct source, (3) the proper concentration of oxygen exists at each outlet, and (4) all equipment conforms to the manufacturer's published specifications. A double check of the pipeline system may detect problems overlooked by other uninterested inspectors.[15] Perhaps outside certification is needed when contractors lack long-term experience in the installation of anesthesia gas pipeline systems. Another benefit is the assumption of medicolegal responsibility of the correct installation of the system by an independent company.

Whenever the pipeline system is modified, the entire system should be rechecked and verified to ensure the correct gas emerges from the specified outlet. Anesthesiologists should pay particular attention to the oxygen outlets in anesthetizing locations and recovery room areas. A personal, second independent check by the anesthesiologist with an oxygen analyzer would certainly be an excellent procedure.

A case of interchanging the oxygen and nitrous oxide hoses to the anesthesia machine occurred in Britain[16] in 1977. An inquiry recommended that a "single-hose test" be done prior to the first daily use of the anesthesia machine. The test involves plugging and unplugging connectors from the wall sockets. In 1978 the Safety Sub-Committee of the Association of Anaesthetists of Great Britain and Ireland recommended that the single-hose test be dropped because of severe limitations.[17] A suggestion was made to support the use of the "whistle discriminator," which changes pitch when blown with gases of different sonic velocity.[17-19] The test where the anesthesiologist breathes oxygen from the patient's circuit was viewed as being very simple and completely reliable; however, some members of the committee viewed the practice "with alarm," since peers might accuse the anesthesiologist of addiction and physicians should not be called on to routinely test equipment on themselves.

Outside each operating room a manually operated shutoff valve similar to the one in

Figure 9-10 must be available for each anesthetic gas.[1, 14] A shutoff valve isolates a section of the pipeline for maintenance, repair, testing, or problems distal to the valve.

Master alarm systems as pictured in Figure 9-11 are placed in the engineering office and one area under constant surveillance by responsible hospital personnel. Area alarms linked to the anesthesia gas pipeline system can be connected to the master alarm (Fig. 9-12). A variety of information can be linked to the master alarm: (1) the oxygen reserve in or out of use, (2) the level of the oxygen liquid, (3) the reserve level of emergency oxy-

gen, (4) high and low oxygen and nitrous oxide line pressures, (5) when the emergency oxygen and/or nitrous oxide reserve is in use, and (6) similar inputs for carbon dioxide, nitrogen, air, and vacuum sources.

Anesthesia gas pipeline systems are subject to the proverb "Nothing can be made foolproof because fools are so ingenious."[20] Pipelines for nitrous oxide and oxygen continue to be crossed,[2, 21-25] despite rigid standards by the NFPA.[1] Patients are still dying from failure to purge the nitrogen from the oxygen pipeline prior to use in a new hospital.[21] Crossing of the connecting lines to the anesthesia

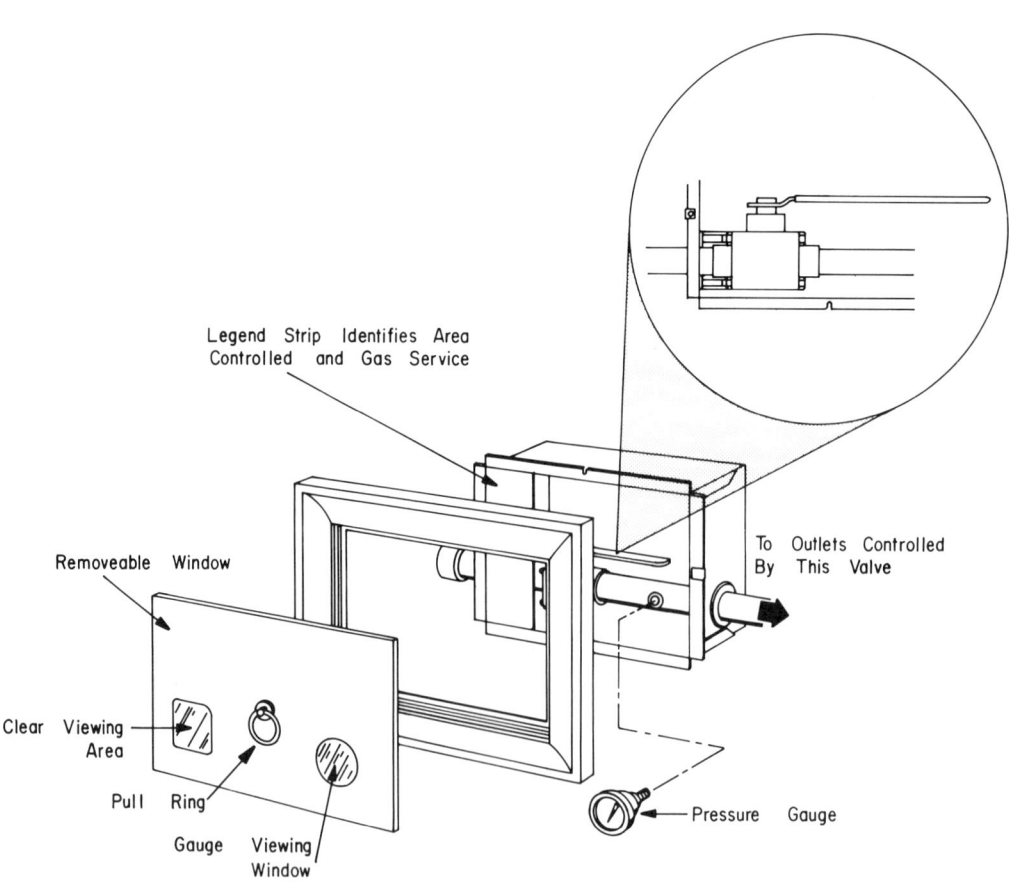

Fig. 9-10 Room zone shutoff valve. One of these valves must be present for each gas entering the operating room from the hospital pipeline. These valves must be readily accessible at all times for use in an emergency. (Redrawn from Single Zone Valve Box Assembly Selection Chart. Allied Healthcare Products, Inc., St. Louis, 1983.)

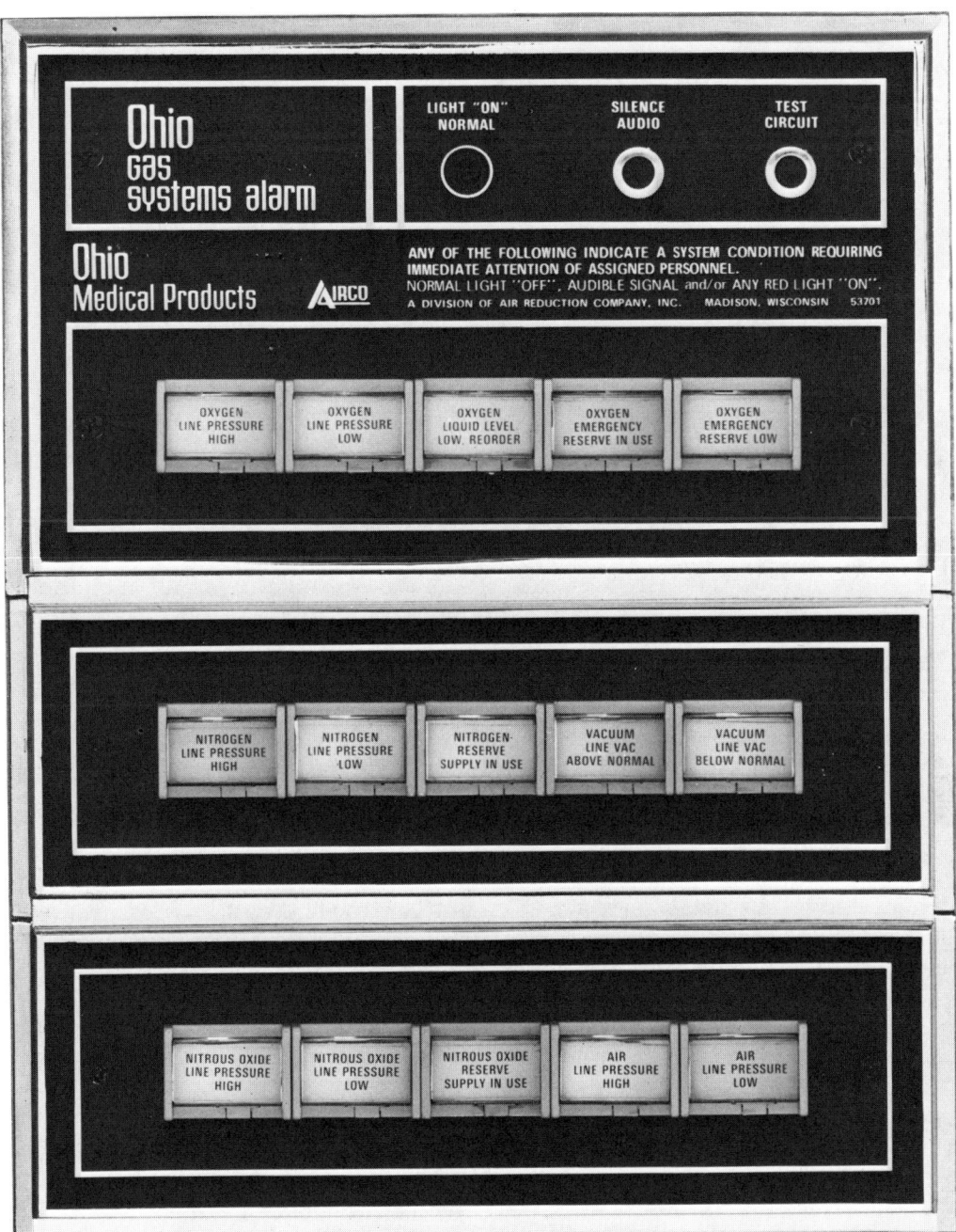

Fig. 9-11 Master alarm system panel connected to various area alarms and the sources of anesthesia gas supply. (Courtesy of Ohmeda, The BOC Group, Inc.)

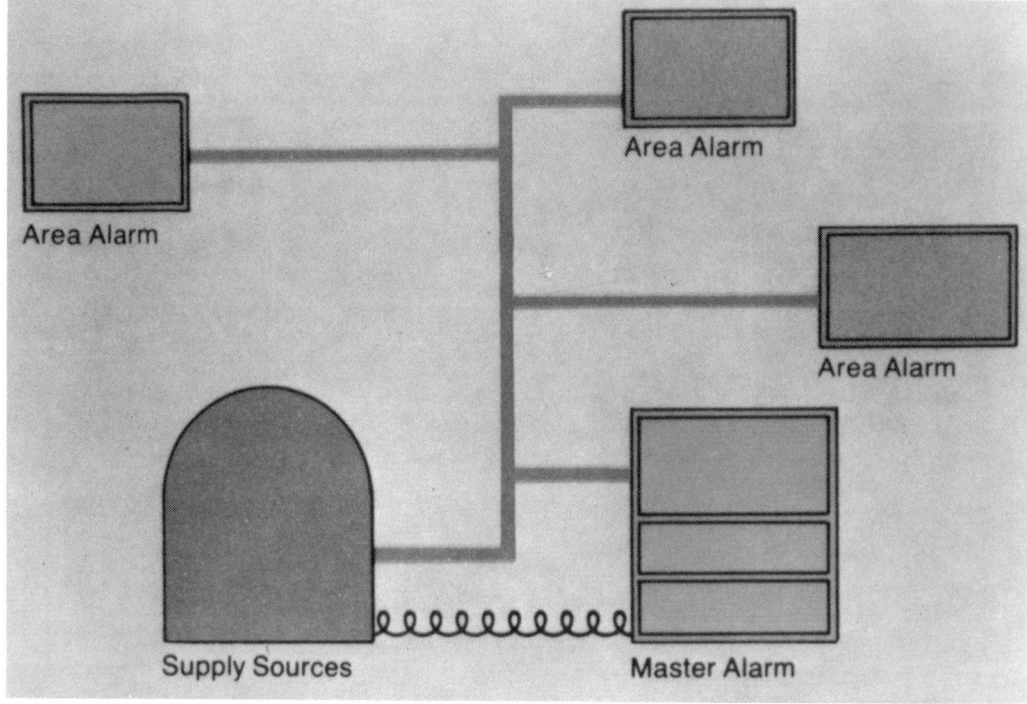

Fig. 9-12 Master alarm system for hospital medical gas pipeline system. All pipeline and supply source alarms are linked to the master alarm panel. (Courtesy of Ohmeda, The BOC Group, Inc.)

machine has occurred after servicing of the anesthesia machine.[16, 25-27] Worn connectors that attach to the central supply system can accept the anesthesia machine hose but fail to seat sufficiently, thus leaving the oxygen valve in the closed position. In one such incident this problem was combined with the compressed oxygen tank on the anesthesia machine having been left in the open position, depletion of the tank oxygen after 90 minutes, and death of the patient.[28] Perhaps the use of an oxygen analyzer in the anesthesia circuit would detect a crossing of the lines if the oxygen flowmeter was turned on prior to the nitrous oxide. It would be good practice to establish the procedure of checking the output of the oxygen flowmeter with an oxygen analyzer after every anesthesia machine servicing and following any maintenance of the hospital pipeline system.

Connections to the Anesthesia Machine

Color-coded hoses (oxygen, green; nitrous oxide, blue; air, yellow) are connected to the anesthesia machine using the CGA's diameter index safety system (DISS).[29] The DISS was introduced in 1959 as a noninterchangeable low-pressure connection system devised for medical gas applications.[29, 30] Nut and nipple fittings of different diameters and threads are assigned to each medical gas. The ANSI requires that every anesthesia machine have DISS threaded body fitting for all pipeline inlet fittings.[31] Each anesthesia gas is given a code number fitting, for example, 1240 for oxygen, 1220 for air, and 1040 for nitrous oxide.[29] Figure 9-13 illustrates the body, nipple, and nut which make up the connector for the oxygen inlet. The DISS is used only for connections with less than 200 psig and does not replace the pin index safety system designed for the compressed gas tank–anesthesia machine connection.

The connector linking the anesthesia machine to the hospital pipeline gas can be mounted on the wall or ceiling. Ceiling connectors can be in columns, on ceiling tracks (Fig. 9-14), or suspended on mobile arms (Figs. 9-15 and 9-16). Either a DISS connector or an automatic quick coupler valve can be used at this interface. A national standard has not been developed for the automatic quick coupler valve system; therefore each individual supplier has a safety-keyed index pin system (see Fig. 9-17). The gas inlet port and the pin engagement mechanism are separated by a specific distance on the male connector. The female portion of the connector has corresponding acceptance ports. A releasable spring mechanism locks the quick coupler valves to-

gether to provide the quick-connect feature.

Quick-connect mechanisms will wear out slowly,[28] making it increasingly difficult to get a proper connection, or fail suddenly[32] during the course of anesthetic administration. Two such instances resulted in cardiovascular collapse, with one patient death.[28, 32] Any connector system requires consistent quarterly maintenance and a keen awareness on the part of the user that equipment can fail.

PIPELINE SYSTEM INTERNAL TO THE ANESTHESIA MACHINE

The anesthesia machine pipeline system connects the high-pressure gas supply, that is, hospital pipeline gases and compressed gas tanks, to the pressure regulators, flowmeters, vaporizers, and common gas outlet. The piping diagram of the North American Drager

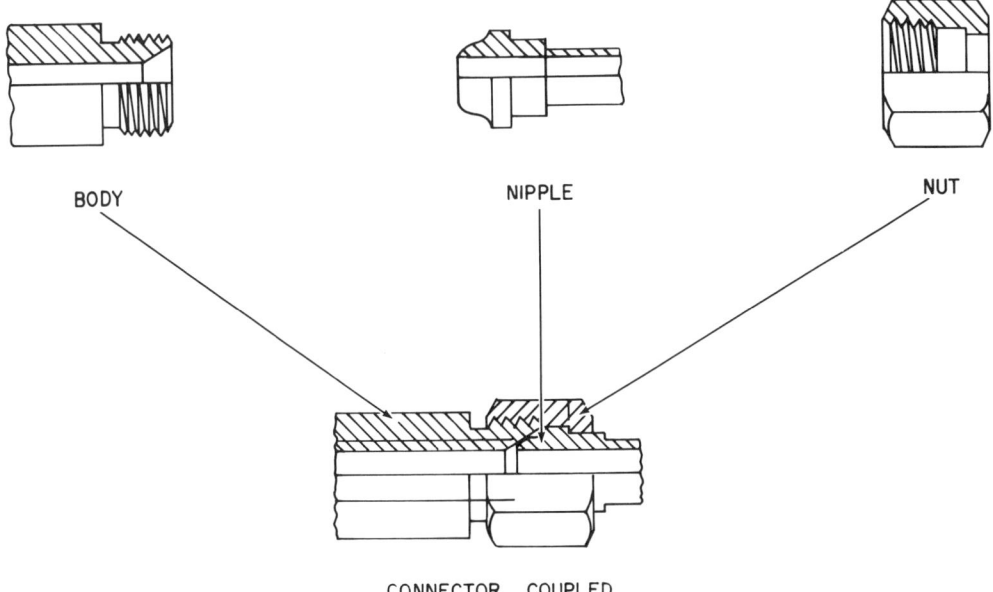

BODY   NIPPLE   NUT

CONNECTOR COUPLED

Fig. 9-13 Standard low-pressure diameter index safety system (DISS) connection for oxygen. The body of the connector is on the top left, the nipple is in the top center, and the connecting nut is on the top right. The lower figure illustrates the assembled connector (CGA Pamphlet G-4: Oxygen. © 1980 By permission of the Compressed Gas Association, 1235 Jefferson Davis Hwy, Arlington, VA 22202.)

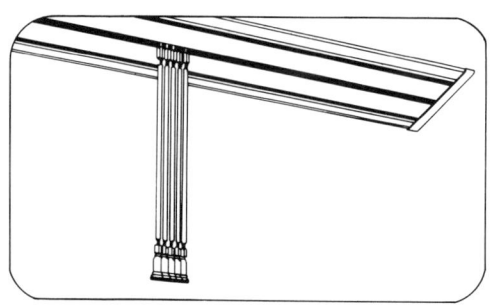
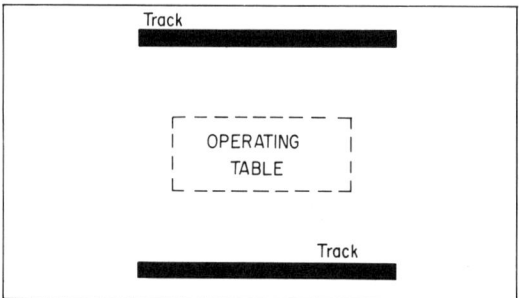

Fig. 9-14 Ceiling gas tracks for hospital pipeline connections to the anesthesia machine. A rolling manifold (left diagram) moves along the track to improve flexibility. The operating table has one track on each side. (Courtesy of Ohmeda, The BOC Group, Inc.)

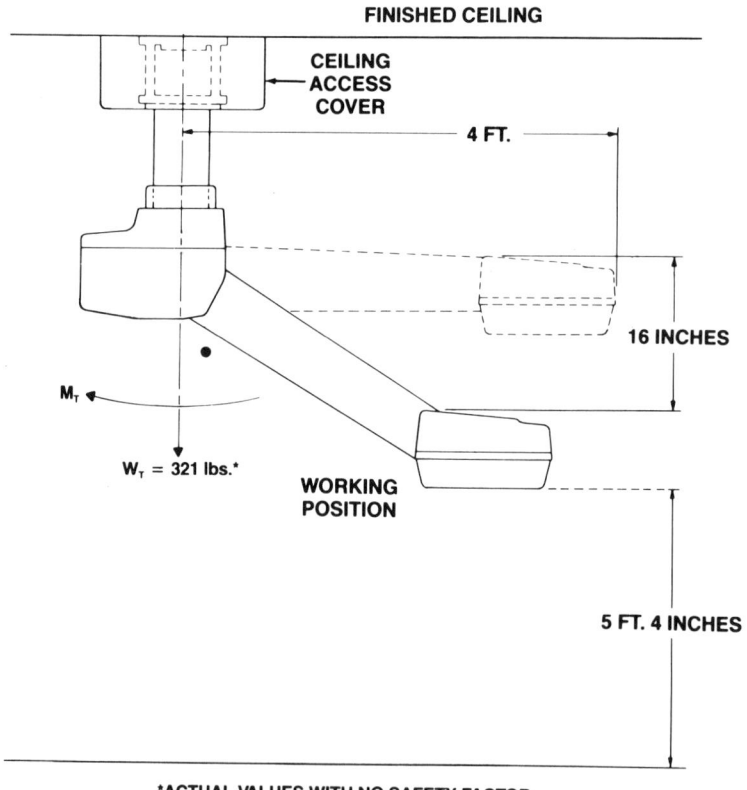

Fig. 9-15 Total articulating service center ceiling mount for anesthesia gases, vacuum, and electrical outlets. The suspended arm is capable of a 350° arc of travel and can be positioned through 16 in. of vertical movement. (Product Specification. TASC 2000. Chemetron Medical Division, Allied Healthcare Products. Inc., St Louis, 1985.)

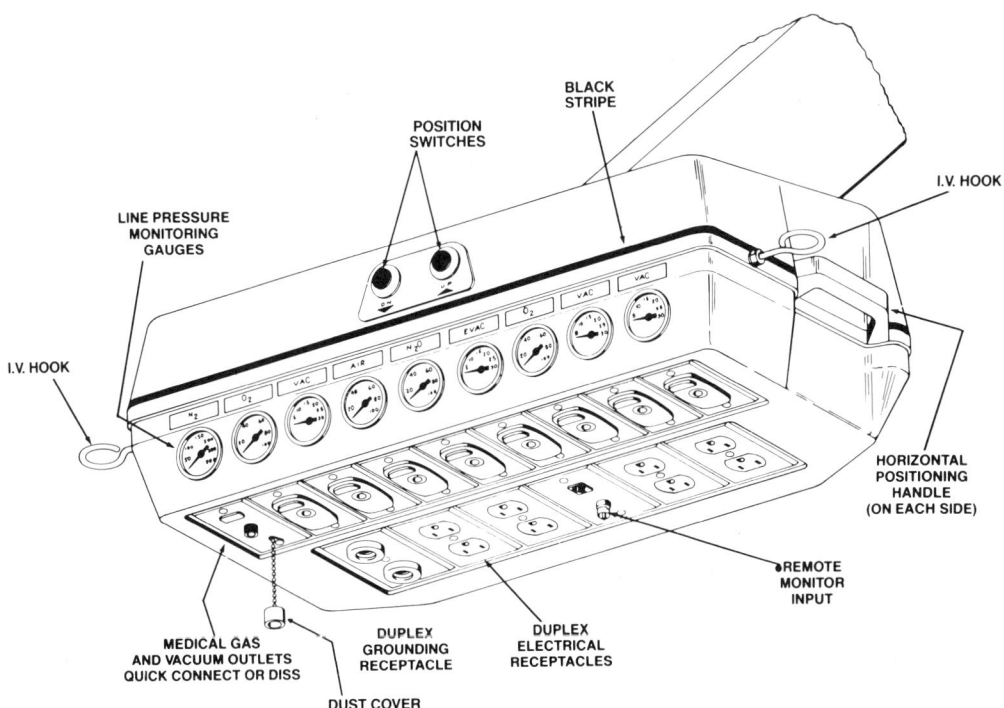

Fig. 9-16 Distribution head for the ceiling mounted total articulating service center. Nine medical DISS or quick connect color-coded gas outlets are available. (Product Specification. TASC 2000. Chemetron Medical Division, Allied Healthcare Products, Inc., St. Louis, 1985.)

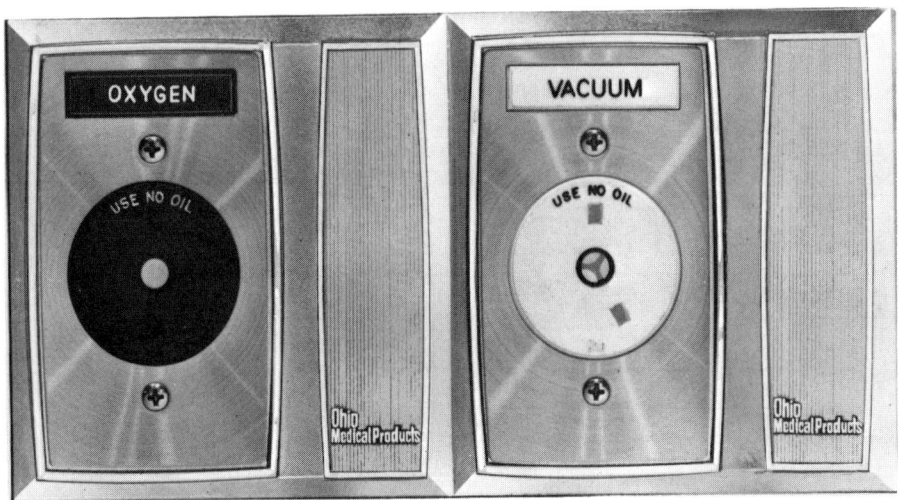

Fig. 9-17 Quick-connect safety-keyed index pin coupler system for oxygen and vacuum. Each double-pin inlet has an assigned space within the circumference of the circle. Vacuum inlet pins are at 1200 and 1700 hours here. (Courtesy of Ohmeda, The BOC Group, Inc.)

Narkomed IIA anesthesia machine is shown in Figure 9-18. Three anesthesia gases—oxygen, nitrous oxide, and air—enter from two sources each: the cylinder yokes and the hospital pipeline DISS. Each gas inlet is provided with a check valve (see Figs. 9-19 and 9-20) which prevents the transfer of gases between cylinders and avoids the release of gas during the exchange of cylinders or when cylinders are not attached to the yoke.[14, 33] A filter is usually placed in the gas inlet to prevent dust and dirt from entering the pipeline. Pressure gauges measure the pipeline pressures of the hospital-supplied gases and the compressed gas cylinder pressures. Standards for all pressure gauges on the anesthesia machine are outlined in detail by the ANSI.[31] The delivery pressure of the regulators for the compressed gas cylinders is preset below the hospital pipeline pressure inlet. The hospital pipeline can

thus supply the anesthesia gases when the cylinders happen to be open.[33] This arrangement avoids depleting the cylinder backup source of anesthesia gases during the administration of anesthesia. Precision control of the pressure in the pipeline is required to power the ventilator and ensure proper function of the anesthesia machine safety alarm systems.

Both the Drager Narkomed IIA and the Ohmeda Modulus II require the main switch of the anesthesia machine to be activated before gas flow can take place. One exception is the availability of oxygen via the oxygen flush valve. A separate line to the oxygen flush valve comes from a common source of the hospital pipeline DISS and the cylinder yokes. As can be seen in Figure 9-21, the line bypasses all alarm systems, flowmeters, and vaporizers and enters directly into the system just proximal to the common gas outlet. Oxygen is

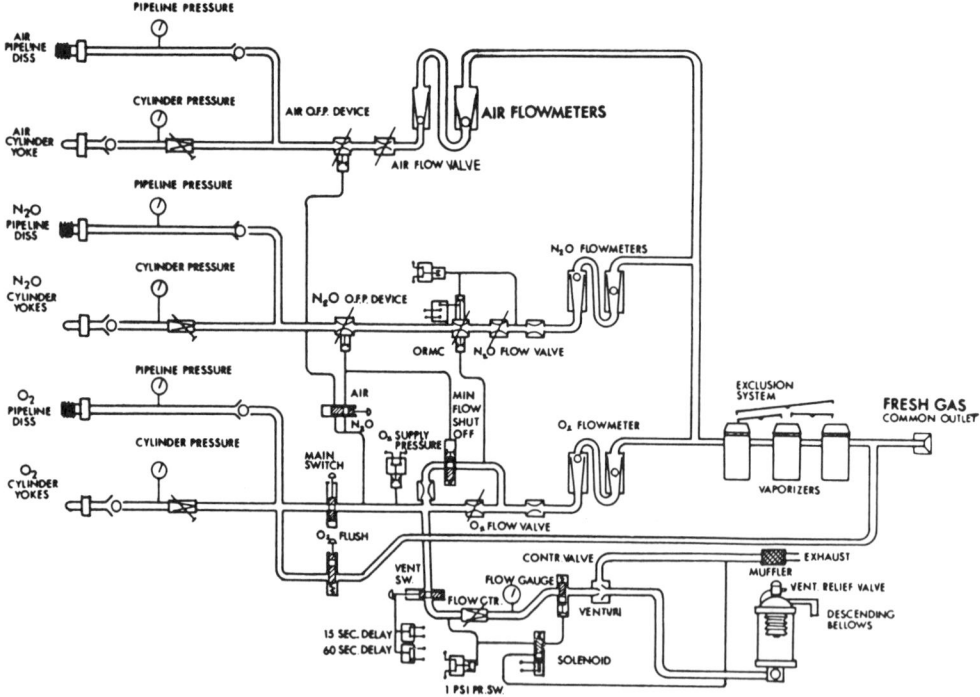

Fig. 9-18 Piping diagram for the Drager Narkomed IIA anesthesia machine. The diagram is for a three-gas anesthesia machine with a ventilator, three vaporizers, and an oxygen ratio monitor controller device. (Technical Service Manual. North American Drager. Telford, PA, 1985.)

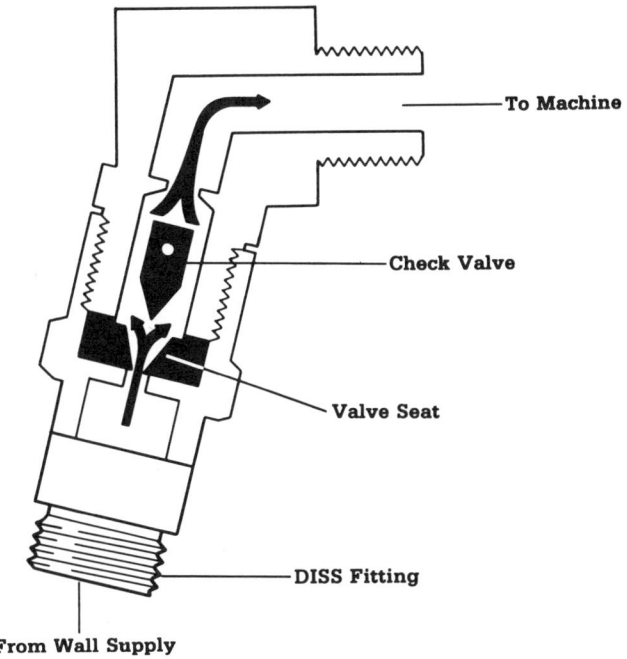

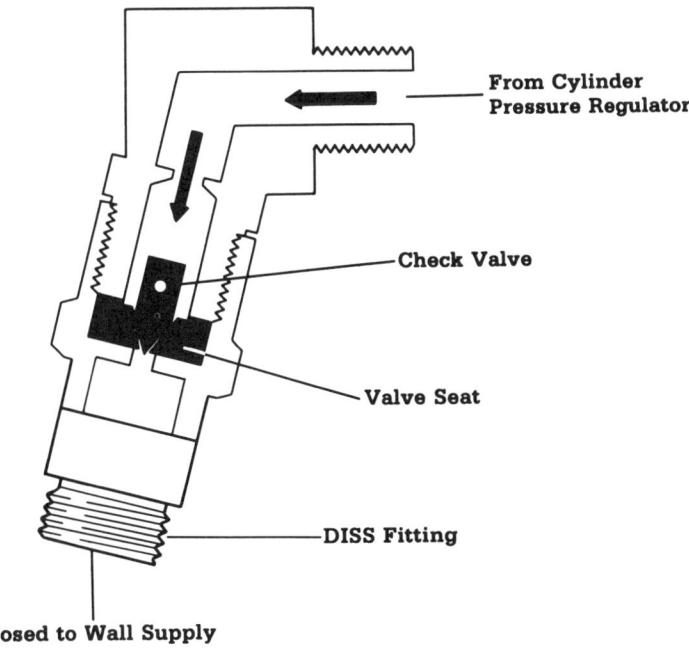

Fig. 9-19 The DISS inlet to the anesthesia machine with check valve and valve seat. The top diagram illustrates the check valve lifted off the valve seat by the gas from the hospital pipeline entering the anesthesia machine. The bottom diagram shows the check valve seated and closed by gravity and the flow of gases from the cylinder pressure regulator. (Reproduced with permission from Bowie E, Huffman LM: The Anesthesia Machine: Essentials for Understanding. Ohmeda, The BOC Group, Inc., 1985.)

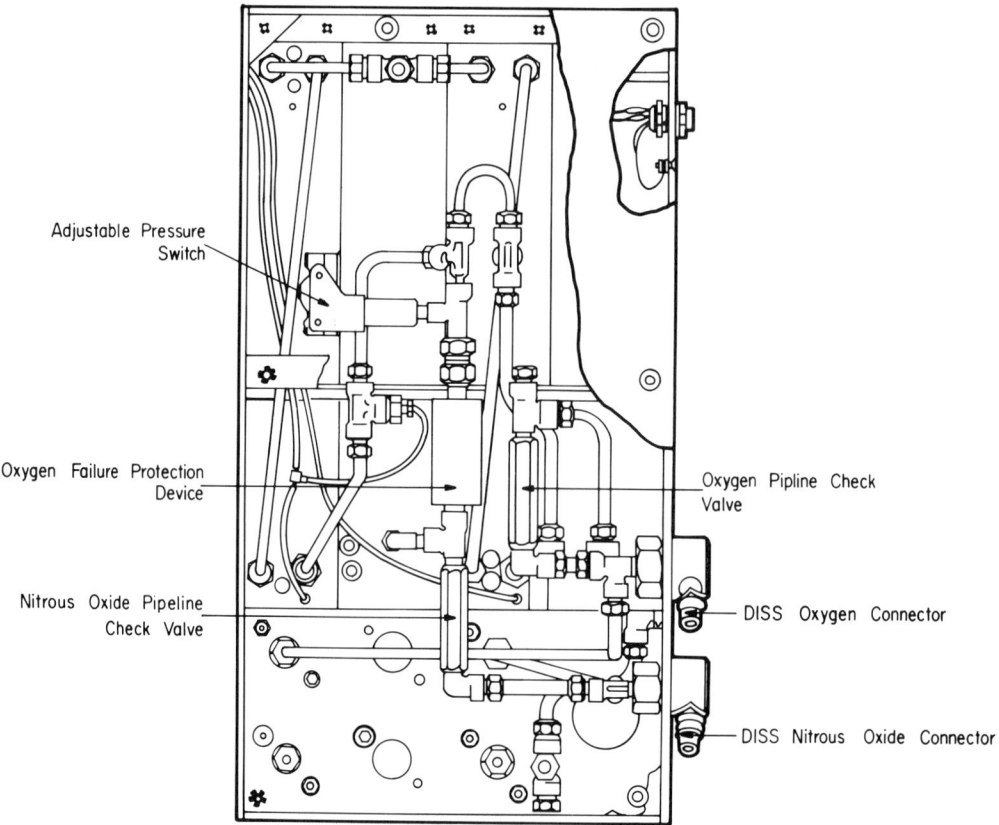

Fig. 9-20 Back view of the anesthesia machine at the level of the flowmeters. Check valves for nitrous oxide and oxygen are near their respective DISS connectors. The oxygen failure protection device ("fail-safe") shuts off nitrous oxide flow when the oxygen pressure decreases to a critical level. (Redrawn from Parts Manual. North American Drager, Telford, PA, 1984.)

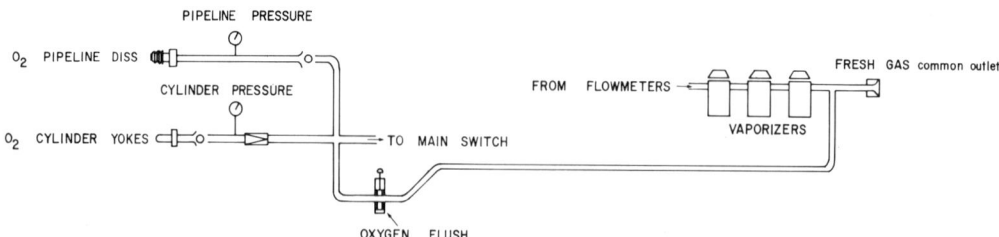

Fig. 9-21 Piping diagram for the oxygen flush valve system. The oxygen flush valve is supplied oxygen directly from the common source of the DISS pipeline and compressed gas yoke. Activation of the flush valve allows oxygen to be delivered at 50 to 70 L/min just distal to the common gas outlet. (Redrawn from Technical Service Manual. North American Drager, Telford, PA, 1984.)

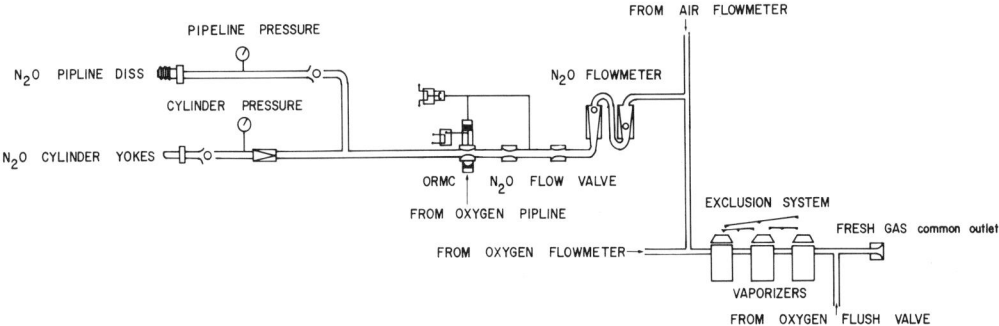

Fig. 9-22 Nitrous oxide piping system in the Drager Narkomed IIA anesthesia machine. The ORMc is located prior to the flowmeter. (Redrawn from Technical Service Manual. North American Drager, Telford, PA, 1985.)

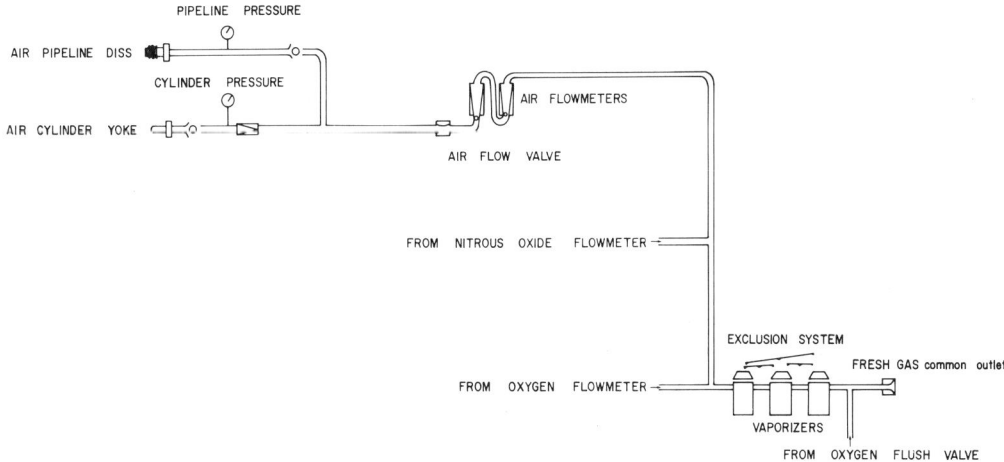

Fig. 9-23 Piping system for air in the Drager Narkomed IIA anesthesia machine. (Redrawn from Technical Service Manual. North American Drager, Telford, PA, 1985.)

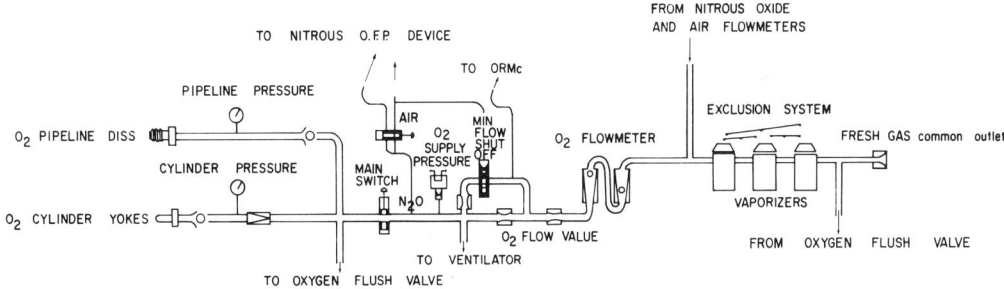

Fig. 9-24 Piping diagram of the portion of the oxygen system which supplies the flowmeter and vaporizers. The main switch must be activated to allow any flow through the flowmeter. Note the many safety features in the oxygen system depicted: the ORMc, the minimum oxygen flow, the oxygen supply pressure alarm, and the nitrous oxygen failure device. (Redrawn from Technical Service Manual. North American Drager, Telford, PA, 1985.)

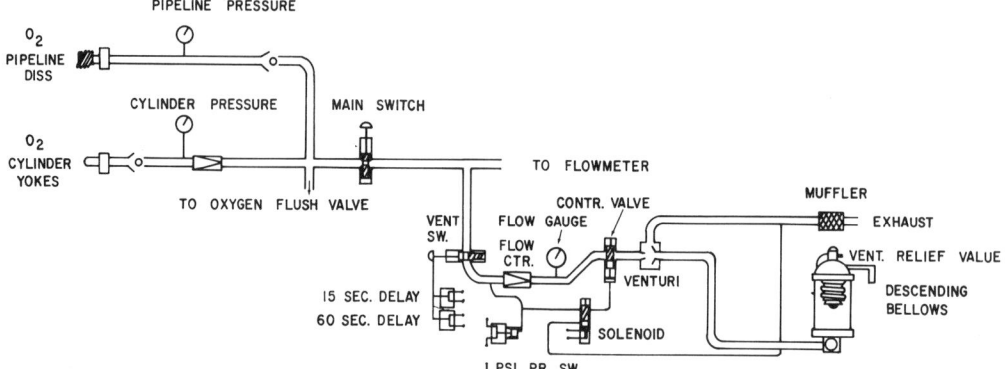

Fig. 9-25 Oxygen supply to drive the ventilator. The main oxygen pipeline is tapped just after the main switch. Oxygen passes through the control box of the ventilator and into the bellows chamber. (Redrawn from Technical Service Manual. North American Drager, Telford, PA, 1985.)

therefore provided for emergencies in the operating room without having to turn on the master switch of the anesthesia machine.

Each gas has a separate pipeline system within the anesthesia machine. The common point of connection for the gases is just proximal to the vaporizers. Pressures generated by the individual gas pipelines may be tapped to activate certain safety control mechanisms such as the oxygen ratio monitor controller (ORMc) of the Drager Narkomed IIA. The isolated piping system for nitrous oxide, air, and oxygen are seen in Figures 9-22 to 9-24. The oxygen source which powers the ventilator comes off the oxygen pipeline just distal to the main switch and flows through the ventilator control box and into the bellows chamber (see Fig. 9-25).

At each piping junction the name, chemical symbol, or appropriate color code must indicate the gas content.[31] In addition, the gas piping system must withstand twice the intended service pressure without rupture.

Only a leak of 5 ml/min is allowed in the pipeline between the cylinders or hospital pipeline inlet and the flow-control valves. From the flow-control valves to the common gas outlet a leak of 30 ml/min at a pressure of 30 cmH$_2$O is permissible.[31] The manufacturer of the anesthesia machine must supply information with each machine which outlines

testing methodology. Standards for the anesthesia machine high-pressure and low-pressure leak tests are well outlined by the ANSI.[31]

Anesthesia machine pipelines have been found to develop leaks in many ways and places. Mismounting the vaporizer,[34] leaks developing in sidearm universal vaporizers,[35, 36] failure to reconnect the output pipeline to the vaporizer after servicing,[37] fine longitudinal cracks in the oxygen pipeline to the ventilator,[38] and kinking of the common outlet gas tubing[39] are just a few of the many complications which can happen within the pipeline system. Many of these problems cannot be detected by preventive maintenance and require vigilance on the part of the anesthesiologist to recognize malfunction.

REFERENCES

1. NFPA 56F: Nonflammable Medical Gas Systems. National Fire Protection Association, Quincy, Mass., 1983
2. Feeley TW, Hedley-Whyte J: Bulk oxygen and nitrous oxide delivery systems: design and dangers. Anesthesiology 44:301, 1976
3. Howell RSC: Piped medical gas and vacuum systems. Anaesthesia 35:676, 1980
4. Chi OZ: Another example of hypoxic gas mixture delivery. Anesthesiology 62:543, 1985

5. Handbook of Compressed Gases. 2nd Ed. Van Nostrand Reinhold, New York, 1981
6. NFPA 50: Bulk Oxygen Systems 1979. National Fire Protection Association, Quincy, Mass., 1979
7. Grant WJ: Medical Gases. Their Properties and Uses. Yearbook Publishers, Chicago, 1978
8. Bancroft ML, du Moulin GC, Hedley-Whyte J: Hazards of hospital bulk oxygen delivery systems. Anesthesiology 52:504, 1980
9. CGA Pamphlet S-1.1: Pressure Relief Device Standards: Part 1—Cylinders for Compressed Gases. Compressed Gas Association, Arlington, VA, 1979
10. Sprague DH, Archer GW, Jr: Intraoperative hypoxia from an erroneously filled liquid oxygen reservoir. Anesthesiology 42:360, 1975
11. Army investigating gas mixup that led to hospital deaths. Am Med News, June 24, 1983
12. CGA Pamphlet G-8.1: Standard for Nitrous Oxide Systems at Consumer Sites. Compressed Gas Association, Arlington, VA, 1979
13. CGA Pamphlet G-4.1: Cleaning Equipment for Oxygen Service. Compressed Gas Association, Arlington, VA, 1977
14. NFPA 99: Health Care Facilities 1984. National Fire Protection Association, Quincy, Mass., 1984
15. Krenis LJ, Berkowitz DA: Errors in installation of a new gas delivery system found after certification. Anesthesiology 62:677, 1985
16. Editorial. The Westminster inquiry. Lancet 2:175, 1977.
17. Robinson JS, Marshall RD, MacWhirter GI: Safety and piped medical gas supplies. Anaesthesia 33:638, 1978
18. Wright BM: Whistle discrimination for oxygen and nitrous oxide. Lancet 2:1008, 1977
19. Dinnick OP: Medical gases—piping problems. Eng Med 8:243, 1979
20. Roth F, Karmann U: Failures in pipeline systems. Anaesthesia 37:1222, 1982
21. American Medicorp, Inc., et al., v Daniel Lord et al., 578 S. W. 2d 837, No. 8186, Ct. Civil App. Texas, Beaumont, 15 February 1979
22. DiPaolo V: Hospital's failure to analyze gases made crossing of gas lines deadly. Modern Healthcare 7:16, 1977
23. Hawkins v Kurlander, 469 N.Y.S. 2d 820. N.Y. Sup. Ct. App. Div., 16 December 1983
24. Goebel WM: Failure of nitrous oxide and oxygen pin-indexing. Anesth Prog, 188, 1980
25. Arrowsmith LWM: Medical gases—piping problems. Eng Med 8:247, 1979
26. Bonsu AK, Stead AL: Accidental cross-connexion of oxygen and nitrous oxide in an anaesthetic machine. Anaesthesia 38:767, 1983
27. Mazze RI: Therapeutic misadventures with oxygen delivery systems: the need for continuous in-line oxygen monitors. Anesth Analg 51:787, 1972
28. Meyer JA: Guest discussion. Anesth Analg 51:790, 1972
29. CGA Pamphlet G-4: Oxygen. Compressed Gas Association, Arlington, VA, 1980
30. Rendell-Baker L: Problems with anesthetic and respiratory therapy equipment. Int Anesthesiol Clin 20:171, 1982
31. American National Standard: Minimum Performance and Safety Requirements for Components and Systems of Continuous-Flow Anesthesia Machines for Human Use. Z79.8-1979. American National Standards Institute, New York, 1979
32. Craig DB, Culligan, J: Sudden interruption of gas flow through a Schrader oxygen coupler unit. Can Anaesth Soc J 27:175, 1980
33. Schreiber P: Anaesthesia Equipment: Performance, Classification and Safety. Springer-Verlag, New York, 1972
34. Jablundki J, Reynolds A, Ridle RT: A potential cause (and cure) of a major gas leak. Anesthesiology 62:842, 1985
35. Eldrup-Jorgensen S: Gas leaks in anesthesia machines. Anesthesiology 46:439, 1977
36. Mulroy M, Ham J, Eger EI: Inflowing gas leak, a potential source of hypoxia. Anesthesiology 45:102, 1976
37. Comm G, Rendell-Baker, L: Back pressure check valves a hazard. Anesthesiology 56:327, 1982
38. Wolf S, Watson CB, Clark P: An unusual cause of leakage in an anesthesia system. Anesthesiology 55:83, 1981
39. Dolan PF: Connections from anesthetic machine to circle system unsatisfactory. Anesthesiology 50:277, 1979

10

Ventilators for Anesthesia

Ventilators for anesthesia were once anesthesia machine add-ons which the anesthesiologist dragged in the room for special cases. Today the ventilator has become an integral component of the modern anesthesia machine. The anesthesiologist uses the ventilator for a number of reasons: (1) for better control of arterial carbon dioxide levels, (2) to accomplish the vital role of ventilation, thus allowing the hands of the anesthesiologist to be available for other tasks, and (3) for reasonable compensation of changes in lung compliance with a volume-limited ventilator.

Ventilators can be divided into two major categories: pressure limited and volume limited (see Fig. 10-1). Pressure-limited ventilators deliver a tidal volume until a preselected pressure limit is achieved in the patient circuit. In contrast, a volume-limited ventilator delivers a set tidal volume up to a preset maximum safety limit, regardless of the pressure in the patient circuit.[1] Initially pressure-limited ventilators were used in anesthesia because of their small size and mobility; however, they were a nuisance because they required frequent adjustments of the tidal volume to compensate for changes in lung compliance. Design changes reduced the size of volume-limited anesthesia ventilators and eventually the volume-limited ventilator became an inte-

gral part of the anesthesia machine. Today the rule is to purchase the anesthesia machine with a built-in volume-limited ventilator rather than adding the ventilator as an optional item.

Volume ventilators designed as an integral part of the anesthesia machine are separated into a *control box* and a *bellows assembly*. A block diagram of the anesthesia ventilator is shown in Figure 10-2. The control box is mounted on the anesthesia machine frame and the bellows assembly is mounted as an appendage to the frame in a manner similar to the carbon dioxide absorber (see Fig. 10-3). Attachments are provided which connect the control box to the oxygen pressure power outlet and connect the bellows assembly to the scavenger system and patient circuit.

Initially volume-limited ventilators designed for anesthesia provided a limited respiratory rate selection, usually a fixed inspiratory/expiratory (I/E) phase time ratio control, no sigh mechanism, and a preset pressure relief valve to vent excessive pressure (65 to 80 cmH$_2$O) in the patient circuit. These functions were easily controlled by a fluidic or Venturi principle, with the ventilator requiring only an oxygen pressure power input. Anesthesiologists then demanded a wide range of respiratory rates, a sigh cycle, and an ad-

165

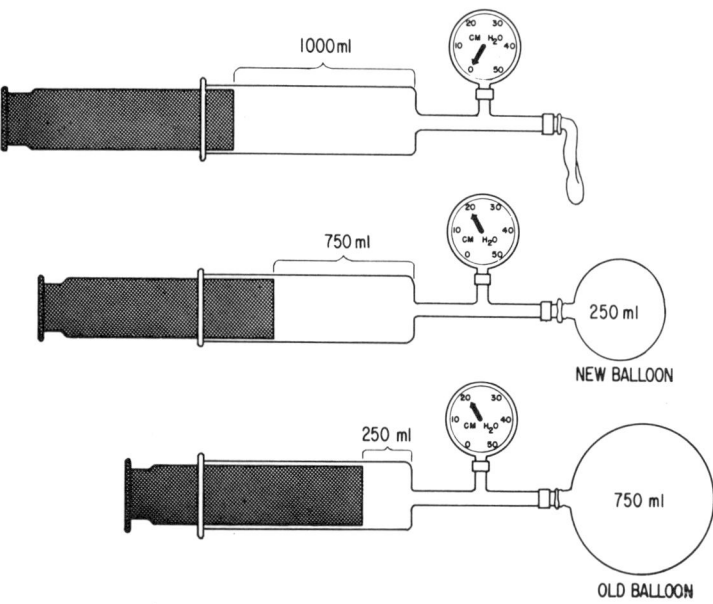

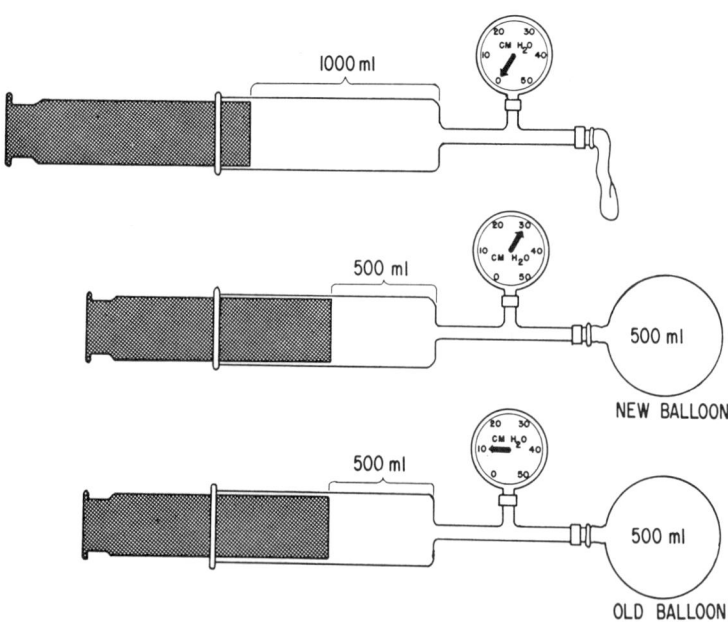

Fig. 10-1 Comparison of pressure-limited and volume-limited generators. A pressure-limited generator (top) blows up the balloon to a preset pressure. When the balloon is new (stiff lung) the pressure is reached at 250 ml; in an old balloon (compliant lung) a volume of 750 ml is achieved before arriving at the same pressure. A volume-limited generator (bottom) delivers the same volume to the new and the old balloon but requires far different pressures to accomplish the task. (From Heironimus TW: The Mechanical Artificial Ventilation: A Manual for Students and Practitioners, 1967. Courtesy of Charles C Thomas, Publisher, Springfield, Illinois.)

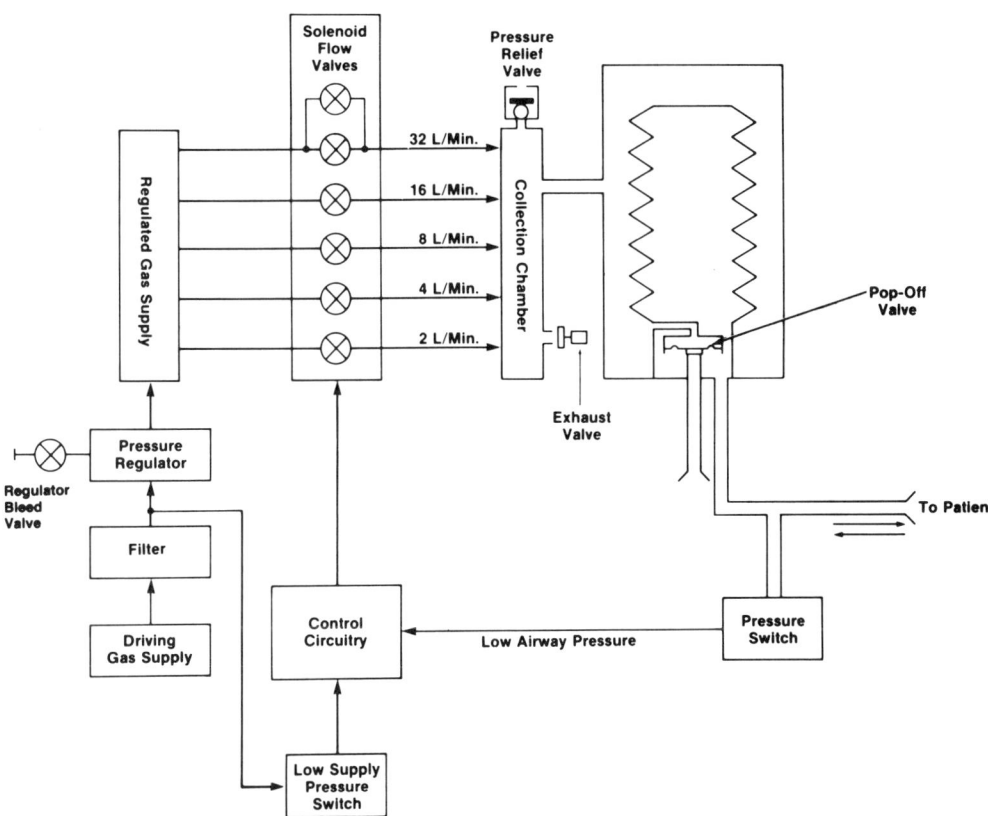

Fig. 10-2 Block diagram of the anesthesia ventilator. Oxygen to drive the ventilator is supplied from the anesthesia machine pipeline. Six solenoid valves control the rate of flow into the chamber outside the bellows. Oxygen used to drive the ventilator exits into the room via the exhaust valve. (Courtesy of Ohmeda, The BOC Group, Inc.)

justable I/E ratio. Such diverse ventilator cycle patterns required the use of computer chips, and thus the electronically controlled ventilator was created. The electronic ventilator requires both an oxygen pressure power input and an electrical power input.

Oxygen is used as the power supply to drive the ventilator because (1) it is inexpensive, (2) it is of high purity and free of dust and particles, (3) it is free of water vapor which can damage the ventilator parts,[2, 3] (4) it is readily available in the operating room, and (5) some ventilators are designed to function only with oxygen.[4] Compressed air is not used, because it contains water vapor and dust particles which can damage the ventilator. Filtered,

compressed dry air is available but it is much more expensive than oxygen and offers no advantages. Any pressurized gas could serve as the driving force to cycle the ventilator, but none have advantages over oxygen.

CONTROL BOX

Inside the control box are the components that integrate the pneumatic and electrical sources to drive the bellows assembly. The external controls seen by the anesthesiologist usually involve a combination of the following: (1) respiratory rate, (2) I/E ratio, (3) an on/

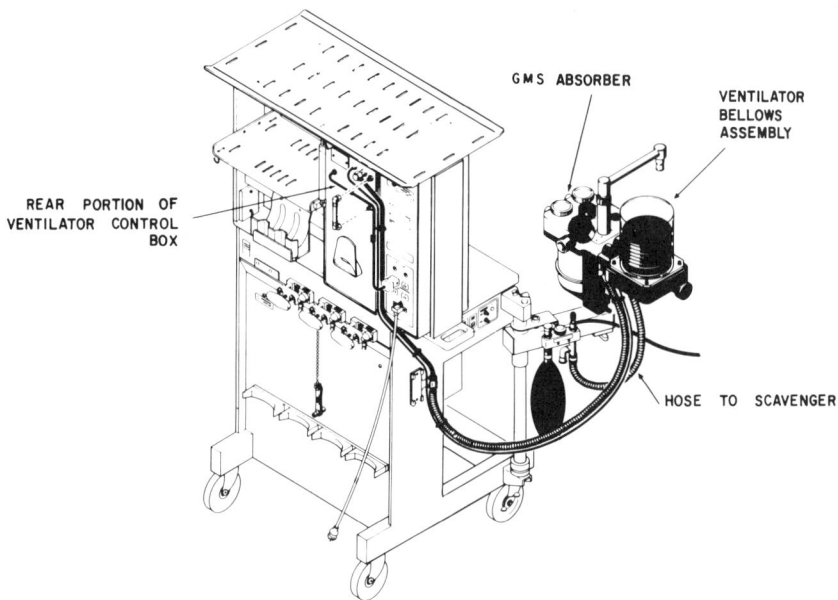

Fig. 10-3 Bellows and control box sections of the anesthesia ventilator. In this instance the bellows assembly is mounted to the GMS absorber; the control box is mounted above the flowmeters of the anesthesia machine. Connecting hoses for waste gas scavenging, oxygen supply, and low airway pressure alarm are provided. (Courtesy of Ohmeda, The BOC Group, Inc.)

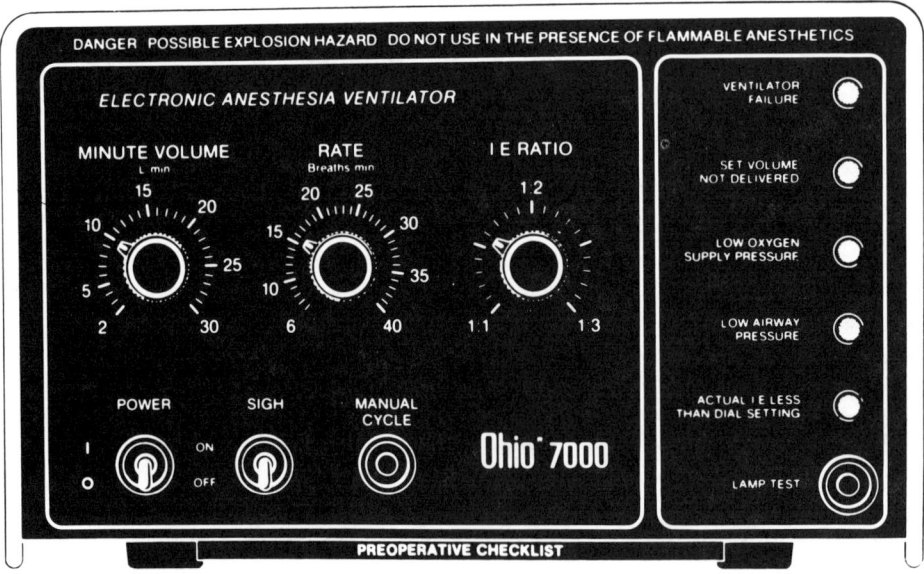

Fig. 10-4 Controls and alarm indicators for the Ohio 7000 anesthesia ventilator. Toggle switches control the power and sigh controls. A push button controls the manual cycle. Pressing the lamp test button will verify the function of the lights. (Courtesy of Ohmeda, The BOC Group, Inc.)

TOP VIEW

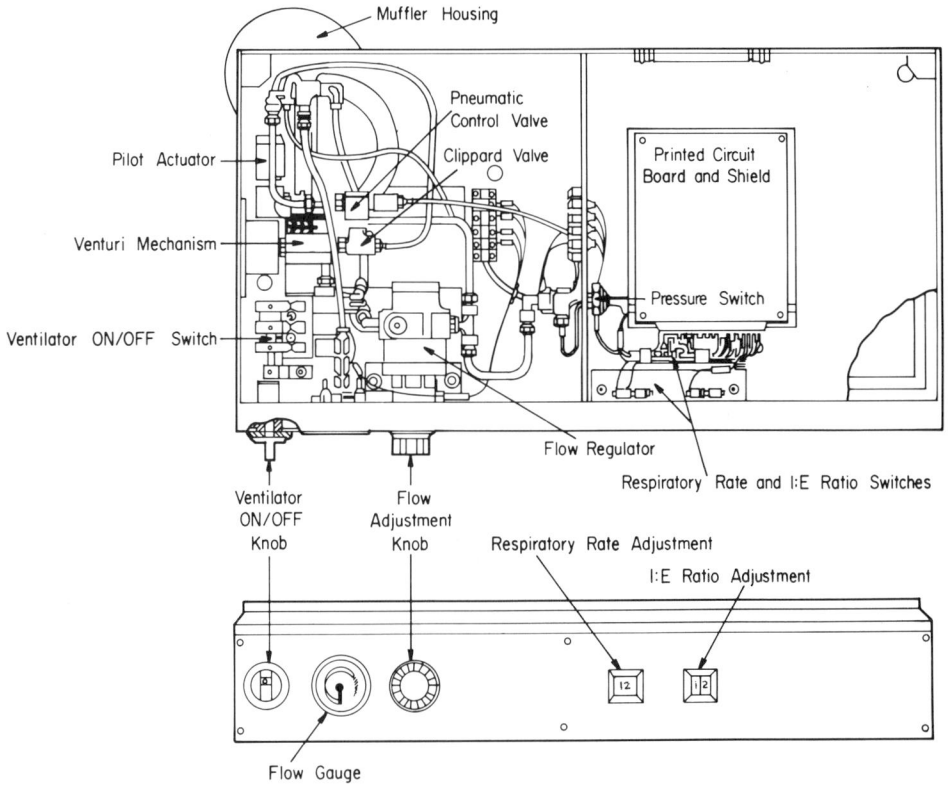

Fig. 10-5 Schematic of the ventilator control box. The top view illustrates the intricate mechanisms required to provide the dial-in functions seen in the front view. Note the printed circuit board which is required to provide control of the ventilator flow rates over wide I/E and frequency ratios. (Redrawn from Parts Manual. North American Drager, Telford, PA, 1984.)

off switch, (4) sigh, (5) flow control, (6) a pressure-limiting device, and (7) a manual switch and/or alarms (see Figs. 10-4 and 10-5). The tidal volume control is sometimes separate from the control box, as an integral part of the bellows assembly.

Electronic circuits inside the control box are matched to their respective pneumatic circuits (see Fig. 10-5). Though complex in appearance (see Fig. 10-6), these electronic circuits are simply solenoid valves which deliver oxygen into the bellows assembly. A parallel series of solenoid valves (see Fig. 10-2), each of which controls a different delivery volume of oxygen, is coordinated to provide flow and

rate combinations over a wide range of selectability.

The Ohmeda 7000 Electronic Anesthesia Ventilator provides certain limits and alarms which sense changes in the electronic circuitry of the control box.[4, 5] A *flow check limit alarm* senses any setting that will exceed the ventilator's capacity of 62 L/min and activates an alarm which notifies the anesthesiologist that the machine is delivering less than the dialed I/E ratio. A *tidal volume sensor* monitors voltages that exceed those required for a tidal volume of 1.5 L and activates an alarm which indicates the set volume is not being delivered. When the solenoid exhaust valve fails to open,

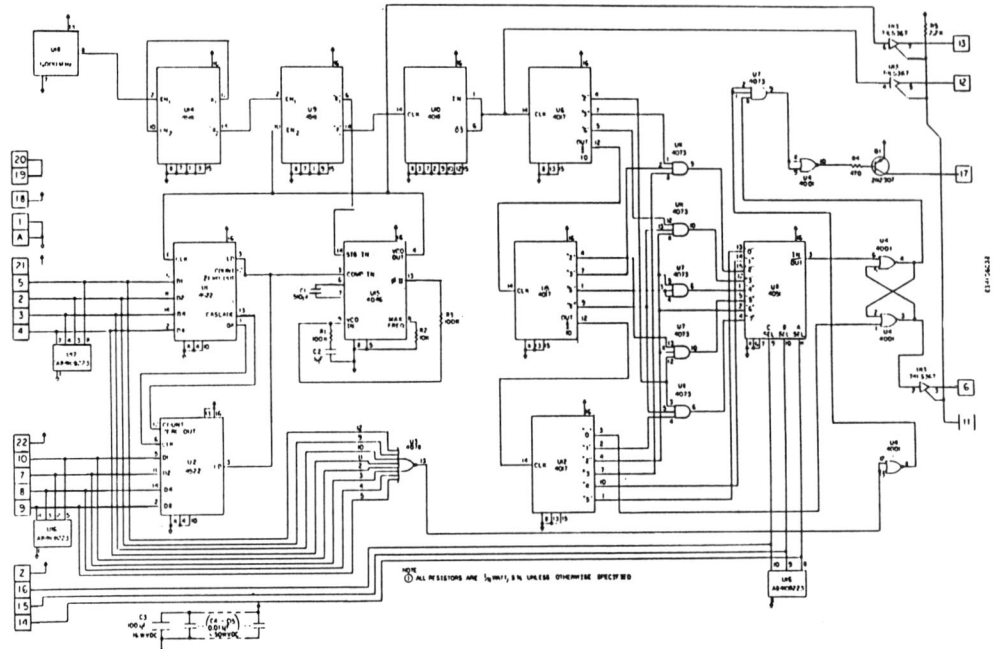

Fig. 10-6 Typical diagram of an electronic control circuitry in an anesthesia ventilator. (Courtesy of North American Drager, Telford, PA.)

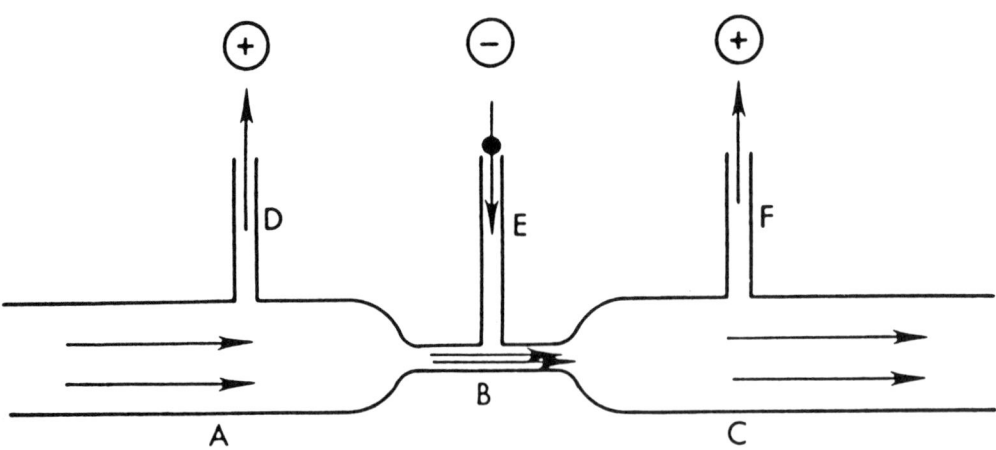

Fig. 10-7 Venturi effect. As a gas flows through a constriction (B) in a laminar fashion, the flow rate increases. Pressure in the constriction becomes less than at points D and F. When the pressure at E is below atmospheric pressure, room air will be entrained into the stream of gas. Mixing of the gas and room air takes place in the distal tube (C). (Technical Service Manual. North American Drager, Telford, PA, 1985.)

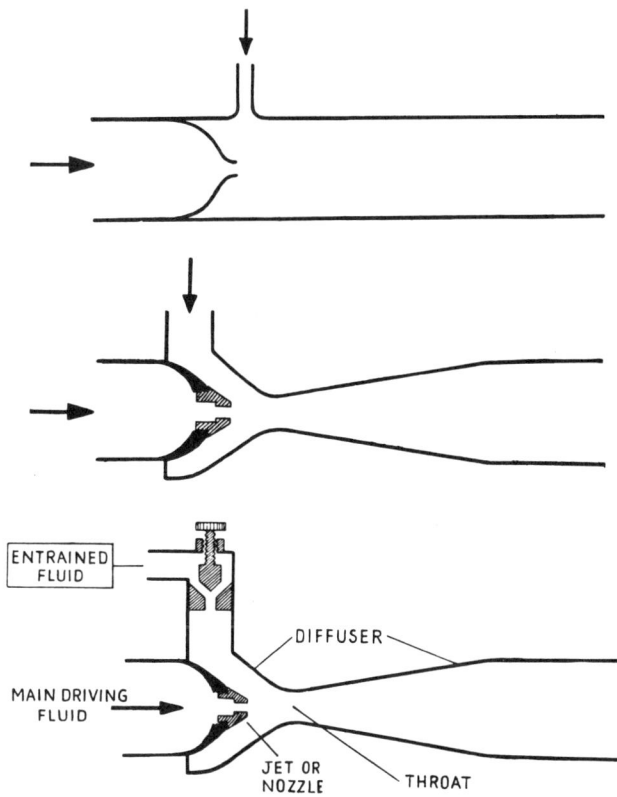

Fig. 10-8 The evolution of the injector from the simple Venturi. Compressed gas, if forced at high speed through the jet and throat, creates a negative pressure in the entrainment port. Ambient air enters and mixes with the compressed gas in the diffuser. A larger gas volume becomes available for driving the anesthesia ventilator. (From MacIntosh R, Mushin WW, Epstein HG: Physics for the Anaesthetist. 3rd Ed. Blackwell, Oxford, 1963.)

ENTRAINED FLUID

DIFFUSER

MAIN DRIVING FLUID

JET OR NOZZLE

THROAT

a *red lamp and audio tone* indicating ventilator failure are activated. A pressure-sensitive switch monitors the oxygen supply pressure and activates a *low oxygen supply pressure alarm* when the oxygen pressure falls below 40 psig. An additional pressure-sensitive device monitors the pressure output inside the patient circuit portion of the bellows assembly. If the pressure in the patient circuit falls below 6 cmH$_2$O during two successive breaths, the *low airway pressure alarm* is activated. An additional feature is the provision of an *altitude compensation circuit,* which can be adjusted for pressures from sea level up to 1,800 m. The electronic circuitry which controls the tidal volume is set at the factory at approximately 270 m above sea level.

The density of anesthesia gases in the bellows changes with elevation—thus the need for an altitude compensator for the electronic circuit.

The North American Drager (NAD) Anesthesia Ventilator AV-E requires electronic circuits to control a solenoid valve but in addition includes a Venturi device in the pneumatic power circuit.[2, 6] A Venturi device diminishes the bobbing effect on the oxygen flow tube, uses less oxygen, and promotes the smooth, quiet delivery of gases into the lungs. Figure 10-7 shows diagrammatically how a Venturi effect is achieved. Gas flows in a laminar fashion along a large-bore tube with a constriction in the center. In order for the same volume of gas to get through the constriction in the same amount of time, the gas must accelerate. The pressure in the constriction is decreased by the accelerated gas flow and can drop below atmospheric pressure. If

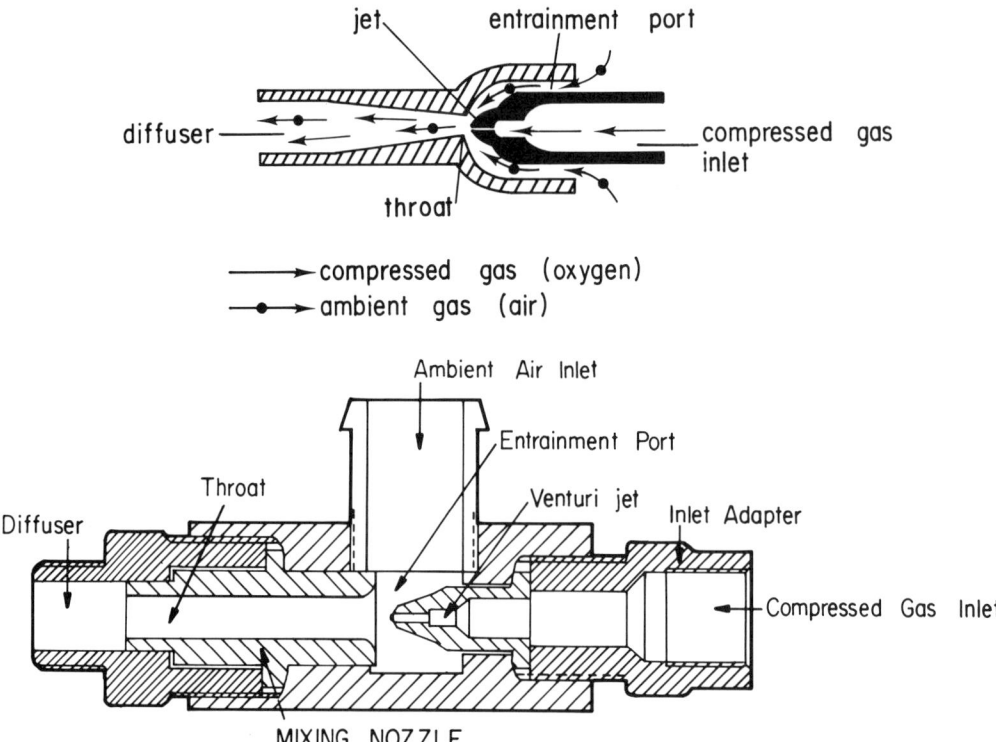

Fig. 10-9 Venturi assembly. The upper diagram shows the flow of compressed gas through the jet and the entry of ambient gas (air) via the entrainment port into the diffuser. The lower diagram is a cross-sectional schematic of the Venturi used in the Drager AV-E ventilator. (Redrawn from Parts Manual, North American Drager, Telford, PA, 1984.)

a hole or inlet is introduced at the constriction, outside air will be entrained by the subatmospheric pressure created by the gas traversing the constriction.[7] Application of the Venturi effect is incorporated into the anesthesia ventilator via an injector. An injector consists of a compressed gas tube, a jet, an entrainment port, a throat, and a diffuser (see Fig. 10-8). A subatmospheric pressure is created at the throat by the flow of compressed oxygen through the jet. Ambient air is entrained by the subatmospheric pressure of the oxygen flowing through the constricted portion of the injection. Both oxygen and air are mixed in the diffuser (see Fig. 10-9).[2, 6] The diffuser reduces turbulence in the gas stream, converts kinetic energy into pressure energy, entrains a large volume of gas, and makes the final

volume independent of fluctuations in resistance or pressure.[7] Gas volumes larger than the original compressed gas source can be supplied by the Venturi system, which is useful when the ventilator settings require a large I/E ratio combined with a rapid respiratory rate.

BELLOWS ASSEMBLY

The bellows assembly can be conceived of as two separate systems: One system, the anesthesia gas for the patient, is contained inside the bellows; a second system, the oxygen which supplies the driving force to power the anesthesia ventilator, is located between the outside wall of the bellows and the inside wall of the container. Bellows can be filled during the expiratory cycle with anesthesia gas from the bottom of the container (ascending bellows) or from the top of the container (descending or hanging bellows). An ascending bellows ventilator is shown in Figure 10-10. The ascending bellows will not fill unless the patient circuit is intact, thus providing a safety feature which can help detect a circuit disconnect. A descending bellows ventilator will continue to cycle during a disconnect because room air can enter the patient circuit at the disconnect point and fill the bellows as it descends via gravity. A hole in the bellows wall will entrain oxygen from the space between the container and bellows. For closed-circuit or low-flow anesthesia techniques the safest design is the ascending bellows.[5, 6, 8, 9]

Ventilator bellows can be set to deliver a range of volumes by control bars or plates, as shown in Figures 10-10 and 10-11. Numbers on the outside of the container wall are only rough estimates of the delivered tidal volume. The tidal volume will vary with a number of factors, for example, lung compliance and peak end-expiratory pressure.[10] When the exact tidal volume delivered becomes critical, it is necessary to interpose a measuring respiratory spirometer.

VENTILATOR CYCLE

Figures 10-12 and 10-13 show the North American Drager Anesthesia AV-E Ventilator with a descending bellows and an injector (Venturi device). Figures 10-12 and 10-13 will both be used to follow the cycle of the ventilator.[6] Component part numbers in parentheses correspond to the legend table of Figure 10-12.

Anesthesia gas flow rates are first determined by the anesthesiologist. Ventilator set-

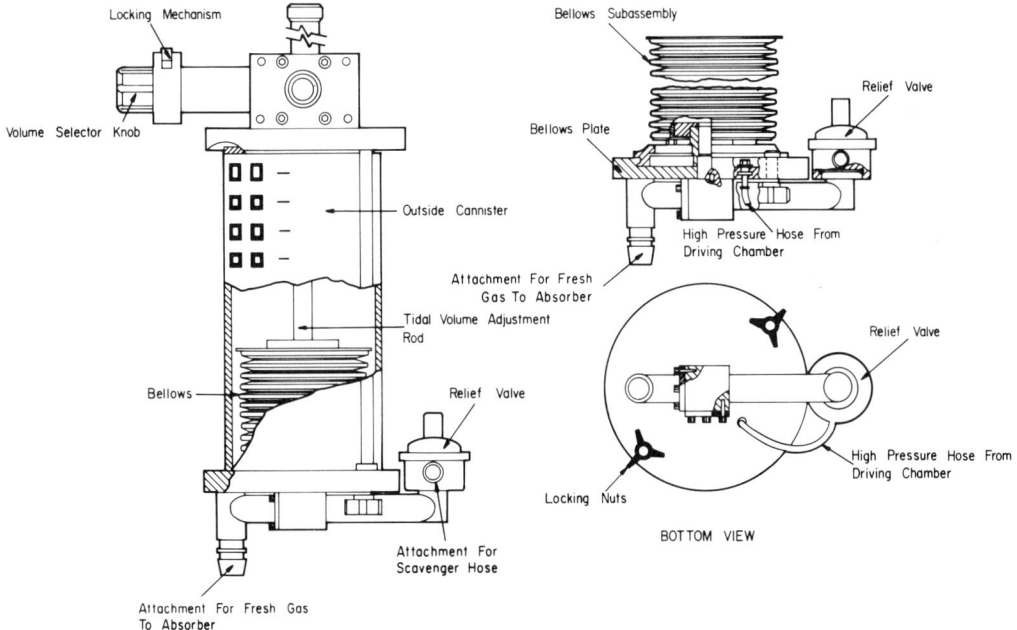

Fig. 10-10 Ascending bellows assembly. A cutaway in the side view shows the bellows inside the canister. The tidal volume adjustment rod is seen limiting the excursion of the bellows. The bottom view shows the high-pressure hose from the driving chamber connecting to the relief valve. The bellows subassembly shows the bellows plate. (Redrawn from Parts Manual. North American Drager, Telford, PA, 1984.)

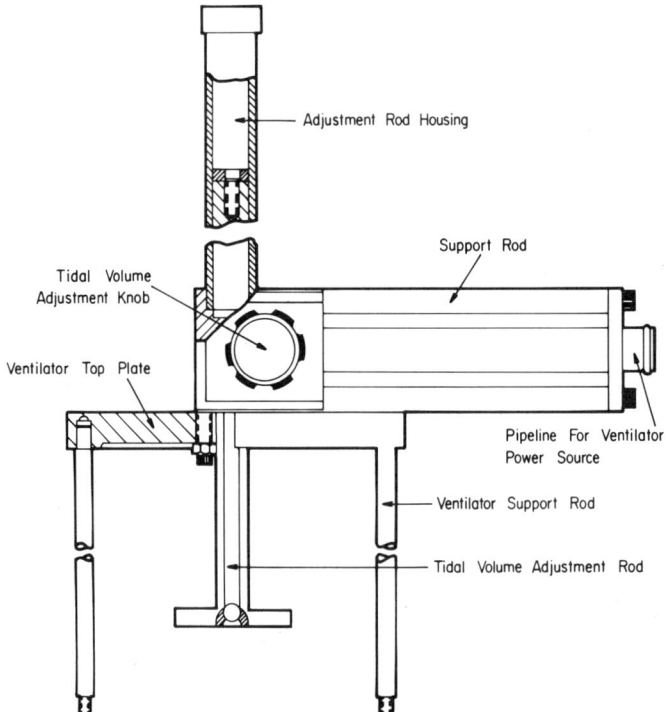

Fig. 10-11 Front view schematic of the ascending bellows adjustment mechanism. The adjustable rod limits the upward excursion of the ascending bellows. (Redrawn from Parts Manual. North American Drager, Telford, PA, 1984.)

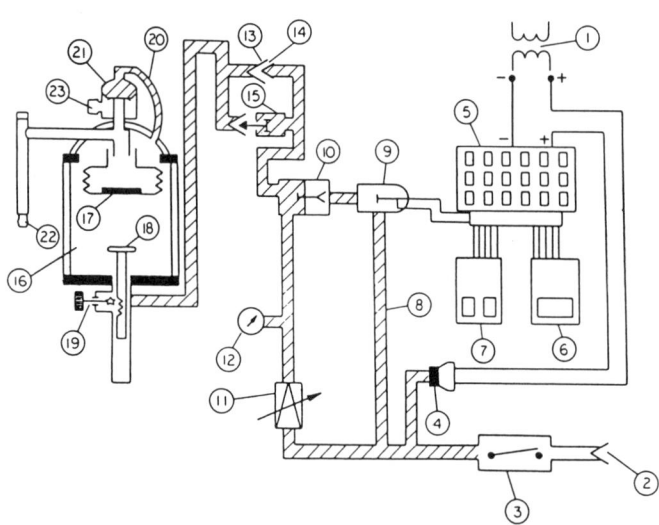

Fig. 10-12 Schematic of the Drager AV-E Ventilator. The two major divisions of the ventilator are the bellows assembly on the left and the control box to the right of the bellows (13). (1) Power supply, (2) oxygen supply, (3) on/off ventilator pneumatics, (4) on/off electrical supply, (5) electronic circuit board, (6) I:E ratio control, (7) respiratory rate control, (8) pressure line to solenoid, (9) solenoid valve, (10) control valve, (11) flow regulator, (12) flow indicator gauge, (13) injector (Venturi), (14) entrainment port, (15) pilot actuator, (16) bellows chamber, (17) bellows, (18) tidal volume adjustment plate, (19) tidal volume control, (20) relief valve pilot line, (21) ventilator relief valve, (22) connect to breathing circuit, (23) connect to scavenger. (Technical Service Manual. North American Drager, Telford, PA, 1985.)

tings are made for respiratory rate (6), tidal volume (18), flow rate (11), and I/E ratio (6). The switchover valve is turned to the setting which places the ventilator bellows in the breathing circuit and allows the inside of the bellows to fill with anesthetic gas. Turning on the on/off switch (3,4) activates the electronic circuits and allows oxygen from the anesthesia pipeline to flow into the pneumatic circuit (2). The solenoid valve is then automatically adjusted for opening time by the electronic circuit.

The inspiratory cycle begins when the solenoid valve (9) opens and oxygen at 50 psig begins to flow toward the bellows chamber (16). The bellows chamber is the space between the outside wall of the bellows and the inside wall of the container. Gas used for compression of the bellows flows through the flow regulator (11), past the control valve (10), and into the injector (13). Back-pressure from the injector closes the pilot actuator (13; see Fig. 10-14). As the oxygen passes through the injector, it entrains ambient air (14; see also Fig. 10-9) and the combined driving gas flows into the bellows. Increasing pressure from the driving gas in the bellows chamber forces the bellows to rise (Fig. 10-13A) and the anesthesia gas inside the bellows flows into the breathing circuit. The pressure increase in the bellows chamber is transmitted via the relief valve pilot line (20) to the ventilator relief valve (21; see also Fig. 10-15). The ventilator relief valve substitutes for the pop-off or APL valve. During inspiration the ventilator relief valve remains closed unless pressure in the bellows chamber exceeds 65 cmH$_2$O.

The inspiratory pause shown in Figure 10-13B occurs after the bellows reach maximal excursion and before the bellows begins to

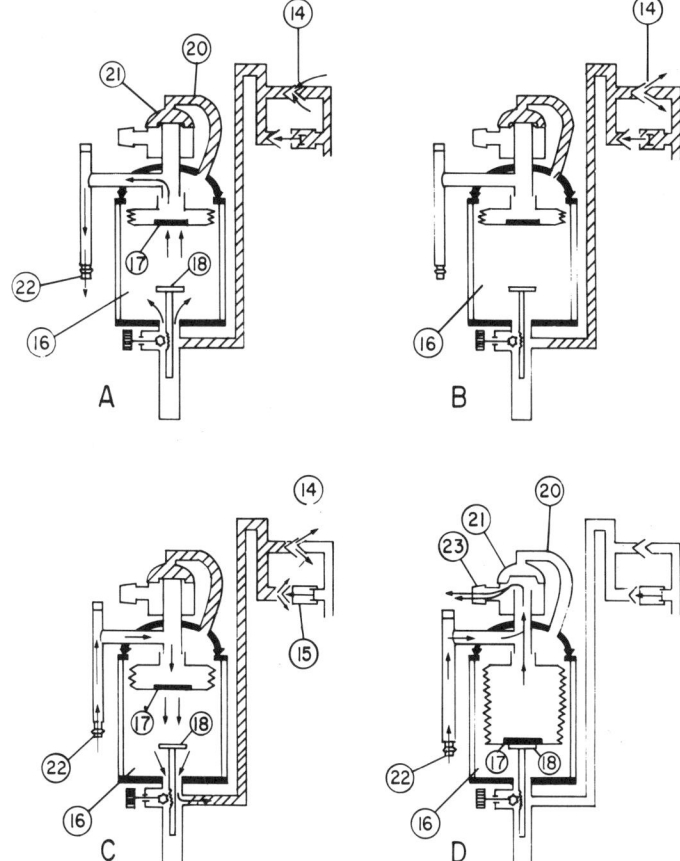

Fig. 10-13 A complete ventilator cycle. The same figure legend numbers apply here as in Figure 10-12. See text for explanation. (Technical Service Manual. North American Drager, Telford, PA, 1985.)

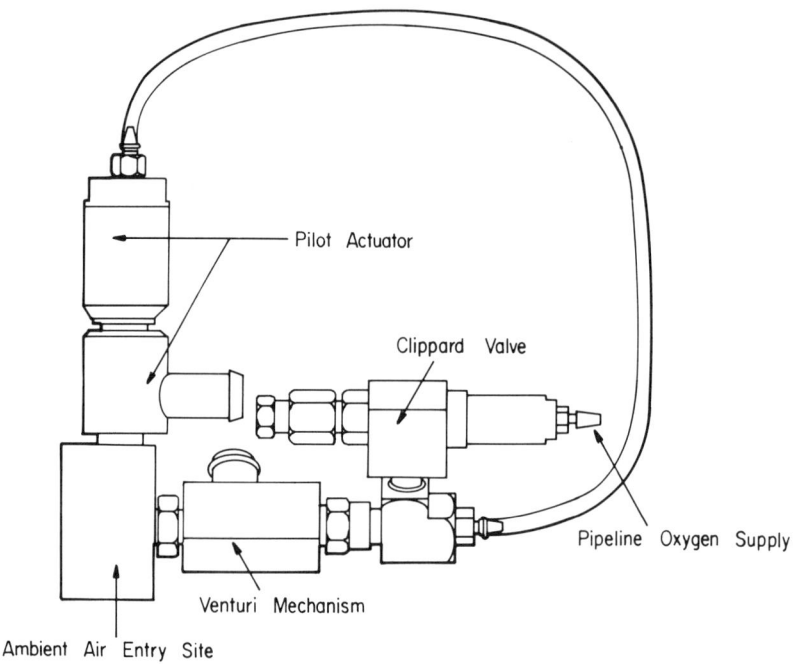

Fig. 10-14 Pilot actuator mounted in the control box of the ventilator. It controls the mixing of ambient air with compressed oxygen via the Venturi mechanism. (Redrawn from Parts Manual. North American Drager, Telford, PA, 1984.)

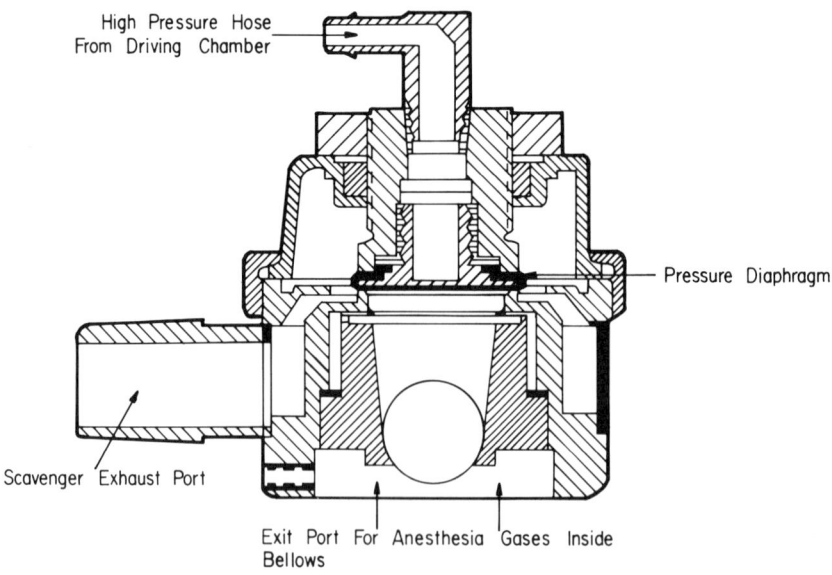

Fig. 10-15 Ventilator relief valve which exits fresh gas and exhaled gas inside the bellows to the scavenger interface. This valve is opened and closed by pressure fluctuations from the ventilator bellows chamber and functions as an automatic pop-off valve when the anesthesia ventilator is being used. (Redrawn from Parts Manual. North American Drager, Telford, PA, 1984.)

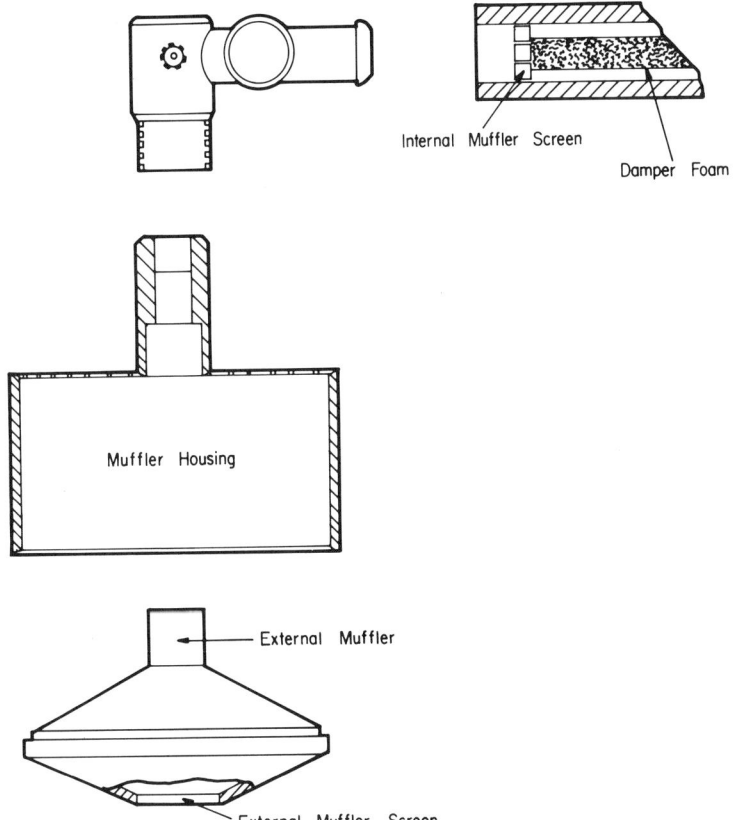

Fig. 10-16 Ventilator muffler exhaust. Ambient air is filtered prior to entering the ventilator control box on its way to the Venturi mechanism. Ventilator noise is also muffled. (Redrawn from Parts Manual. North American Drager, Telford, PA, 1984.)

move downward. During the inspiratory pause excess driving gas in the bellows chamber (16) exits through the entrainment port (14).

The expiratory cycle (Fig. 10-13C) begins as the solenoid valve is deactivated by the electronic circuit, which closes the penumatic circuit and stops all oxygen from going past the control valve. An immediate pressure drop occurs at the injector outlet, which allows the pilot actuator to open. All the driving gas in the bellows chamber discharges through the pilot actuator (15) and the entrainment port (14) of the injector into the muffler system. The muffler system shown in Figures 10-16 and 10-17 is a device which filters the ambient air entering the entrainment port and serves as an outlet for the driving gas in the bellows

chamber. As the pressure in the bellows chamber reaches atmospheric, the bellows descends by gravity and fills with the anesthetic gases in the breathing circuit.

When the bellows rests on the tidal volume adjustment plate (18), as shown in Figure 10-13D, the ventilator relief valve opens. Residual exhaled gases from the patient and excess fresh gas flow are discharged from inside the bellows to the waste gas-scavenging interface (23; see Fig. 10-17).

In summary, oxygen which supplies power to drive the anesthesia ventilator is exited to room air and does not enter the inside of the bellows. Excess anesthesia gas mixtures from the anesthesia machine flowmeters and exhaled gases from the patient are exited into the scavenger system.

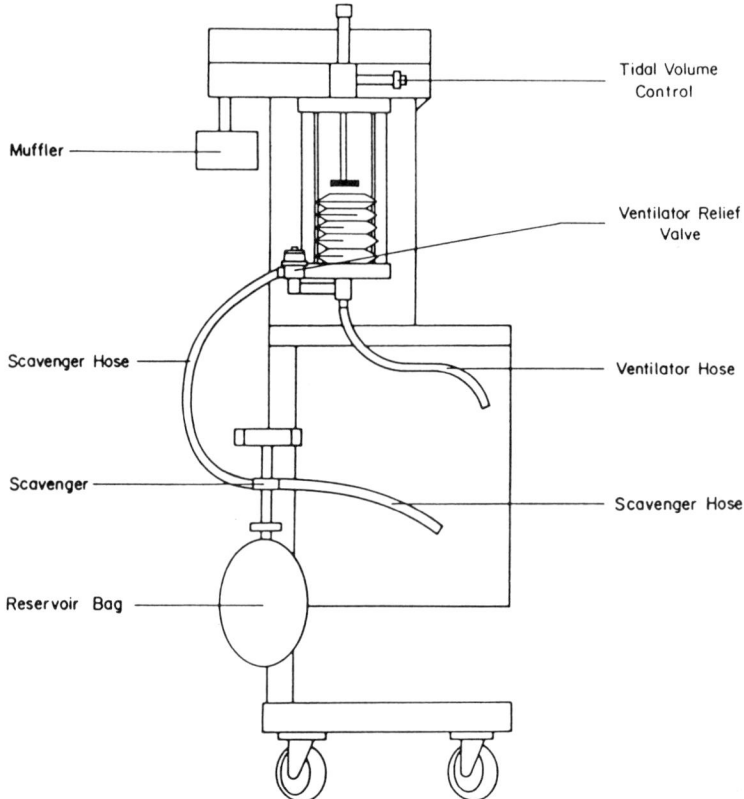

Fig. 10-17 Side view of the Drager Narkomed IIA anesthesia machine. Note the position of the muffler and the connections of the ventilator bellows assembly to the scavenger interface and breathing circuit. (Technical Service Manual. North American Drager, Telford, PA, 1985.)

LIMITATIONS AND FEATURES

Mathematical analyses of different ventilator cycles and their physiologic implications have been reviewed in a number of excellent sources.[11-13] A great deal has been said about the type of cycle, for example, sine wave versus square wave, and the duration of I/E. Current anesthesia ventilators are designed to maximize simplicity and yet remain functional in the role played in the operating room. In general, mechanical ventilation replaces a negative intrathoracic pressure with a positive intrathoracic pressure.[14] A rise in intrathoracic pressure can cause pulmonary capillary compression with a concomitant decrease in pulmonary perfusion.[15] Ventilation perfusion ratios are altered and physiologic dead space increases, requiring larger tidal volumes during mechanical ventilation to prevent carbon dioxide retention.[14] Patients taking sympathetic blocking drugs or with a low blood volume may not be able to compensate for the increase in mean intrathoracic pressure and may develop hypotension. On occasion, it will be necessary to bring in other ventilators for unusual cases, for example, a patient with adult respiratory distress syndrome requiring a pressure of 85 cmH_2O to ventilate in the intensive care unit.

Peak end-expiratory pressure (PEEP) valves can be placed in a number of positions in the expiratory limb of the patient anesthesia circuit. The NAD AV-E Ventilator has a PEEP valve built into the circuit (see Fig. 10-18). This valve is magnetically controlled and adjustable over a range of 0 to 20 cmH₂O. Function of the PEEP valve should be monitored by observing the pressure gauge in the

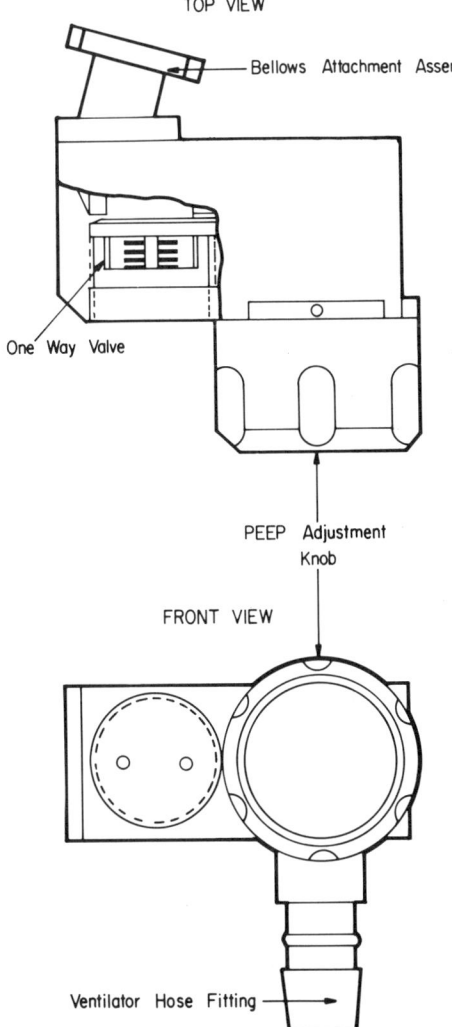

Fig. 10-18 The PEEP adjustment valve for the Drager AV-E ventilator. The valve attaches to the bellows assembly of the ventilator. The PEEP can be varied from 0 to 20 cmH₂O. (Redrawn from Parts Manual. North American Drager, Telford, PA, 1984.)

patient breathing circuit.

Auxiliary power supplies for the anesthesia machine alarm systems can be connected to the electronic circuitry and allow the ventilator to function during emergency conditions.

One must be aware that use of the compressed E oxygen cylinders on the anesthesia machine to power the ventilator will result in rapid depletion of the cylinder contents. A good rule of thumb is the following: Oxygen consumption to drive the ventilator is approximately the same as the minute volume delivered to the patient circuit.[4, 5] One testing source[10] found the Ohio fluidic ventilator to consume 22.3 L/min, the Air-Shields Controller ventilator to consume 12.9 L/min, and the Drager AV ventilator to consume 6.1 L/min.

The on/off switch of the NAD AV-E Ventilator has an upper (1200 hours position) and a lower (1800 hours position) on position. Positioning the on switch at 1800 hours activates a 60-second disconnect alarm, which allows the anesthesiologist to set the ventilator at extremely low frequency and high I/E ratios with an expiratory phase in excess of 15 seconds.[16] This ventilator will not function when the pipeline pressure is less than 28 psig.

The sigh volume on the Ohmeda 7000 Ventilator is set to deliver 150 percent of the tidal volume up to a 1.6-L maximum every 64 breaths. The number 64 was convenient for the logic circuit to achieve a sign every 6 to 7 minutes at a respiratory rate of 8 to 10 per minute. A regulator is placed between the solenoid valves and the anesthesia pipeline to reduce the pressure from 50 to 38 psig. The ventilator will not function when the pressure in the pipeline is less than 30 to 35 psig and flow is limited to 62 L/min.

Delivered ventilator volumes are dependent on the viscosity of the carrier anesthetic gas delivered to the lung. Oxygen is more viscous than nitrous oxide. The calibration of a ventilator will determine the output accuracy. One clinical study using a pressure-limited anesthesia ventilator suggested that factory calibration be done with a 3:1 mixture of nitrous oxide and oxygen.[17]

MAINTENANCE

All anesthesia ventilators should be included in the anesthesia machine quarterly preventive maintenance contract. Bellows and tubing will thus be cleaned at least every 3 months. Some individuals feel that since the inside of the bellows is within the patient breathing circuit, the bellows should be taken out and cleaned between every case or at least once a day. In fact, a disposable bellows assembly designed for one 24-hour use period is available.[18] I suspect the majority of anesthesiologists clean the inside of the bellows when they happen to think of it rather than on a routine schedule. It is prudent to at least disconnect the ventilator hose to the patient circuit at the end of the day to allow the inside of the bellows to air-dry overnight. Up to 1 pint of water has been found[2] in descending bellows by service personnel! Water left in the breathing circuit will lead to the growth of bacteria and molds.

COMPLICATIONS

Standards for anesthesia ventilators define minimal testing but are otherwise vague when compared to standards for rebreathing bags or anesthesia machines.[19] Some reasonable suggestions regarding ventilator performance testing have been made.[10] These suggestions might serve as the beginning of concise standards defining the function and purpose of anesthesia ventilators.

Between 1976 and 1980 the Device Experience Network (DEN) established by the Food and Drug Administration through the Division of Compliance Programs, Bureau of Medical Devices, collected 280 reports of problems with mechanical ventilatory devices.[20] The breathing circuit accounted for nearly 40 percent of the problems. Electrical circuit failures comprised 14 percent, mechanical failures 14 percent, and failures of controls, indicators, and alarms 14 percent.

Total electrical failure can easily be detected. Partial electrical failure can be very serious because of resultant insidious alveolar hypoventilation.[10] On/off switches for the ventilator have been discovered in the intermediate position with the potential for reverting to the off position spontaneously.[21] Switch design should eliminate any possibility of such an event.

Electromagnetic interference from sources such as cooling blankets, electrocautery, hemodialysis machines, and paramagnetic oxygen anaylzers has been reported to alter the function of the anesthesia ventilator.[10] Further research is necessary to define the type of electromagnetic interference present in the operating room environment. Appropriate data would then allow the ventilator manufacturer to correct the interference problem in a cost-effective manner.

High airway pressure from a malfunctioning pressure relief valve or a hole in the bellows can cause barotrauma.[20, 22] The high pressure from the bellows chamber is transmitted to the patient circuit and into the alveoli. Remember: When 50 psig is released directly into the lung, this represents approximately 3,500 cmH_2O! Gases will leak directly into the surrounding interstitial tissue to produce pulmonary emphysema. High pressures will allow the gas to dissect to the hilum of the lung, escape into the mediastinum, and finally into the fascial planes of the neck, where the gas will be manifest as subcutaneous emphysema.[15, 23] Compression of gas bubbles on the pulmonary capillaries, the pulmonary vessels, and the heart via cardiac tamponade in the mediastinum can result in marked alterations in cardiac output.

A hole in the bellows can lead to alveolar hyperventilation.[20] Oxygen from the driving chamber enters the inside of the bellow, causing hyperinflation of the lungs during the inspiratory cycle. An in-line oxygen analyzer reflects a rise in the concentration of oxygen in the circuit and may alert the anesthesiologist of an anesthetic machine malfunction. When air serves as the driving gas, the anesthesia gas in the breathing circuit will be diluted and could lead to hypoxemia in a compromised patient.

In one reported complication the breathing tubes of the patient circuit were extended. A portion of the tubes lay on the cold floor, allowing the water from the expired air to condense and accumulate from a number of patients. The internal expiratory valve of the ventilator was intermittently jammed by the water backflow. The last patient developed pneumothorax, mediastinal emphysema, and pneumoperitoneum.[24]

Rigid metal pipes in the ventilator can develop insidious leaks, causing ventilator malfunction.[25, 26] Paint flakes can blister off the base of the bellows assembly and enter the breathing circuit.[27] Sarnquist and Demas[28] recommend the use of an esophageal stethoscope for monitoring ventilator respirations. They report the failure of a ventilator timing valve in a very quiet ventilator. Pressure did not decrease in the breathing circuit, so the disconnect alarm did not sound. White noise in the operating room sufficiently masked changes in the sounds of ventilator function. Only the change in respiratory sounds in the esophageal stethoscope reflected the malfunction. The esophageal stethoscope "ventilator ear" is an extremely important monitor for the anesthesiologist to cultivate.

REFERENCES

1. Heironimus TW: Mechanical Artificial Ventilation: A Manual for Students and Practitioners. Charles C Thomas, Springfield, IL, 1967
2. Technical Service Seminar. North American Drager, Telford, PA, 4-9 April 1983
3. Howell RSC: Piped medical gas and vacuum systems. Anaesthesia 35:676, 1980
4. Operation Maintenance Manual. Ohio 7000 Electronic Anesthesia Ventilator. Ohmeda, Madison, WI, 1984
5. Service Manual. Ohio 7000 Electronic Anesthesia Ventilator. Ohmeda, Madison, WI, 1984
6. Technical Service Manual. North American Drager, Telford, PA, 1985
7. MacIntosh R, Mushin WW, Epstein HG: Physics for the Anaesthetist. 3rd Ed. Blackwell, Oxford, 1963
8. Graham DH: Advantages of standing bellows ventilators and low-flow techniques. Anesthesiology 58:486, 1983
9. Lin CY, Mosert JW, Benson DW: Closed circle systems: a new direction in the practice of anesthesia. Acta Anaesthesiol Scand 24:354, 1980
10. ECRI: Anesthesia Ventilators. Health Devices 8:151, 1979
11. Spearman CB, Saunders HG: Physical principles and functional design of ventilators. In Kirby RR, Smith RA, Desautels DA (eds): Mechanical Ventilation. Churchill Livingstone, New York, 1985
12. Schreiber P: Anaesthesia Equipment: Performance, Classification and Safety. Springer-Verlag, New York, 1972
13. Robinson JS: Principles of mechanical ventilation of the lungs. p. 132. In Gray TC, Nunn JF (eds): General Anaesthesia. 3rd Ed. Butterworths, London, 1971
14. Sellery GR: Hazards of artificial ventilation in the operating room. Can Med Assoc J 10:421, 1972
15. Newton NI: Safety in the operating theatre: the meaning of excessive airway pressure. Br J Hosp Med 25:504, 1981
16. Instruction Manual. Drager AV-E ventilator. North American Drager, Telford, PA, 1984
17. Jones CS: Gas viscosity effects in anesthesia. Anesth Analg 59:192, 1980
18. Disposable bellows. Air Shields Ventimeter®. Healthdyne, Hatoboro, PA, 1984
19. American National Standard for Breathing Machines for Medical Use. Z79.7-1976. American National Standards Institute, New York, 1976
20. Feeley TW, Bancroft ML: Problems with mechanical ventilators. Int Anesthesiol Clin 20:83, 1982
21. Ciobanu M, Meyer JA: Ventilator hazard revealed. Anesthesiology 52:186, 1980
22. Rendell-Baker L, Meyer JA: Accidental disconnection and pulmonary barotrauma. Anesthesiology 58:286, 1983
23. Newton NI, Adams AP: Excessive airway pressure during anaesthesia: Hazards, effects and prevention. Anaesthesia 33:689, 1978
24. Hilton PJ, Clement JA: Surgical emphysema

resulting from a ventilator malfunction. Anaesthesia 38:342, 1983

25. Rolbin S: An unusual case of ventilator leak. Can Anaesth Soc J 24:522, 1977

26. Wolf S, Watson CB, Clark P: An usual cause of leakage in an anesthesia system. Anesthesiol-ogy 55:83, 1981

27. Wald A, Mercurio A: Blistering of epoxy mate-rial of Narco Airshields® ventilator. Anesthe-siology 58:390, 1983

28. Sarnquist FH, Demas K: The silent ventilator. Anesth Analg 61:713, 1982

11

Safety Features of the Anesthesia Machine

Safety features for the anesthesia machine have achieved their present state through a long process of evolution. Anesthesia machines were initially an assembly of desired apparatus in one complex, for example, carbon dioxide absorber, gas pressure regulator, and flowmeters. Successful efforts have been made to standardize fittings, color-code compressed gas tanks, and so on. The combined efforts of industry, medicine, and government resulted in the formation of the American National Standards Institute, Inc. (ANSI). At present the ANSI "implies" a consensus of the members and is "intended as a guide to aid the manufacturer, the consumer, and the general public."[1] Perhaps, the next step in putting some teeth into minimum standards for anesthesia machines is to mandate ANSI standards as law.

The majority of safety features on the Drager Narkomed IIA and the Ohmeda Modulus II anesthesia machines are a result of the manufacturers' desire to provide a safe machine. Many of the features were suggestions from anesthesiologists. Safety features are an attempt to defeat the truism that if anything can go wrong, it will, and when it goes wrong it will probably cause the greatest damage possible.

Many of the safety features of the anesthesia machine are described in detail in other chapters, including such things as the pin index safety system for compressed gas tanks, see-through chambers for the carbon dioxide absorber, addition of ethyl violet to the carbon dioxide granules, vaporizer interlock systems, single-agent vaporizers, positive- and negative-pressure relief valves in the scavenger interface, key-index filling systems for vaporizers, baffles in vaporizers, and ascending bellows ventilators.

OXYGEN ANALYZERS

Many have expressed grave concerns about anesthesiologists who do not routinely use oxygen analyzers.[2-8] The causes of low oxygen concentrations in the breathing circuit are numerous but the end result to the patient exposed to long periods of hypoxia is the same. Oxygen analyzers are certainly not without fault. If they are properly maintained and calibrated, they can be used to assist the anesthesiologist in the detection of a very serious condition. Clinical signs, such as blood and skin color, heart rate, and blood pressure, are not reliable methods to detect hypoxia.[9] Some

183

states require the anesthesia machine to be equipped with a "device to measure the oxygen component of the gas being inhaled by the patient."[6]

Will the uniform adaptation of oxygen analyzers by anesthesiologists in the United States be as slow as the adoption of the pin index safety system? A survey[5, 10] in 1970 indicated 25 percent of anesthesia machines in use in the United States were not equipped with the pin index safety system, despite its being adopted as the standard in 1953. Any anesthesiologist in practice for more than 5 years can recall one or more times when the nitrous oxide was turned on instead of the oxygen or some other incident which could have led or did lead to a severe hypoxic episode. Oxygen analyzers are not the panacea of protection from hypoxia for the patient but they serve as an aid in detecting episodes of hypoxia.

Standards for oxygen analyzers have been established by the ANSI.[11] Each analyzer must read oxygen accurately within ±3 percent and maintain stability for at least 8 hours after calibration. When an alarm is present, it must activate within ±2 percent of the set alarm level. Illuminated alarms must be flashing or nonflashing red and audio alarms must have a frequency of 200 to 4,000 Hz, with a repetitive cycle of 1 to 5 seconds. Detailed expectations for testing, characteristics, and manufacture documentation are outlined in the ANSI standards.

Operating Principles

Oxygen can be analyzed by numerous methods but the two most practical for use in anesthesia have been the oxygen galvanic cell sensor and the polarographic oxygen sensor. Presently North American Drager and Ohmeda have chosen the oxygen galvanic sensor cell for oxygen analysis.[12, 13]

An *oxygen galvanic cell sensor* is an electrochemical device which converts the energy from a chemical reaction into an electrical sig-

nal. Output voltage is proportional to the oxygen pressure in the breathing circuit. The galvanic cell sensor has been called a microfuel cell, but in reality it does not regenerate itself.[14, 15]

Figure 11-1 illustrates the necessary components of an oxygen galvanic cell sensor. The sensor contains two electrodes, a lead anode and a gold cathode, surrounded by an electrolyte bath of CsOH or KOH. Oxygen molecules diffuse through a Teflon membrane and are reduced at the gold anode to hydroxyl ions.[12, 15, 16] The hydroxyl ions react with the lead cathode to form lead oxide and in the process release electrons. The output voltage is created by the electron flow through the external load resistor connecting the lead anode and the gold cathode. The voltage is proportional to the number of oxygen molecules reduced at the gold cathode, which is in turn dependent on the partial pressure of the oxygen at the Teflon membrane.

Oxygen galvanic cell sensors have a response time of 15 to 20 seconds to 90 percent of the total change in oxygen concentration.[12, 13, 16] Following a 10-minute warmup, sensors have been found to be extremely stable over a 7-hour period,[17] with an average drift of less than 0.5 percent. Life expectancy is dependent on the amount of exposure time to various concentrations of oxygen. Sensor cell lifetime is usually expressed in percent-hours; most cells have a lifetime[16] of 180,000 to 240,000 percent-hours. This means sensor cells continuously exposed to 21 percent oxygen will last 12 to 15 months, and those exposed to 100 percent oxygen will last 2 to 3 months. In addition, carbon dioxide can significantly reduce the life expectancy of the sensor cell.[12] An oxygen galvanic sensor cell placed in the expiratory limb of the breathing circuit and exposed to 80 to 100 percent oxygen and 2 to 4 percent carbon dioxide will have a markedly reduced lifetime. Simply removing the sensor from the circuit at the end of the day and placing the protective cap over the end can prolong the life of the sensor. Temperature changes in the monitored gas can

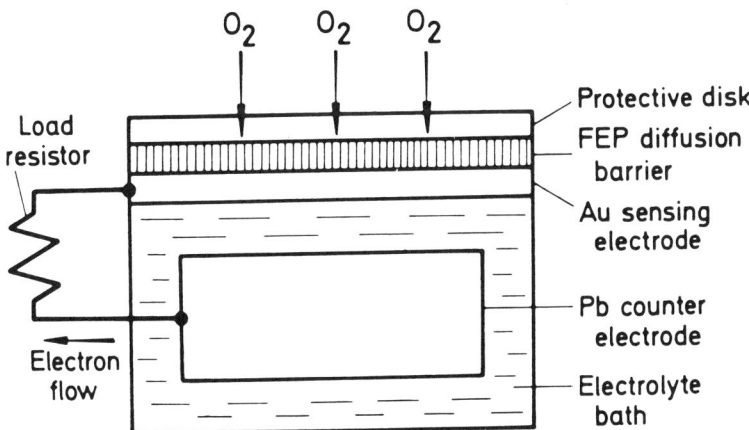

Fig. 11-1 Oxygen galvanic cell sensor. Oxygen molecules selectively pass through the Teflon diffusion barrier and are reduced to hydroxyl ions at the gold (Au) cathode. Hydroxyl ions react with the lead (Pb) anode to form lead oxide and release electrons. The output voltage across the external load resistor is proportional to the number of oxygen molecules reduced at the gold cathode. (Schreiber P: Anaesthesia Equipment. Performance, Classification and Safety. Springer-Verlag, New York, 1972.)

affect the output voltage of the sensor cell.[12, 13] Usually a thermistor is placed in the sensor housing to compensate for any temperature changes. Fluctuations in pressure may be seen when a ventilator is being used.[15] Moisture content in the breathing circuit will not affect the performance of the cell unless the water vapor condenses on the sensor membrane. The condensate functions as a diffusion barrier to oxygen molecules and may lower the actual oxygen concentration display.[12, 15] Sensors should be pointing down in order to reduce moisture buildup. Halothane and nitrous oxide do not significantly affect a galvanic sensor cell.[17]

Numerous safety features can be built into the oxygen galvanic sensor analyzer. Each analyzer can be equipped with two identical independent sensor cells which detect oxygen simultaneously and allow a sensor error detection signal to alert the operator should the difference between the two signals exceed a predetermined percentage. The likelihood of both sensors failing at exactly the same moment is extremely remote; thus, when the first sensor fails, the second sensor can continue monitoring until the exhausted sensor is replaced. Both low and high alarms which are preset by the anesthesiologist are available. Connecting the on switch of the oxygen analyzer to the main switch of the anesthesia machine will ensure that the oxygen monitor is turned on whenever the machine is in use. Autocalibration, which establishes zero and scaling constants for 12 hours, allows the anesthesiologist to calibrate the machine once in a normal operating day.[13] Shielding the analyzer with stainless steel will limit the radiofrequency interference created by equipment in the operating room.

Polarographic oxygen analyzers are similar to the common Clark oxygen electrode in the blood gas machine. Polarographic oxygen sensors depend on the chemical reduction of oxygen at an electrode surface. Oxygen molecules must first pass through a Teflon membrane and into a electrolyte solution of KCl. Electrolysis occurs at the polarized surface of the platinum (cathode) electrode. A reference silver (anode) electrode provides a fixed potential. The cathode is polarized negatively between -0.5 and -0.8 V with respect to the anode. Reduction of the dissolved oxygen to hydroxyl ion at the cathode produces an electric current directly proportional to the tension of the oxygen in the electrolyte solution.[15]

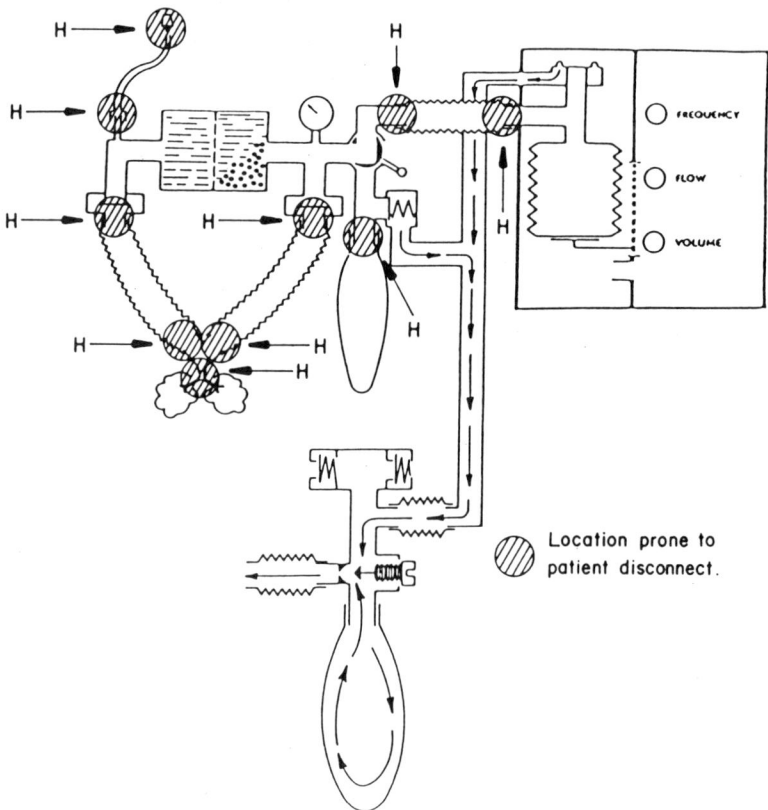

Fig. 11-2 Possible disconnect points in a circle breathing circuit: The need for a disconnect alarm and an ascending bellows instead of a descending bellows is readily apparent. (Schreiber P: Safety Guidelines for Anesthesia Systems. North American Drager, Telford, PA, 1984.)

Fig. 11-3 Fresh gas hose locking device for the Drager Narkomed IIA anesthesia machine. The spring-loaded device maintains a constant pressure at the standard 15-mm fresh gas outlet from the anesthesia machine pipeline. (Schreiber P: Safety Guidelines for Anesthesia Systems. North American Drager, Telford, PA, 1984.)

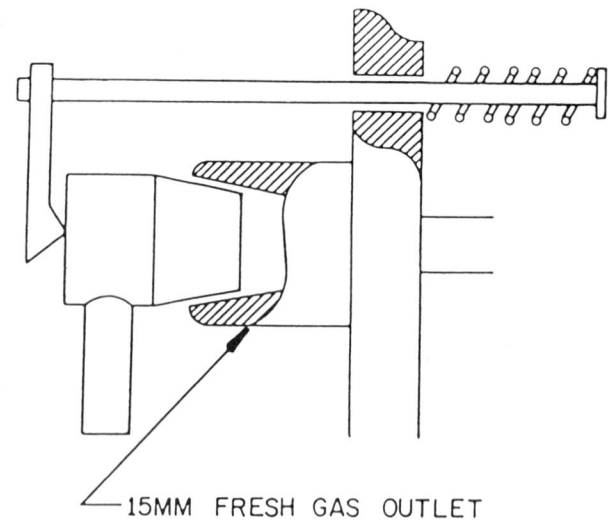

Polarographic oxygen sensors are capable of rapid responses, but the faster the response the shorter the sensor life.[18] Electrode response time is not limited by the electrode chemical reaction time but by the diffusion time of oxygen through the membrane and electrolyte.[19] A rapid response should make the electrode ideal for anesthesia. However, the polarographic analyzers are not widely used because of the demands for daily checkup procedures and extensive maintenance. Many technical problems associated with the polarographic analyzers have made the slower but more stable galvanic sensor cell the most popular analyzer.[15]

Small amounts of halothane can alter the readings of the polarographic analyzers by variable amounts.[20] In one instance, nitrous oxide was sensed as oxygen when the battery in the analyzer failed.[21] As the battery failed, the voltage threshold to the electrode was raised enough to reduce nitrous oxide. The increase in pressure in the breathing circuit caused by the ventilator during inspiration can also cause fluctuations in oxygen readings.[15]

Polarographic sensors are stable during storage because the diffusion of electrolyte through the 1-mil Teflon membrane is extremely slow.[18] Once the sensors are committed to use, the electrolyte gel must be changed regularly. The Teflon membrane does not require frequent changes. Sensors can be maintained for long periods of time with appropriate gel and membrane changes. Disposable units that last about 6 months[15] are also available.

DISCONNECTS IN THE BREATHING CIRCUIT

Disconnects in the breathing circuit are frequent and represent one of the highest areas of adverse incidents in the practice of anesthesia. Figure 11-2 shows a number of possible sites for disconnect in a circle breathing circuit. Most of the sites identified in Figure 11-2 are subject to standard recommendations by the ANSI.[1, 22] Much attention has been given to minimizing the number of disconnects and detecting a disconnect early when it does occur.

One of the most dangerous disconnects occurs when either end of the fresh gas hose comes off. Since the orifice of the inlet to the breathing system is small, this disconnect is very difficult to detect. Occasionally an oxygen analyzer will pick up the disconnect.[23] In the situation where an oxygen analyzer is not present and a descending ventilator is being used, the disconnect may go undetected. In order to limit this disconnect, the fresh gas hose has been designed to mate in a locking fashion with the carbon dioxide absorber inlet and the anesthesia machine outlet. Figure 11-3 shows the design of the fresh gas hose locking mechanism for the Drager Narkomed IIA anesthesia machine. A spring-loaded device maintains pressure against the standard 15-mm connection. Figure 11-4 shows the Ohmeda Modulus II fresh gas hose design. The spring-loaded attachment for the anesthesia machine outlet is shown in an enlarged view in Figure 11-5. The spring device must be completely engaged before the connection can be secured. Incomplete engagement of the fresh gas hose at the machine outlet will cause the internal spring to actually propel the fresh gas hose to the floor. The absorber end is antidisconnect and is provided with a push-button release mechanism. These two attempts to lock securely two mated components of the anesthesia machine appear to be advances in the right direction.

Various monitors of the breathing circuit have been developed to detect disconnects. Three of the most common disconnect alarms are pressure monitors, respiratory volume monitors, and end-tidal carbon dioxide monitors. Utilization of one alarm or all three alarms at once will not guarantee the detection of every disconnect.[24-26] We must realize the limitations of our equipment and be ever vigilant during the administration of anesthesia. When the patient is breathing spontaneously,

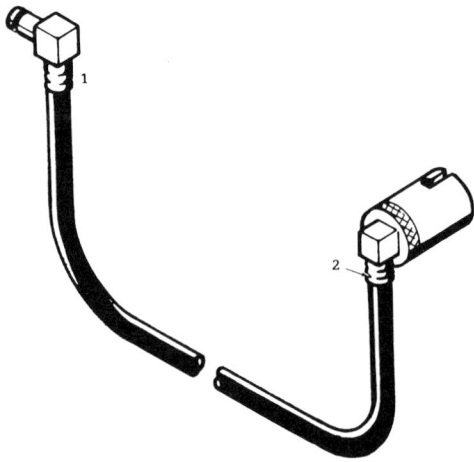

Fig. 11-4 Fresh gas hose designed for the Modulus II anesthesia machine: (1) attachment to the GMS absorber inlet and (2) attachment to the common gas outlet of the anesthesia machine. (Redrawn from illustration. Courtesy of Ohmeda, The BOC Group, Inc.)

movement of the reservoir bar is an excellent indicator of an intact circle system. When the ventilator is introduced into the circle system, a disconnect alarm becomes a necessity. A survey of Canadian anaesthetists in 1983 found that 87 percent of respondents used a disconnect alarm in the anesthesia circuit.[27]

Pressure disconnect alarms function by monitoring the amplitude of ventilator-generated pressure in the breathing circuit. An electrical pulsatile signal is generated from the pressure wave and compared to a preset alarm or reset point.[28] A small-diameter tube in the breathing circuit (Fig. 11-6), usually at the carbon dioxide absorber, transfers pressure waves to a common pressure manifold located in the main frame of the anesthesia machine. Figure 11-7 shows the female adapter end which accepts the tube from the carbon dioxide absorber sensing point. Figure 11-8 shows the multipurpose pressure alarm subassembly unit of the Drager Narkomed IIA containing

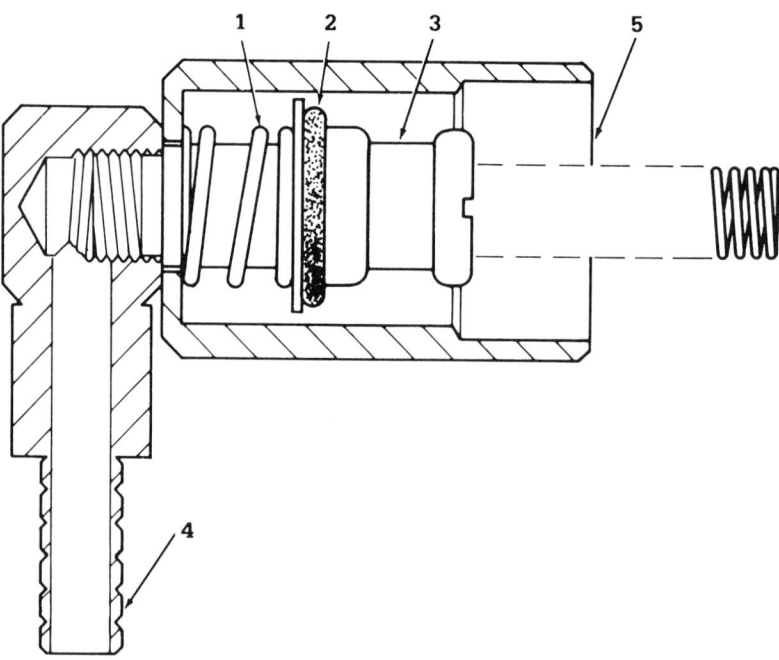

Fig. 11-5 Connector assembly for the fresh gas hose to the Modulus II anesthesia machine: (1) spring, (2) O-ring for a tight fit, (3) piping for fresh gas flow, (4) serrated nipple to attach the fresh gas hose, and (5) sleeve with bayonet slots (not shown) to provide positive engagement between this connector hose assembly and the common gas outlet. (Courtesy of Ohmeda, The BOC Group, Inc.)

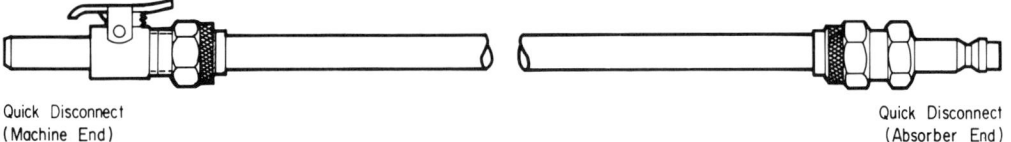

Quick Disconnect
(Machine End)

Quick Disconnect
(Absorber End)

Fig. 11-6 Pressure alarm hose. Both ends feature a quick connect–disconnect fitting. (Redrawn from Parts Manual. North American Drager, Telford, PA, 1984.)

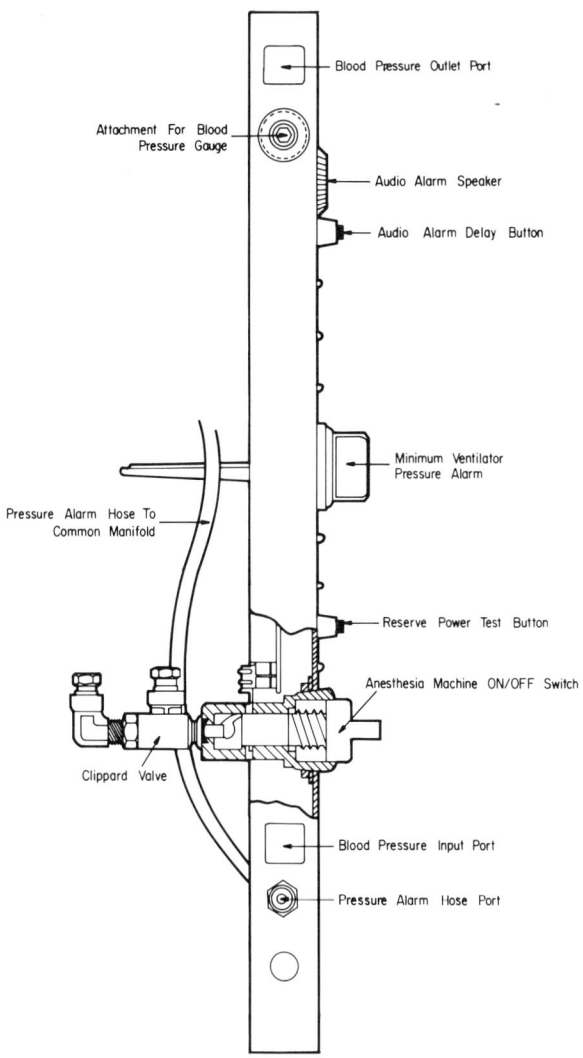

Blood Pressure Outlet Port

Attachment For Blood Pressure Gauge

Audio Alarm Speaker

Audio Alarm Delay Button

Minimum Ventilator Pressure Alarm

Pressure Alarm Hose To Common Manifold

Reserve Power Test Button

Anesthesia Machine ON/OFF Switch

Clippard Valve

Blood Pressure Input Port

Pressure Alarm Hose Port

Fig. 11-7 Side schematic of the central alarm panel for the Drager Narkomed IIA anesthesia machine. The pressure alarm hose from the breathing circuit is inserted at the pressure alarm hose port. Pressure waves are then transferred to the common manifold through the pressure alarm hose on the left. Turning the on/off switch to on activates the Clippard valve and allows gas to flow in the pneumatic circuit. (Redrawn from Parts Manual. North American Drager, Telford, PA, 1984.)

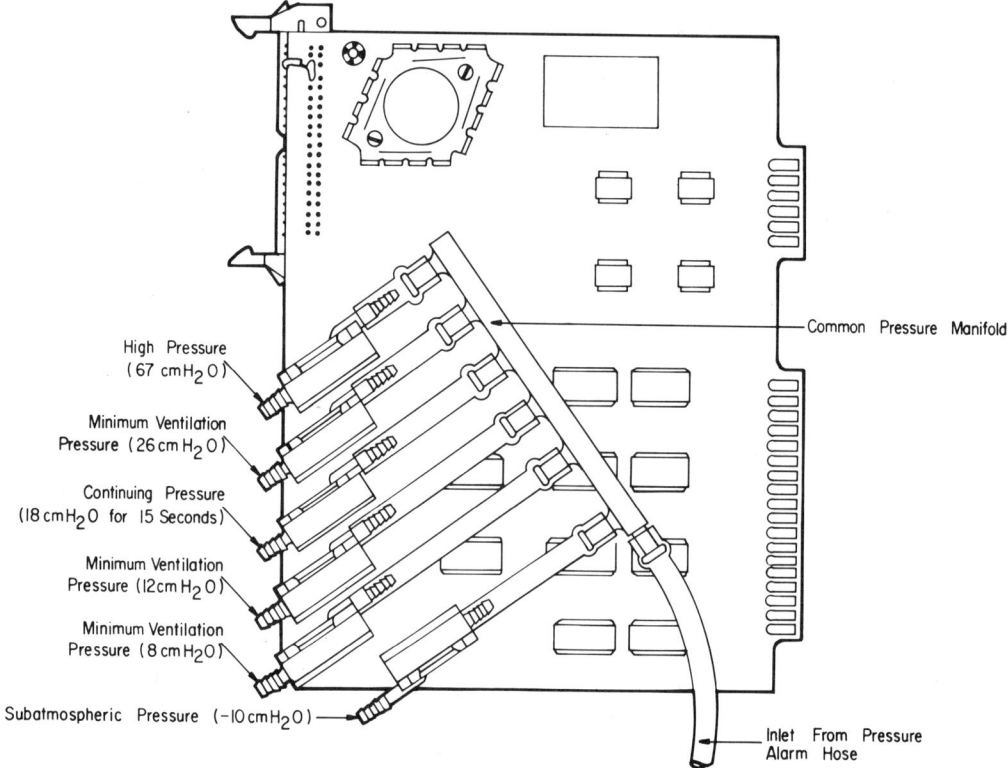

Fig. 11-8 Pressure alarm subassembly unit of the printed circuit board for the Drager Narkomed IIA anesthesia machine. Pressure waves from the breathing circuit enter the common pressure manifold. Specific sensory monitor numerous pressures. Alarm conditions for each pressure monitor are shown. See text for explanation. (Redrawn from Parts Manual. North American Drager, Telford, PA, 1984.)

three sensors ("pots") which detect pressures less than 26, 12, and 8 cmH_2O respectively, in the breathing circuit. Only one of these sensors is chosen by the anesthesiologist. Monitoring pressure should be set as close as possible below the expected peak of the ventilator cycle. If the monitoring pressure of 25 cmH_2O is chosen and the breathing circuit pressure does not reach 25 cmH_2O during a 15-second period or the frequency of ventilation is less than four a minute, the disconnect alarm will sound.[29] A switch is present on the Drager AV-E Ventilator which allows the delay time to be extended to 50 seconds. Use of this switch setting is to be discouraged except under very unusual circumstances, when ex-tremely low frequency respiratory rates or high I/E ratios are required.

Respiratory volume monitor disconnect alarms measure the total volume and rate of respiration in the expiration limb of the breathing circuit. An optical volume sensor is used on the Ohmeda Modulus II anesthesia machine. Figure 11-9 shows the two components of the system. The sensor clip is placed around the cartridge after it has been positioned in the expiration limb of the breathing circuit. Gas flows through the cartridge and spins a vane, as shown in Figure 11-10. An infrared light beam is passed from one arm of the horseshoe-shaped sensor clip to the other arm (see Fig. 11-11). Each time the light

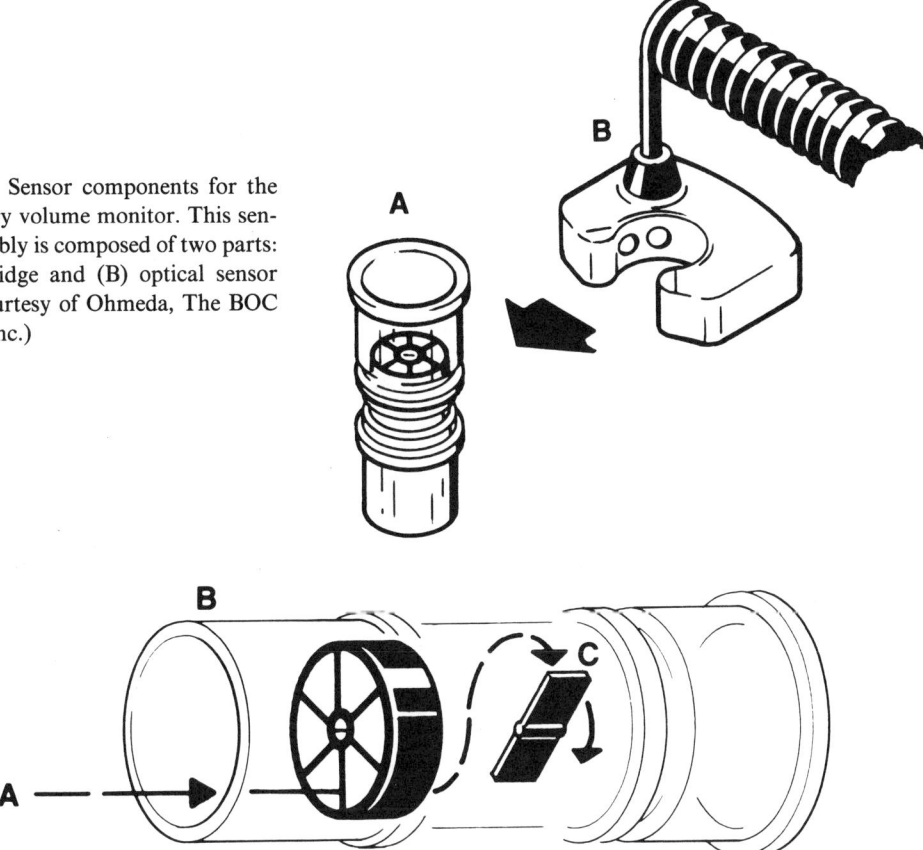

Fig. 11-9 Sensor components for the respiratory volume monitor. This sensor assembly is composed of two parts: (A) cartridge and (B) optical sensor clip. (Courtesy of Ohmeda, The BOC Group, Inc.)

Fig. 11-10 Cartridge (B) of the respiratory volume monitor. Gas flows from the expiratory limb of the breathing circuit through A and spins vane C. (Courtesy of Ohmeda, The BOC Group, Inc.)

Fig. 11-11 Schematic of the optical sensor clip of the respiratory volume monitor. The optical sensor (A) generates a voltage pulse (B) each time a light beam (C) is blocked by the spinning vane (D). A computer in the monitor counts the voltage pulses, processes the data, displays the information, and triggers an alarm if the tidal volume or respiratory rate fall outside the preset levels. (Courtesy of Ohmeda, The BOC Group, Inc.)

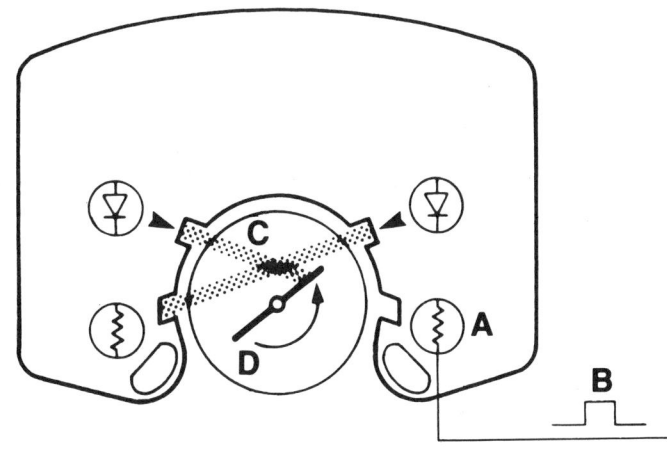

is interrupted by the spinning vane the optical sensor in the arm of the sensor clip generates a voltage which is proportional to the gas flow volume through the sensor. A computer in the monitor control box counts the voltage pulses, and if the tidal volume or respiratory rate is less than a critical preset number the alarm is triggered.

End-tidal carbon dioxide monitors can be used as disconnect alarms. Infrared carbon dioxide analyzers are extremely rapid and can easily detect breath-by-breath changes in carbon dioxide. The measurement technique is based on the absorption of infrared radiation by gases having polyatomic asymmetric molecules (see Chap. 7 for a detailed explanation). The selected wavelength for carbon dioxide is 4.26 μm because of the presence of a strong absorption band which avoids water vapor interference. Figure 11-12 is a picture of a carbon dioxide monitor with features allowing the monitoring of end-tidal, inspiratory mini-

mum, or instantaneous carbon dioxide levels in the breathing circuit. High and low alarms are available. End-tidal carbon dioxide levels rapidly decrease when there is total lack of ventilation, complete obstruction of the endotracheal tube, or presence of the endotracheal tube in the esophagus.[28] The carbon dioxide monitor at present may be the best means to detect a patient disconnect.[22]

OXYGEN SOURCE FAILURE

As the oxygen pressure in the anesthesia machine pipeline decreases, a number of systems begin to function to alert the anesthesiologist of a low oxygen pressure and stop the flow of all gases other than oxygen.

An *oxygen supply pressure alarm* will trigger an audio and/or visual alarm on the Narkomed IIA when the oxygen supply pressure decreases below 30 psig.

One of the first systems adapted to the an-

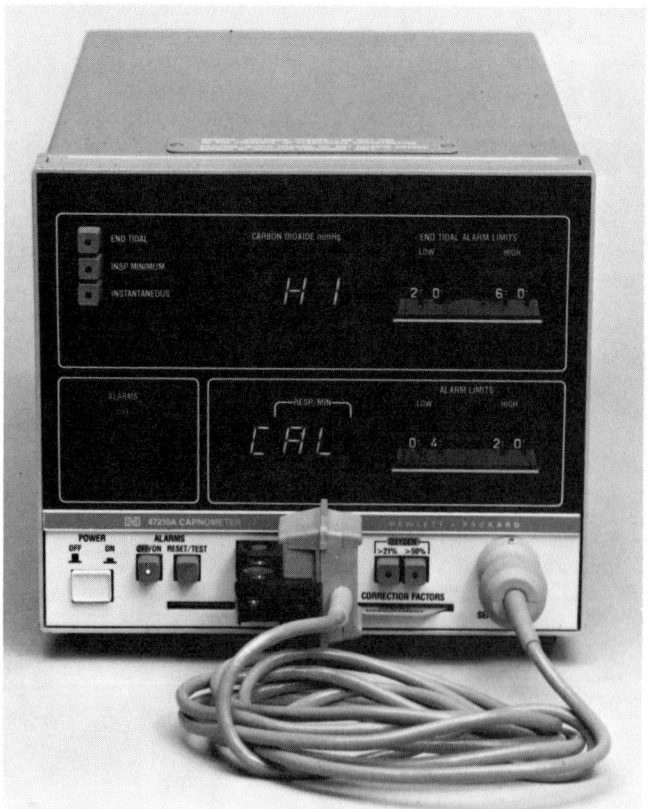

Fig. 11-12 End-tidal carbon dioxide monitor. The instrument is useful in detecting certain breathing circuit disconnects. (Courtesy of Hewlett-Packard, Co., Waltham, MA, 1985. Reproduced with permission.)

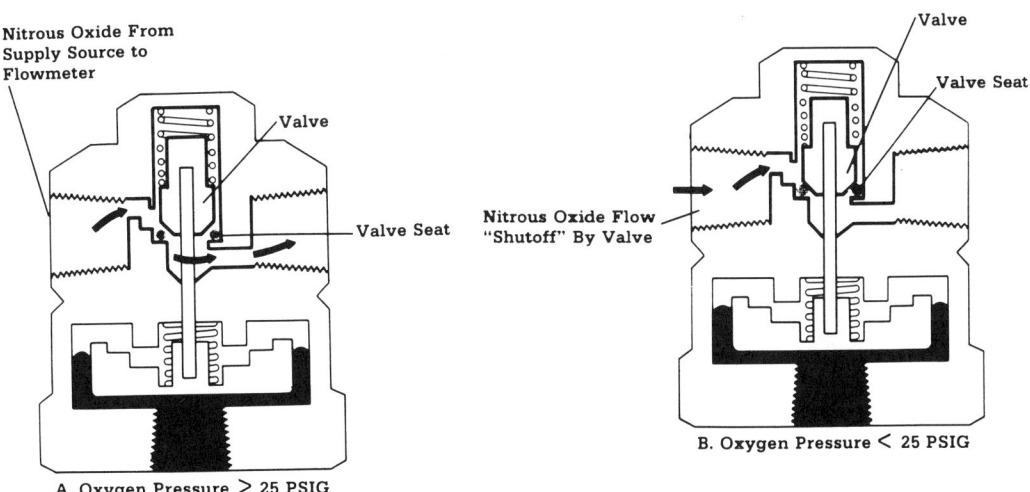

Fig. 11-13 Pressure sensor shutoff valve commonly referred to as the fail safe valve. When oxygen line pressure exceeds 25 psig (left) the pressure on the diaphragm will keep the valve open and allow nitrous oxide to flow. A decrease in oxygen line pressure to below 25 psig (right) will allow the spring tension to engage the valve on the valve seat and shut off all nitrous oxide flow. (Reproduced with permission from Bowie E, Huffman LM: The Anesthesia Machine: Essentials for Understanding. Ohmeda, The BOC Group, Inc., 1985.)

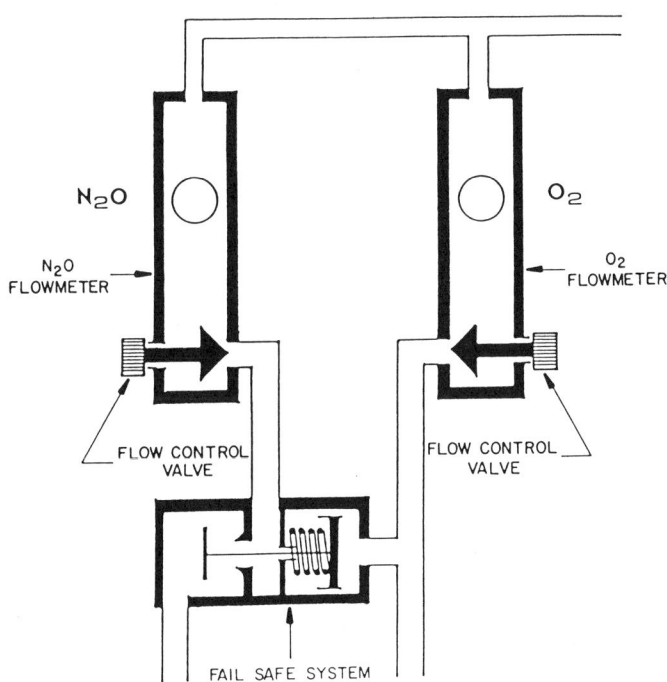

Fig. 11-14 The oxygen failure protection system for the Narkomed IIA anesthesia machine. Oxygen line pressure forces the diaphragm against the spring, opening the orifice to the flow of nitrous oxide. When the oxygen line pressure reaches a critical low level, the spring tension pushes the diaphragm against the orifice and completely stops the flow of nitrous oxide. (Schreiber P: Safety Guidelines for Anesthesia Systems. North American Drager, Telford, PA, 1984.)

esthesia machine was the oxygen failure protection device, or so-called *fail-safe system,* which has been and still is widely overestimated.[22, 30, 31] The purpose of the fail-safe system is to stop the flow of nitrous oxide when the oxygen pressure reaches a critical level. Figures 11-13 and 11-14 illustrate the fail-safe systems of the Ohmeda Modulus II and the Drager Narkomed IIA anesthesia machines. In principle, a diaphragm separates nitrous oxide from oxygen. Pressure in the oxygen line pushes against a diaphragm and opens an orifice through which the nitrous oxide can flow. At pressures greater than 25 psig, nitrous oxide will continue to flow. When the oxygen line pressure drops below 25 psig, a spring pushes a shutoff valve onto a valve seat and stops all nitrous oxide flow into the distal portion of the pipeline. The nitrous oxide compressed tank or hospital source is still on but flow has ceased. All gas systems in the anesthesia machine—air, carbon dioxide,

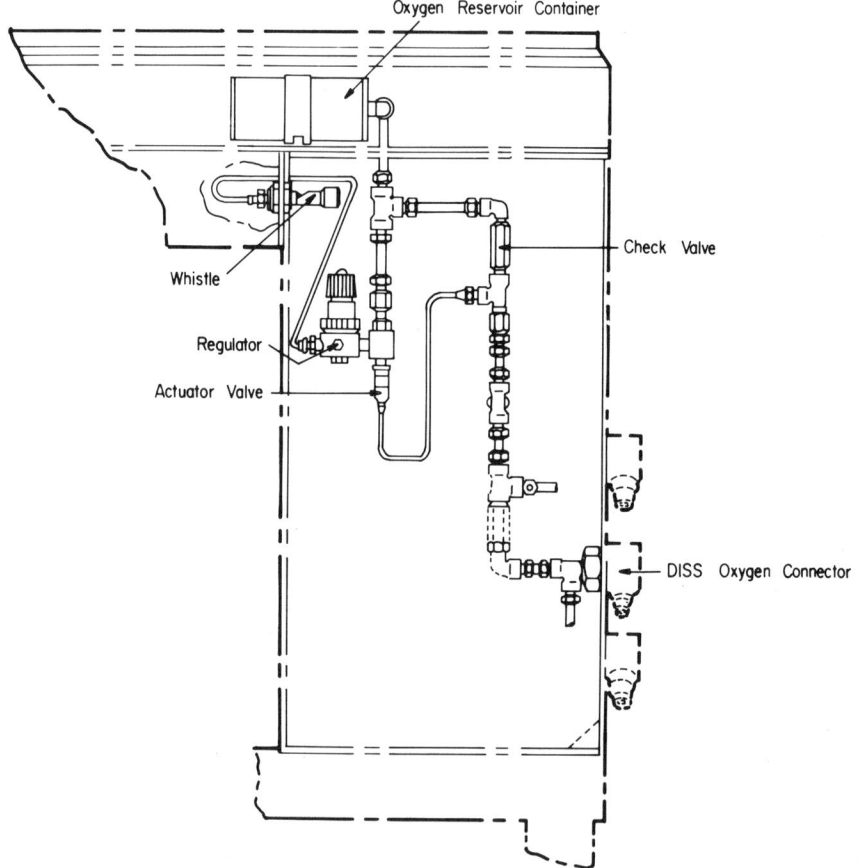

Fig. 11-15 Oxygen whistle alarm for the Drager Narkomed IIA anesthesia machine. The oxygen reservoir container and whistle alarm are mounted behind the back panel of the anesthesia machine's main frame. The oxygen reservoir container is filled when the anesthesia machine is turned on. When oxygen pressure falls below 30 to 35 psig, the oxygen in the container bleeds through the whistle alarm. (Redrawn from Parts Manual. North American Drager, Telford, PA, 1984.)

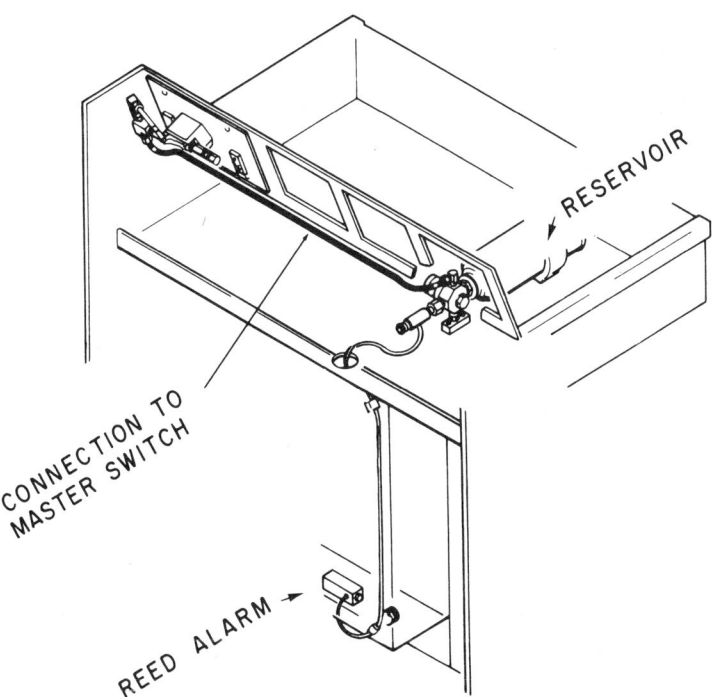

Fig. 11-16 Oxygen Supply Failure Alarm system for the Modulus II anesthesia machine. (Courtesy of Ohmeda, The BOC Group, Inc.)

and so forth—are activated by oxygen pressure in a similar fashion. Hypoxic mixtures can still be given with the fail-safe system in place.[32] It is important to remember that the system only stops the flow of nitrous oxide and other gases when the oxygen supply reaches a critical level.

The last alarm to sound indicating a decreased oxygen line pressure will be the *oxygen whistle alarm*. When the anesthesia machine is turned on, a thermoslike reservoir container is filled with oxygen from the anesthesia pipeline (see Fig. 11-15 to 11-17). A decrease in oxygen line pressure below 30 to 35 psig allows the container to release its contents of oxygen through a reed which makes a whistle sound[29] for approximately 10 seconds. The whistle can sometimes be heard when the anesthesia machine is turned off and the oxygen line pressure decreases.

OXYGEN FLUSH VALVE

Oxygen is required rapidly and in large amounts in the everyday practice of anesthesia. The oxygen flush valve has been designed to deliver 45 to 70 L/min of oxygen with immediate push-button on and off capabilities. Since oxygen may be required in emergency situations, the oxygen flush valve is connected directly to both the wall oxygen source and the compressed oxygen tanks (Fig. 11-18). Once the flush valve is engaged, the oxygen goes directly to the fresh gas common outlet.

An oxygen flush valve assembly is shown in the schematic of Figure 11-19. Pushing the oxygen flush button lifts a ball valve off the valve seat and allows oxygen to enter the fresh gas outlet (Fig. 11-20). As the oxygen under high pressure (45 to 50 psig) passes into the fresh gas hose, it must first pass through a

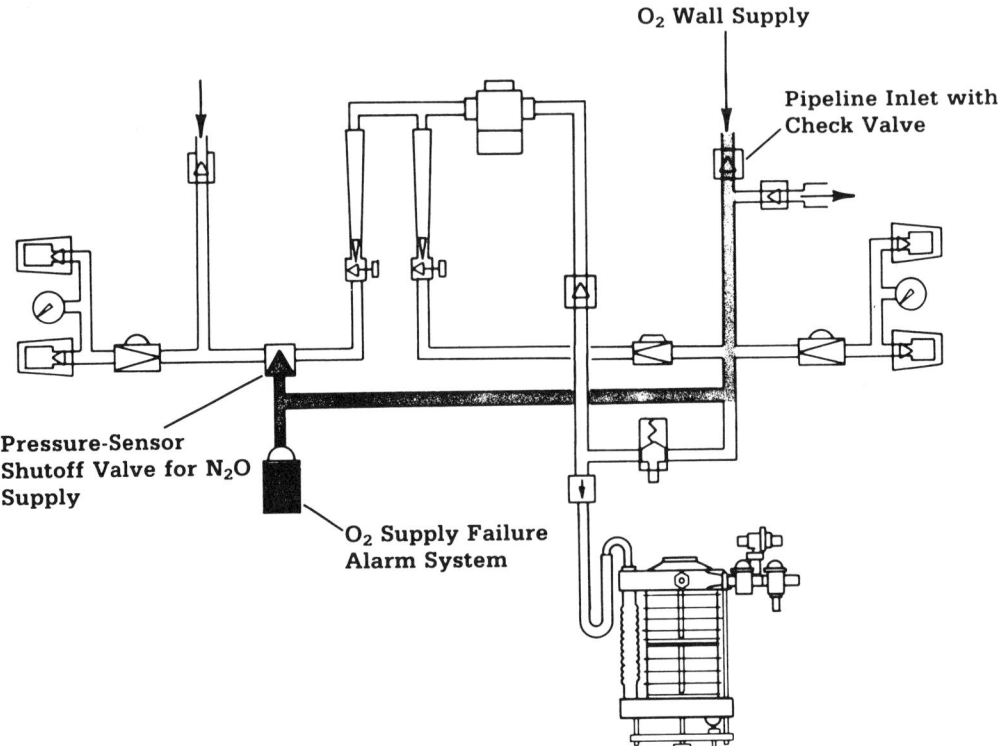

Fig. 11-17 Piping diagram of the oxygen supply failure alarm system in the anesthesia machine. A direct line comes from the wall oxygen supply or compressed gas cylinder(s) to the "whistle alarm" and pressure sensor shutoff valve. (Reproduced with permission from Bowie E, Huffman LM: The Anesthesia Machine: Essentials for Understanding. Ohmeda, The BOC Group, Inc., 1985.)

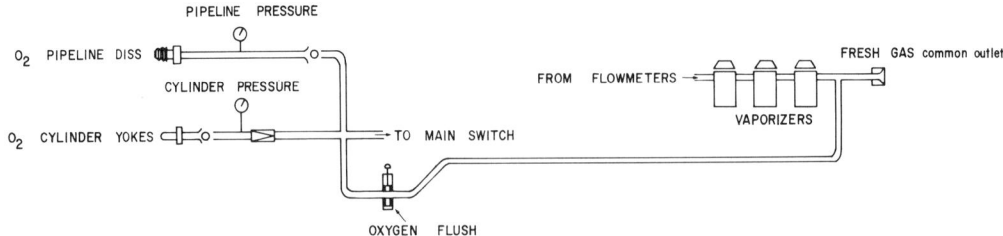

Fig. 11-18 Pipeline diagram for the oxygen flush valve on the Drager Narkomed IIA anesthesia machine. A direct line goes to the oxygen flush valve from the oxygen hospital pipeline and the oxygen cylinders. Oxygen flow from the flush valve bypasses flowmeters and vaporizers to enter directly into the fresh gas common outlet. (Redrawn from Technical Services Manual. North American Drager, Telford, PA, 1985.)

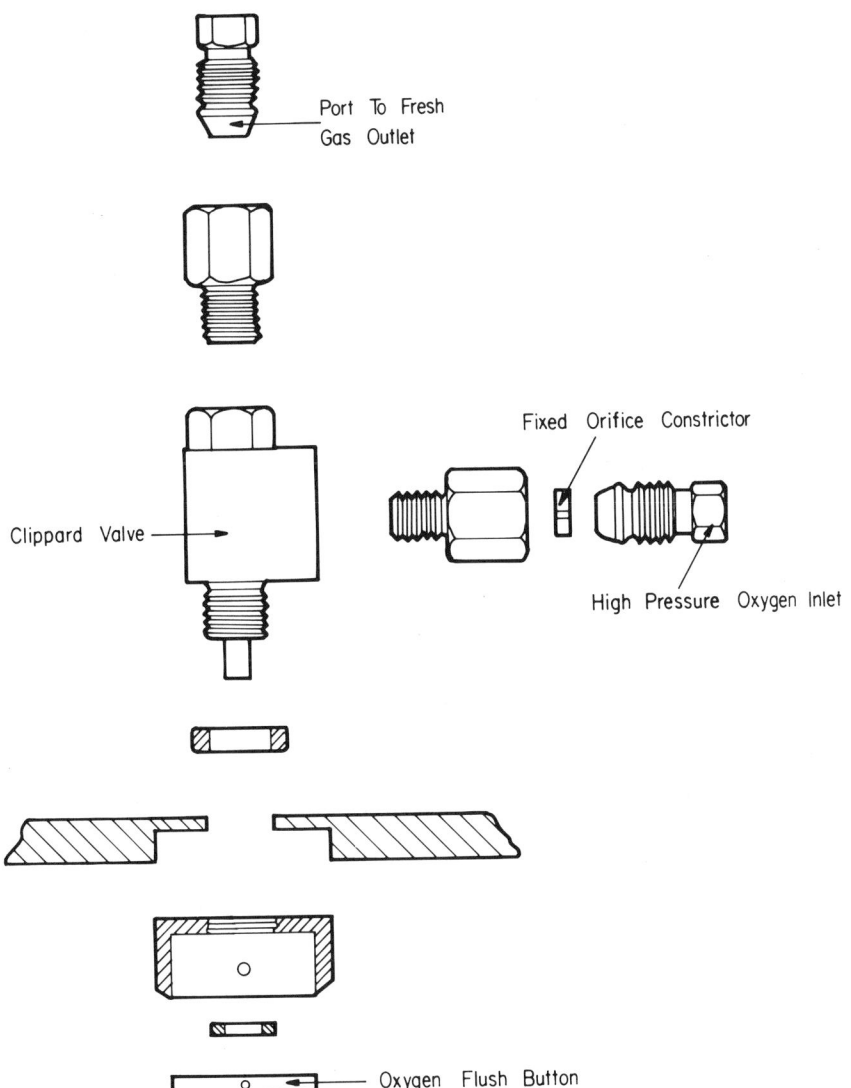

Fig. 11-19 Oxygen flush valve assembly for the Drager Narkomed IIA anesthesia machine. The fixed orifice constrictor limits the oxygen flow into the fresh gas outlet to 50 to 70 L/min. (Redrawn from Parts Manual. North American Drager, Telford, PA, 1984.)

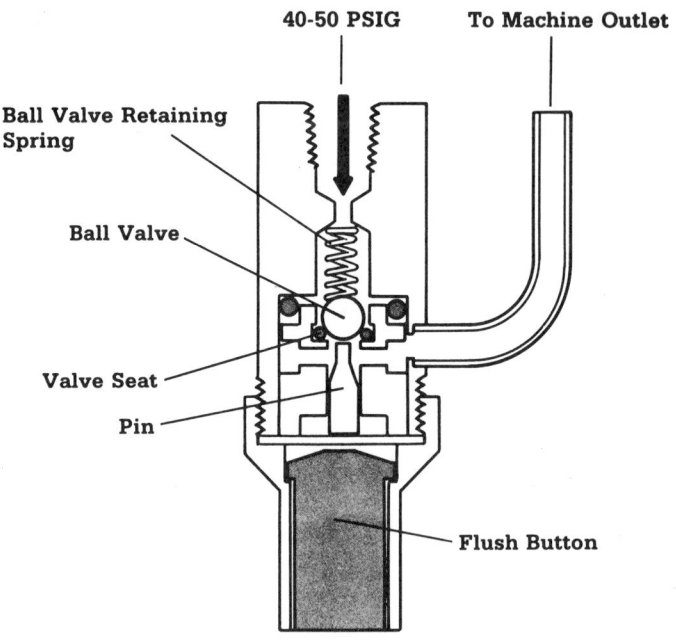

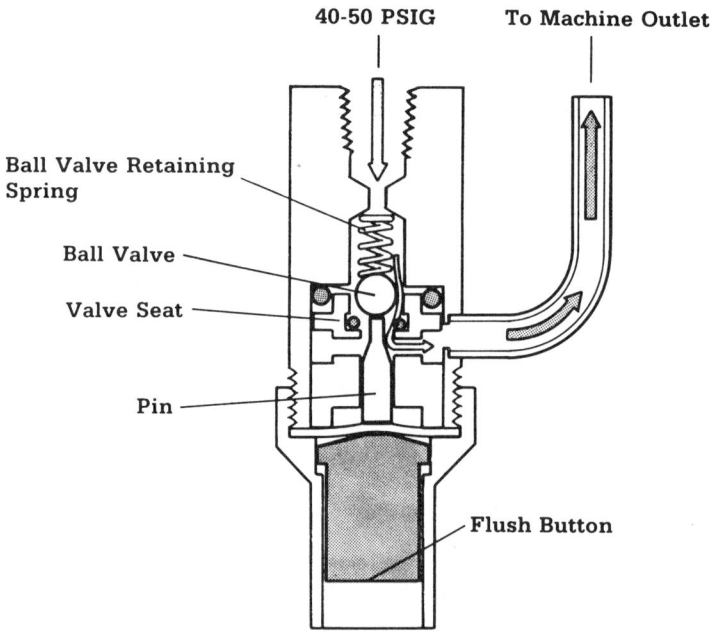

Fig. 11-20 Oxygen flush valve for the anesthesia machine. A spring holds the ball valve against the valve seat when the oxygen flush valve is in the closed position (top; note neutral position of flush button). Pushing the oxygen flush button inward forces the ball valve off the valve seat and oxygen with a pressure less than 40 to 50 psig flows to the machine outlet at flow rates between 35 and 70 L/min (bottom). (Reproduced with permission from Bowie E, Huffman LM: The Anesthesia Machine: Essentials for Understanding. Ohmeda, The BOC Group, Inc., 1985.)

fixed orifice constrictor (see Fig. 11-19) which limits the oxygen flow to a range of 45 to 70 L/min. Removal of the orifice constrictor[33] will allow oxygen flow rates of up to 250 L/min.

The ANSI standard states the oxygen flush valve "shall be clearly and permanently marked to show its function."[1] On the Drager Narkomed IIA and the Ohmeda Modulus II anesthesia machines the oxygen flush button is painted green, placed at the front of the machine for easy access, and surrounded by a protective rim. The rim protects the oxygen flush valve from accidental damage and serves as a tactile signal to the anesthesiologist so the oxygen flush button can be found while maintaining eye contact with the patient.

OXYGEN–NITROUS OXIDE MIXTURES

Alarm systems are available which will alert the anesthesiologist when a mixture of oxygen and nitrous oxide is potentially hypoxic. One such device is the oxygen ratio monitor (ORM) shown in Figures 11-21 to 11-23. Resistors between the nitrous oxide and oxygen flowmeter control valves and the fine flow tubes create a back-pressure. The back-pressure from each gas passes into a chamber containing a diaphragm, as seen in Figure 11-21. An electrical switch contact is attached to a movable shaft connecting the two diaphragms. High oxygen pressure opens the switch contacts. Increased back pressure from a high ni-

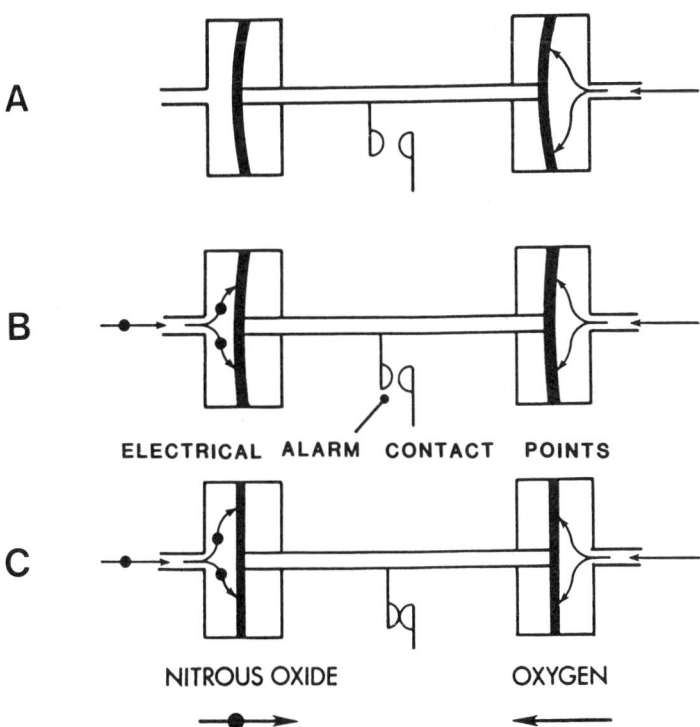

Fig. 11-21 Principle of the oxygen ratio monitor (ORM) alarm of the Drager Narkomed IIA anesthesia machine. Oxygen flow back-pressure pushes against a diaphragm connected by a shaft to a second diaphragm. (A) Oxygen pressure breaks the electrical switch contact. (B) Nitrous oxide is introduced and creates a counter-back-pressure to oxygen. (C) Oxygen flow has decreased to less than 30 ± 5 percent of the combined oxygen–nitrous oxide flow. The switch contacts close and activate the ORM audio and/or visual alarms. (Redrawn from Technical Service Manual. North American Drager, Telford, PA, 1985.)

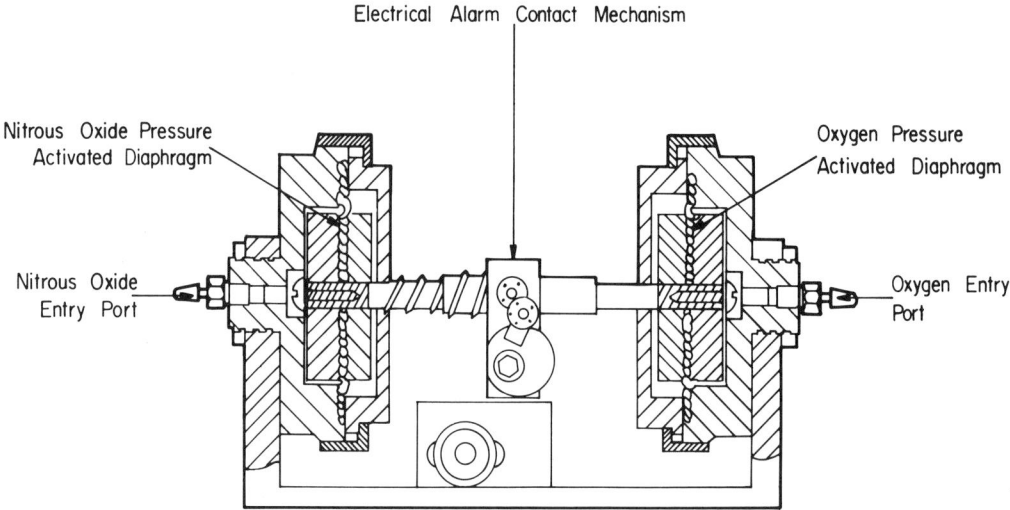

Fig. 11-22 Schematic of the oxygen ratio monitor of the Drager Narkomed IIA anesthesia machine. Note the nitrous oxide and oxygen pressure-activated diaphragms connected by a shaft to the electrical alarm contact mechanism. (Redrawn from Parts Manual. North American Drager, Telford, PA, 1985.)

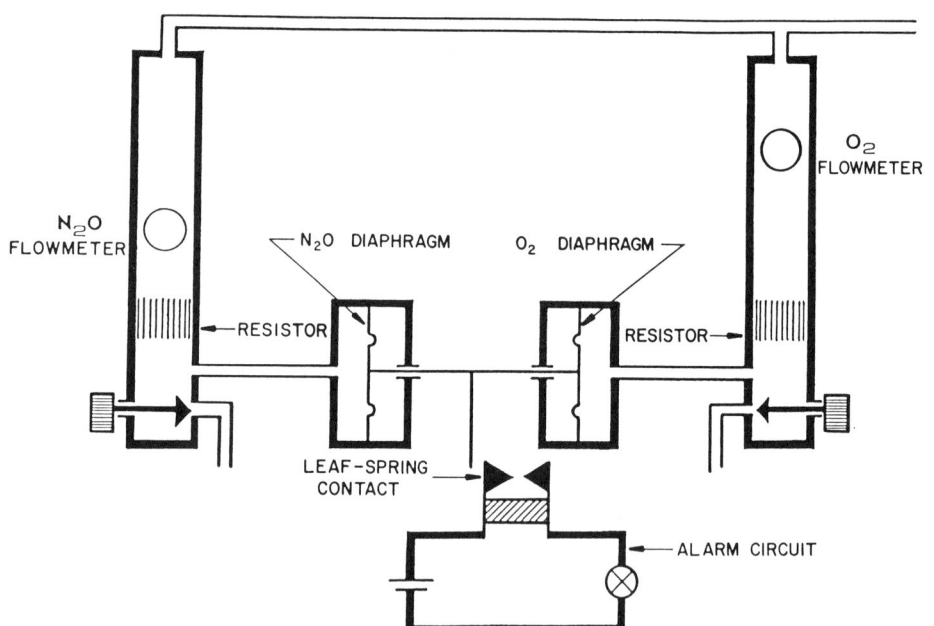

Fig. 11-23 Schematic of the placement of the oxygen ratio monitor in the Narkomed IIA anesthesia machine. The resistor in the nitrous oxide and oxygen flowmeters produces a back-pressure representative of the gas flow. The ratio of the backflow against the two diaphragms determines the position of the electric switch contact on the shaft connecting the diaphragms. When oxygen decreases below the preset safety level, the alarm circuit is activated. (Schreiber P: Safety Guidelines for Anesthesia Systems. North American Drager, Telford, PA, 1984.)

TOP VIEW

ORM Reference Control Box

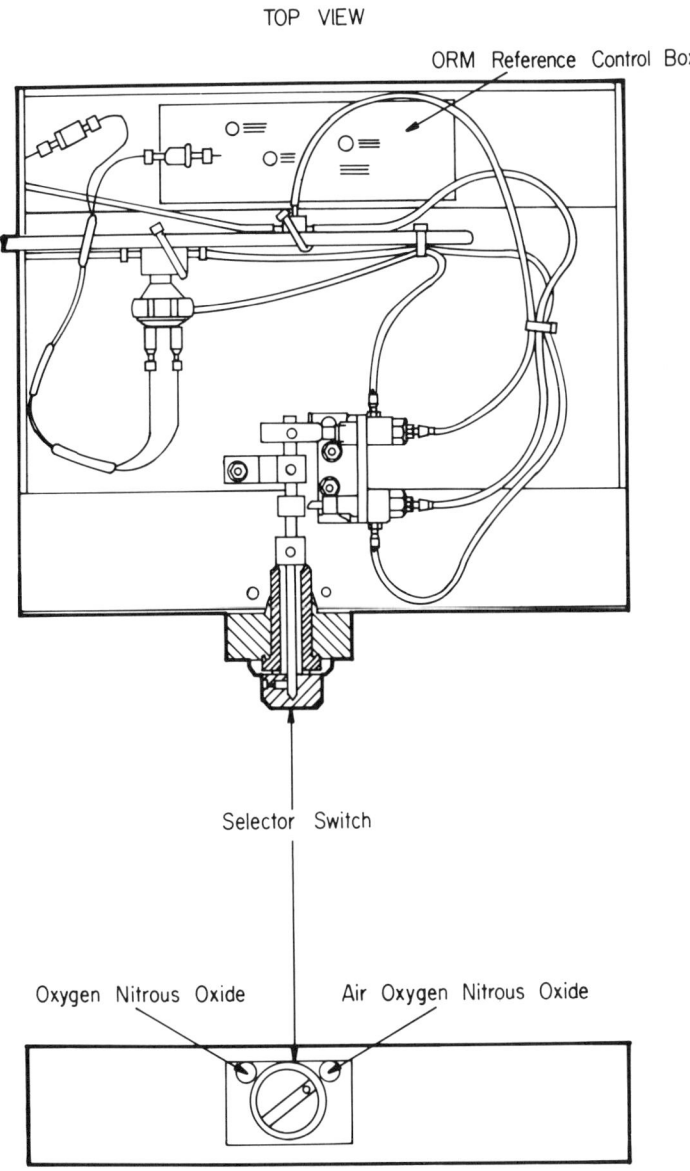

Selector Switch

Oxygen Nitrous Oxide   Air Oxygen Nitrous Oxide

FRONT VIEW

Fig. 11-24 Selector switch assembly for the Drager Narkomed IIA anesthesia machine. Placing the switch in the air–oxygen–nitrous oxide position (front view) will deactivate the ORM (top view—reference control box) or ORMc and stop the minimal oxygen flow. (Redrawn from Parts Manual. North American Drager, Telford, PA, 1984.)

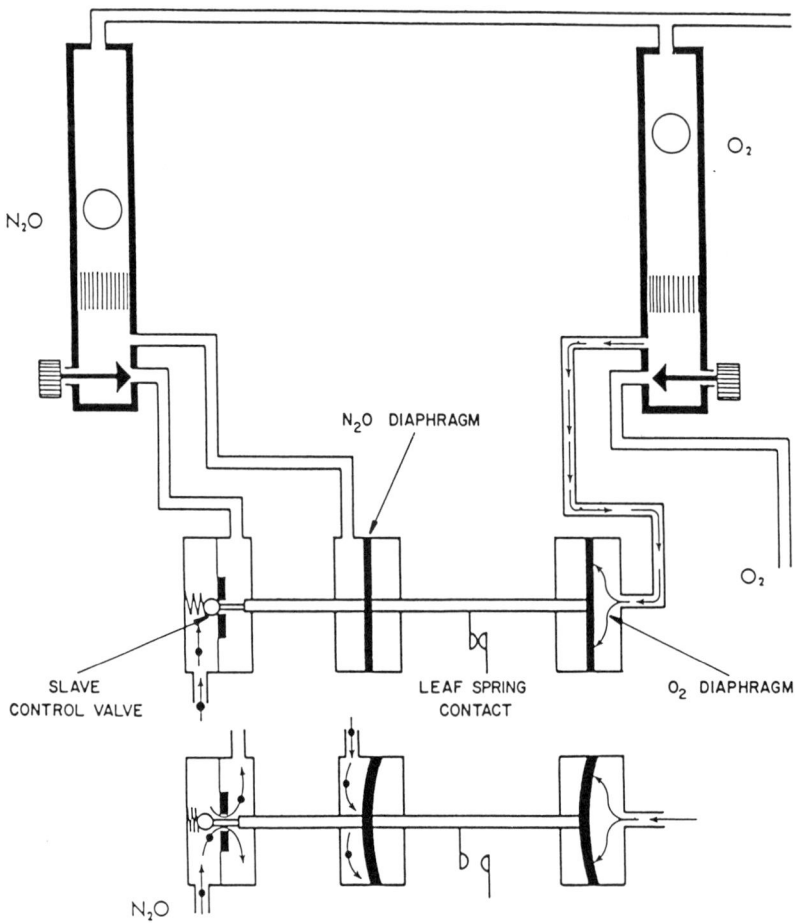

Fig. 11-25 Oxygen ratio monitor controller (ORMc) for the Drager Narkomed IIA anesthesia machine. The basic design principles are the same as for the ORM in Figures 11-21 to 11-23. An ORMc uses a slave control valve to control the flow of nitrous oxide through a spring-loaded orifice (bottom). The ORMc automatically responds to reductions in oxygen pressure and maintains the oxygen concentration at 28 ± 3 percent. (Schreiber P: Safety Guidelines for Anesthesia Systems. North American Drager, Telford, PA, 1984.)

trous oxide flow rate will move the diaphragm switch contacts closer together. When the oxygen flow decreases to 30 ± 5 percent of the combined oxygen–nitrous oxide flow, the switch contacts touch and an audio and/or visual alarm is activated. The ORM functions best at oxygen flow rates between 700 ml/min and 5 L/min. At flow rates below 700 ml/ min, hysteresis of the diaphragm makes the alarm inaccurate.

Introduction of a third gas to the oxygen–nitrous oxide mixture will make the ORM sys-

tem inaccurate and could yield a hypoxic mixture. The Drager Narkomed IIA anesthesia machine has a selector switch assembly which allows the anesthesiologist to choose a setting for oxygen–nitrous oxide or air–oxygen–nitrous oxide (see Fig. 11-24). Placing the switch in the air–oxygen–nitrous oxide setting deactivates the ORM system and shuts off the minimum oxygen flow.[29]

Controlling the oxygen–nitrous oxide mixture at a minimum of 25 to 30 percent oxygen is possible with the Drager Narkomed IIA oxygen ration monitor controller (ORMc) and the Ohmeda Modulus II proportion-limiting control system (Link 25 system).

An ORMc incorporates the basic design features of the ORM. The shaft connecting the two diaphragms of the ORM is extended and connected to a slave control valve, as shown in Figure 11-25. This valve controls the flow of nitrous oxide as the diaphragms and shaft move left or right. When the oxygen pressure is proportionally higher than the nitrous oxide pressure, the valve opens, and vice versa. As nitrous oxide flow is manually increased at the flowmeter valve, the pressure from the nitrous oxide forces the shaft toward the oxygen diaphragm, making the valve opening restrictive and limiting the nitrous oxide flow.[22, 29, 34]

The ORMc will actively lower the proportional flow rate of nitrous oxide as the flow rate of oxygen is manually decreased. Anytime the mixture reaches the predetermined 28 ± 3 percent oxygen limit, an alarm will be activated. The ORMc is nullified if any gas other than oxygen and nitrous oxide is used in the system. Placing the selector switch assembly in the air–oxygen–nitrous oxide mode deactivates the ORMc.

The Ohio Link 25 system mechanically links the nitrous oxide flow control valve to the oxygen flow control valve, as shown in Figure 11-26. Each flow control valve has a sprocket secured to the needle valve stem. A cable chain of 100 lb tensile strength interconnects the two sprockets.[35] At a prescribed minimum of 25 percent oxygen concentration the oxygen sprocket engages the collar of the needle valve stem and links the nitrous oxide and oxygen flow control valves. Independent adjustment of either the nitrous oxide or oxygen is possible but the link system automatically intercedes to maintain a 25 percent minimum oxygen concentration. Initially the link system had a few mechanical problems, but these appear to have been corrected.[35, 36]

OXYGEN FLOWMETER

Special considerations and standards have been given to the design and placement of the oxygen flowmeters[1, 22] The oxygen flow control knob has a design different from all the other flow control knobs on the anesthesia machine (see Fig. 11-27). In addition, the oxygen flow control is green and is located nearest the common gas outlet (Fig. 11-28). These design features provide the anesthesiologist with tactile, positional, and color identification of the critical oxygen flow control knob. Positioning the oxygen flowmeter on the far right of the anesthesia machine can help eliminate hypoxia resulting from leaks in other flowmeter tubes.[1, 37] Leaks within the oxygen flowmeter tube can cause hypoxia despite the position of the oxygen flowmeter.[38-40]

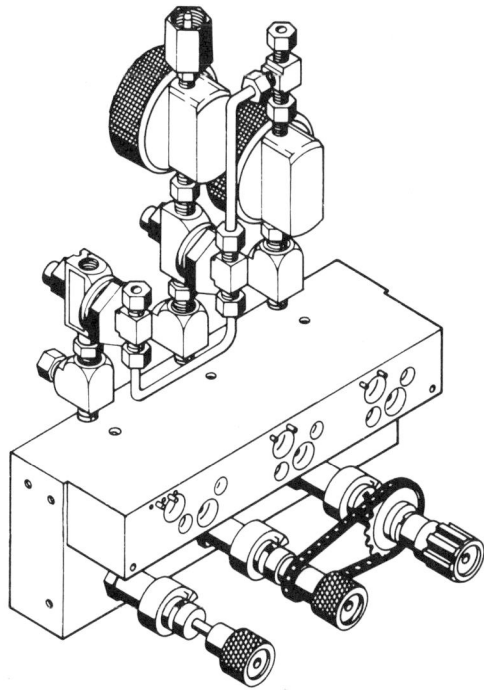

Fig. 11-26 The proportion-limiting control system (Link 25) for the Modulus II anesthesia machine. A sprocket system interconnects the flow control valves for oxygen and nitrous oxide and automatically intercedes to maintain a 25 percent minimum oxygen concentration. (Courtesy of Ohmeda, The BOC Group, Inc.)

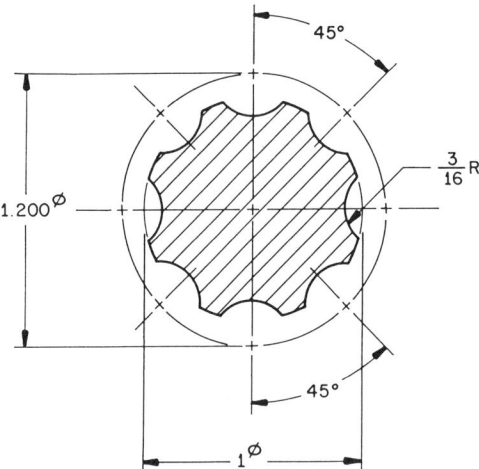

Fig. 11-27 Design of the oxygen touch control flowmeter knob. (Schreiber P: Safety Guidelines for Anesthesia Systems. North American Drager, Telford, PA, 1984.)

Low and high flow rates of oxygen are now provided by a single flow control valve. A low- and a high-flow tube with separate floats are mounted in series, as shown in Figure 11-29. Arranging the flowmeters in this fashion has eliminated the inadvertent use of low-flow oxygen in the presence of high-flow nitrous oxide.[5, 41]

Pressure gauges reflecting the hospital pipeline and compressed tank pressure for each anesthetic gas are positioned below the flow control valve of the specific gas. Figure 11-28 shows the position of the oxygen hospital pipeline and oxygen reserve cylinder pressure gauges directly below the oxygen flowmeter control knob. On older machines the pressure gauges were located in almost inaccessible places! Now the pressure gauges have been moved to a safer position for easy repeated visual confirmation of line pressures.

A minimum oxygen flow has been incorporated into safe anesthesia machines. The flow rate can be set between 200 and 450 cc/min at a pipeline pressure of 50 psig. A resistor placed in the T-piece of the 50-psig oxygen pipeline decreases the gas flow to approximately 250 cc/min and diverts this flow up-stream of the oxygen flowmeter control valve (see Fig. 11-30).[34] Closing the oxygen flowmeter needle valve completely will not eliminate the minimum oxygen flow. Placing the selector switch assembly on the air–oxygen–nitrous oxide setting will disable the minimum oxygen flow safety feature.

Flowmeter lights are an optional safety feature which can be advantageous during surgical procedures which require a darkened room. A flowmeter pin indexing system has been suggested by the ANSI as a mechanism to prevent the inadvertent interchange of flowmeter tubes.[1] A protective bar can be mounted in front of the flowmeter control knobs to protect the knobs from accidental bumping by items placed on top of the anesthesia cabinet (Fig. 11-28).

MISCELLANEOUS FEATURES

Breathing circuit pressure alarms are available which not only monitor disconnect conditions but also detect conditions of high pressure, continuous pressure, and subatmospheric pressure.

High pressure in the anesthesia circuit can result from a kinked endotracheal tube, among other things, and result in barotrauma to the lungs.[42-44] The high-pressure alarm (see Figs. 11-8 and 11-31) of the Drager Narkomed IIA anesthesia machine responds when pressure in the breathing circuit exceeds 65 to 70 cmH_2O. A continuous audio and/or visual alarm will sound as long as the pressure remains in excess.

Continuous pressure in the breathing circuit is possible when the pop-off valve is closed off and the patient attempts to breathe from a grossly overinflated reservoir bag. Numerous malfunctions of the anesthesia machine can result in continuous-pressure conditions.[29, 43, 44] The continuous-pressure monitor (see Figs. 11-8 and 11-31) designed for the Drager Narkomed IIA anesthesia machine activates an audio and/or visual alarm[19] when a positive pressure of more than 18 cmH_2O is present for longer than 10 seconds.

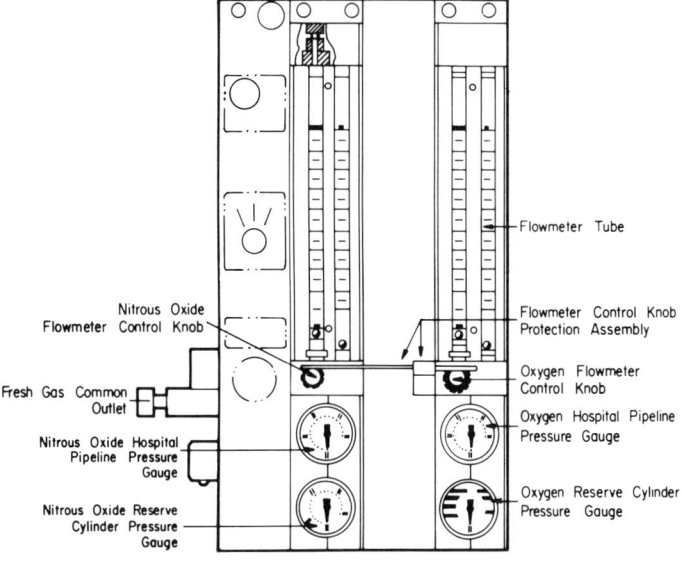

FRONT VIEW

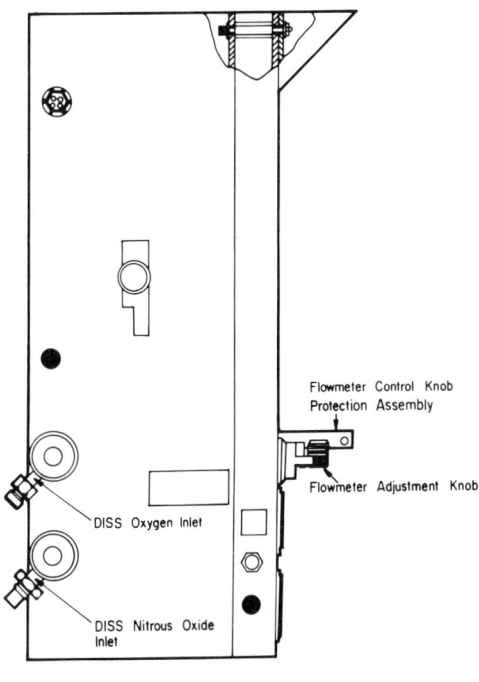

SIDE VIEW

Fig. 11-28 Flowmeter housing for the Drager Narkomed IIA anesthesia machine. Oxygen flowmeters are positioned on the right. Pressure gauges are located below each specific gas. Note the flowmeter control protection assembly in the side view. (Redrawn from Parts Manual. North American Drager, Telford, PA, 1984.)

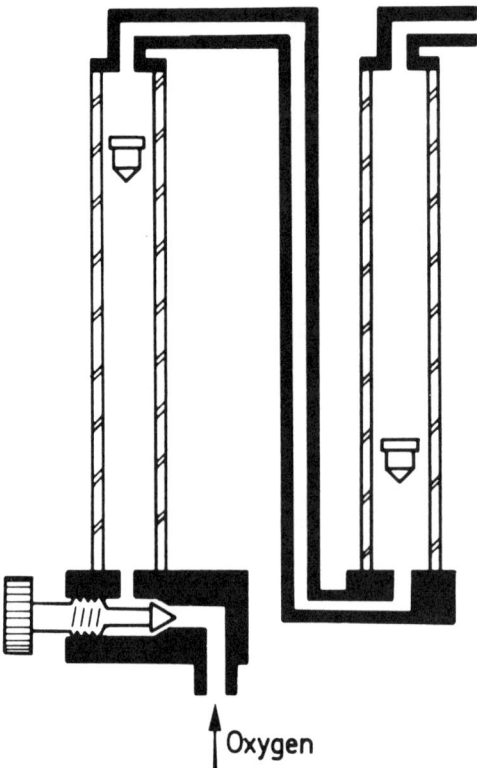

Fig. 11-29 Low and high oxygen flowmeters arranged in series. A single flowmeter knob controls the oxygen flow rate. (Schreiber P: Anaesthesia Equipment: Performance, Classification and Safety. Springer-Verlag, New York, 1972.)

Subatmospheric pressure can occur in the breathing circuit when the negative-pressure relief valve for the scavenger interface system malfunctions.[29] The subatmospheric pressure monitor (see Figs. 11-8 and 11-31) for the Drager Narkomed IIA anesthesia machine alarms[34] when the breathing circuit pressure goes below −10 cmH₂O.

Let us not forget the inclusion of the breathing circuit pressure gauge. This visual gauge is diaphragm activated and covers the pressure range of −20 to +80 cmH₂O in 2-cmH₂O increments. Gauge accuracy[29] for the Narkomed IIA is 3 percent of full scale between

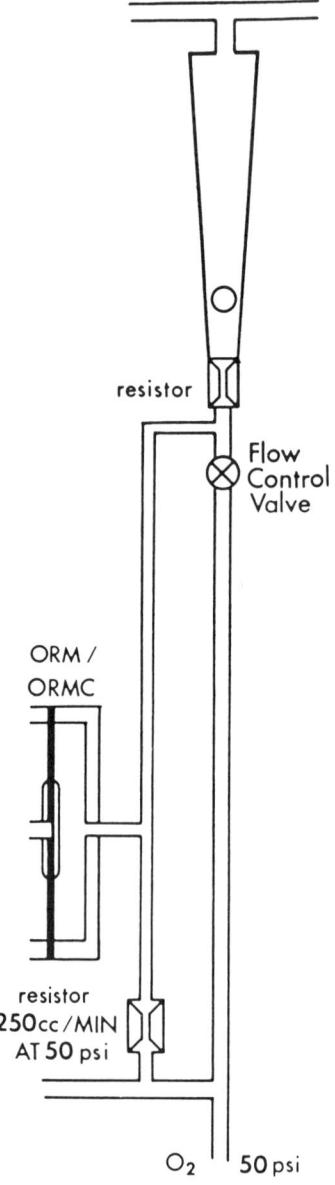

Fig. 11-30 Minimum oxygen flow safety feature on the Drager Narkomed IIA anesthesia machine. A 250-cc/min resistor is placed in the 50-psig oxygen line. The resultant gas flow enters the flowmeter tube downstream of the flow control valve but prior to the reduction resistor in the flowmeter tube. (Technical Service Manual. North American Drager, Telford, PA, 1985.)

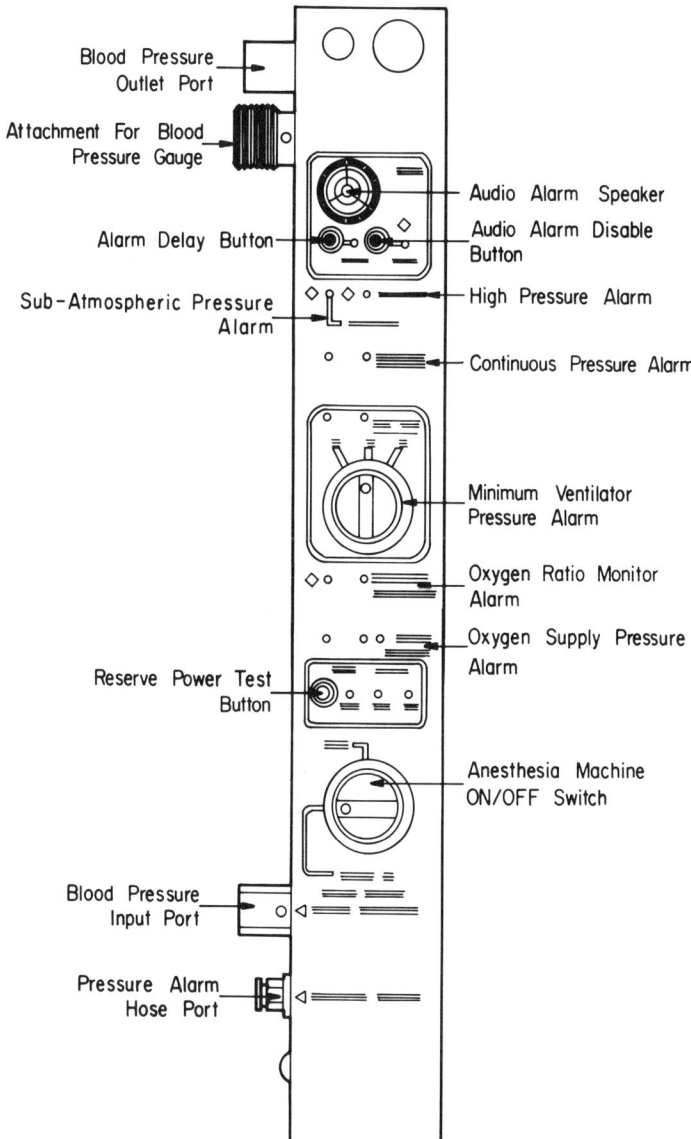

Blood Pressure Outlet Port

Attachment For Blood Pressure Gauge

Alarm Delay Button

Sub-Atmospheric Pressure Alarm

Reserve Power Test Button

Blood Pressure Input Port

Pressure Alarm Hose Port

Audio Alarm Speaker

Audio Alarm Disable Button

High Pressure Alarm

Continuous Pressure Alarm

Minimum Ventilator Pressure Alarm

Oxygen Ratio Monitor Alarm

Oxygen Supply Pressure Alarm

Anesthesia Machine ON/OFF Switch

Fig. 11-31 Central alarm panel for the Drager Narkomed IIA anesthesia machine. Audio alarms can be deactivated for those alarms with diamonds. The visual portion of the alarm has a flashing light-emitting diode (LED) which is on when an alarm situation exists. (Redrawn from Parts Manual. North American Drager, Telford, PA, 1984.)

TOP VIEW

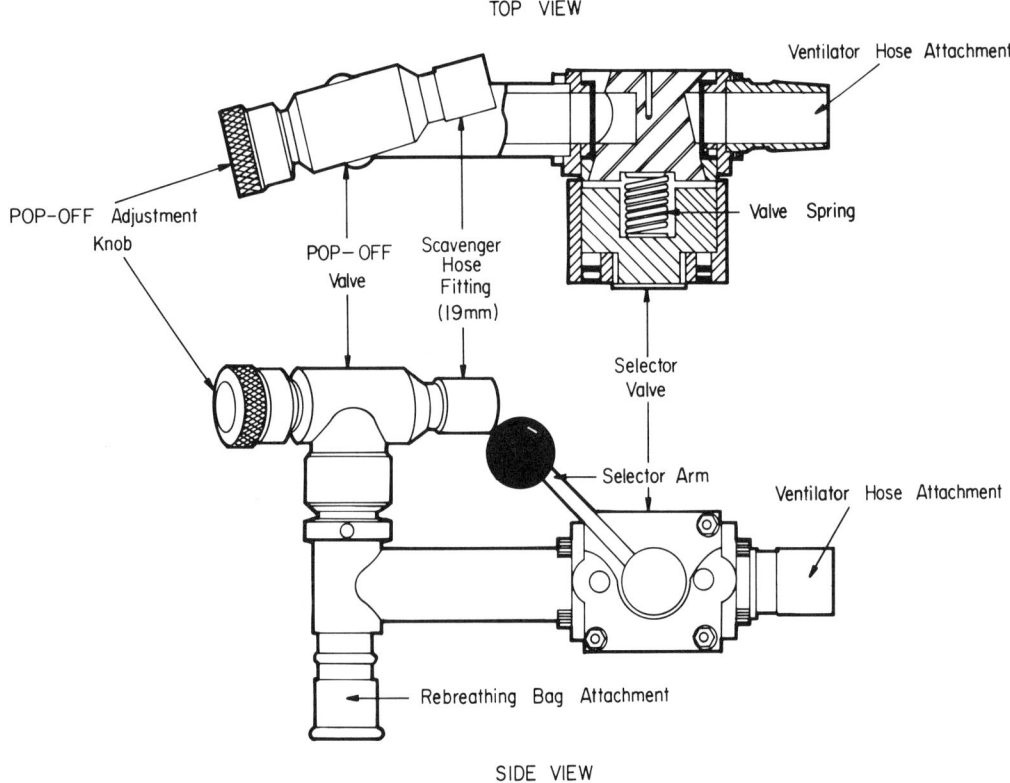

Ventilator Hose Attachment

POP-OFF Adjustment Knob

POP-OFF Valve

Scavenger Hose Fitting (19mm)

Valve Spring

Selector Valve

Selector Arm

Ventilator Hose Attachment

Rebreathing Bag Attachment

SIDE VIEW

Fig. 11-32 The selector valve for the Drager Narkomed IIA anesthesia machine. The selector arm is in the Bag mode, isolating the ventilator connector hose and ventilator relief valve from the breathing circuit. Moving the selector arm to the right (Auto mode) excludes the pop-off valve and reservoir bag from the breathing circuit. (Redrawn from Parts Manual. North American Drager, Telford, PA, 1984.)

−20 and +5 cmH$_2$O, 2 percent of full scale between +5 and +55 cmH$_2$O, and 3 percent of full scale between +55 and +80 cmH$_2$O. A large dial face and excellent location allow the anesthesiologist to check it frequently.

A selector valve isolates the pop-off valve and reservoir bag from the breathing circuit when the ventilator is functioning. The presence of the selector valve eliminates the need to remove the reservoir bag and replace it with the ventilator hose. Figure 11-32 illustrates the features of the selector valve. In the Auto mode the pop-off valve and reservoir bag are not in the breathing circuit. In the Bag (spontaneous/manual) mode the ventilator connec-

tor hose and ventilator relief valve are isolated from the breathing system.

Both the Ohmeda Modulus II and the Drager Narkomed IIA anesthesia machines depend on an uninterrupted electric supply for proper function. Hospitals are required to have emergency power systems, but even these have been known to fail. Both anesthesia machines have a reserve power supply. For instance, the Narkomed IIA has a 12-V lead–acid battery which will provide power to operate the entire anesthesia machine, including the ventilator, should the main power fail or disconnect. These power supplies are designed to go on automatically when the main power fails and return to reserve status as soon as the main power comes on.

Any mechanical, electrical, or pneumatic device on an anesthesia machine or monitor can malfunction. Alarms, batteries, and so forth, have been found to be defective during anesthesia.[24, 25, 32, 45-49] Sometimes the problem is that the anesthesiologist does not know the alarm limitations.[28, 50] However, even the simplest things, such as a red–green colorblind anesthesiologist, who cannot see the red LED alarm displays, can be overlooked and must be rectified.[51]

Anesthesiologists have a difficult problem in establishing a line of sight for the efficient and effective monitoring of the anesthesia machine and patient monitors. A commercial pilot sits on the runway prior to takeoff and can see almost all the essential instruments monitoring the airplane with a narrow range of vision. However, at best, anesthesiologists are 90° away from their monitors. Their attention must include what is behind, to the side, and in front of them. Anesthesia machines are finally showing some design characteristics which incorporate line-of-sight principles. The ANSI has an entire appendix explaining line of sight, vertical and horizontal visual fields, and a host of related items.[1] Tasks performed by anesthesiologists have not been examined by ergonomic experts. Ergonomic studies need to be done on the layout of the anesthesia machine, the monitors, and the relationship of the anesthesiologist to both.[52]

Present-day technology has provided the anesthesiologist with improvements in the anesthesia machine which can make the delivery of anesthesia safer. Too many anesthesia machines are in service in the United States that are 15 to 20 years old. An update of these machines is usually impossible. Every attempt should be made to put these machines where they ought to be: at the bottom of an elevator shaft! Outdated, unsafe anesthesia machines should be replaced.

The relationship of safety features on anesthesia machines to the overall incidence of anesthetic morbidity and mortality is impossi-ble to determine. Epstein[32] feels the simple systems to prevent the administration of hypoxic gas mixtures in anesthesia may be more important than the complex monitoring devices used for critically ill patients. A fine line exists between distracting the anesthesiologist from the patient and providing valuable information on patient care. Anesthesiologists who fail to understand their equipment are easily distracted, while those who understand the limitations of the equipment are less distracted. Safety features and alarms should be looked on as valuable additional precautions which are desirable but not absolutely essential. No warning device can be 100 percent effective. The use of any or all devices does not excuse the anesthesiologist from maintaining constant vigilance.

REFERENCES

1. American National Standard: Minimal Performance and Safety Requirements for Components and Systems of Continuous-Flow Anesthesia Machines for Human Use. Z79.8-1979 American National Standards Institute, New York, 1979

2. Monitors avert injury but must be properly maintained. Manage Rep 1:1-2, 1982

3. Oxygen analyzers create liability if not used consistently. Hosp Risk Manage 4:152, 1982

4. McGarrigle RE: General anesthesia without O_2 analyzer—a substandard practice. Anesthesiology 65:116, 1985

5. Mazze RI: Therapeutic misadventures with oxygen delivery systems: the need for continuous in-line oxygen monitors. Anesth Analg 51:787, 1972

6. Marks WE, Jr: A plea for the routine use of oxygen analyzers. Anesthesiology 59:159, 1983

7. Dorsch SE, Dorsch JA: Use of oxygen analyzers should be mandatory. Anesthesiology 59:161, 1983

8. Rendell-Baker L, Meyer JA: Failure to use O_2 analyzers to prevent hypoxic accidents. Anesthesiology 58:287, 1983

9. Knill RL, Gelb AW: Peripheral chemoreceptors during anesthesia: are the watchdogs sleeping? Anesthesiology 57:151, 1982

10. U.S. Department of Commerce. National Bu-

reau of Standards. Handbook H-28, Part III, Washington, DC, 1957

11. American National Standard: Requirements for Oxygen Analyzers for Monitoring Patient Breathing-Mixtures. Z79.10-1979. American National Standards Institute, New York, 1979

12. Operation Maintenance. Model 5100 Oxygen Monitor. Ohmeda, Madison, WI, 1985

13. Instruction Manual. Oxymed PM. Oxygen Analyzer. North American Drager, Telford, PA, 1984

14. Raia E: Fuel cells: spark utilities' interest. High Technol, 52, 1984

15. Figallo EM, Smith RB, Pautler S et al: Continuous oxygen analyzers in clinical anesthesia: a review. Anesthesiol Rev, 25, 1978

16. Schreiber P: Anaesthesia Equipment. Performance, Classification and Safety. Springer-Verlag, New York, 1972

17. Westenskow DR, Jordan WS, Jordan R et al: Evaluation of oxygen monitors for use during anesthesia. Anesth Analg 50:53, 1981

18. Rost GA: Recent improvements in hypoxia warning systems. Aerospace Med 41:865, 1970

19. Vogel HR, Harth O, Thews G: Continuous recording of PO_2 in respiratory air by a rapid platinum electrode. Prog Respir Res 3:42, 1969

20. Severinghaus JW, Weiskopf RB, Nishimura M et al: Oxygen electrode errors due to polarographic reduction of halothane. J Appl Physiol 31:640, 1971

21. Piernan S, Roizen MF, Severinghaus JW: Oxygen analyzer dangerous—senses nitrous oxide as battery fails. Anesthesiology 50:146, 1979

22. Schreiber P: Safety Guidelines for Anesthesia Systems. North American Drager, Telford, PA, 1984

23. McGarrigle R: Oxygen analyzers can detect disconnections. Anesth Analg 63:422, 1984

24. McEwen JA, Small CF, Saunders BA et al: Hazards associated with the use of disconnect monitors. Anesthesiology 53:S391, 1980

25. Reynolds AC: Disconnect alarm failure. Anesthesiology 58:488, 1983

26. McEwen JA, Jenkins LC: Complication of and improvements to breathing circuit monitors for anesthesia ventilators. Med Instrum 17:70, 1983

27. Neufeld PD, Johnson DL: Results of the Canadian Anaesthetists' Society opinion survey on anaesthetic equipment. Can Anaesth Soc J 30:469, 1983

28. Murray IP, Modell JH: Early detection of endotracheal tube accidents by monitoring carbon dioxide concentration in respiratory gas. Anesthesiology 59:344, 1983

29. Instruction Manual. Narkomed 2A. Anesthesia System. North American Drager, Telford, PA, 1984

30. Scurlock JE: More failsafe failsafes. Anesthesiology 42:226, 1975

31. Craig DB, Longmuir J: An unusual failure of an oxygen fail-safe device. Can Anaesth Soc J 18:576, 1971

32. Epstein RA: Nitrous oxide delivery systems. p. 69. In Eger E: Nitrous Oxide/N_2O. Elsevier, New York, 1985

33. Petty C: Measurements done on a Drager Narkomed IIA anesthesia machine. (Unpublished data) 1985

34. Technical Service Manual. North American Drager, Telford, PA, 1985

35. Davis TM: Failure of a new system to prevent delivery of hypoxic gas mixture: a reply. Anesthesiology 54:437, 1981

36. Malone BT: Failure of a new system to prevent delivery of hypoxic gas mixture. Anesthesiology 54:436, 1981

37. Eger EI, II, Hylton RR, Irwin RH et al: Anesthetic flow meter sequence—a cause for hypoxia. Anesthesiology 24:396, 1963

38. Chung DC, Jing QC, Prins L et al: Hypoxic gas mixtures delivered by anaesthetic machines equipped with a downstream oxygen flowmeter. Can Anaesth Soc J 27:527, 1980

39. Powell J; Leak from an oxygen flow meter. Br J Anaesth 53:671, 1981

40. Wilson ME, Burleton AS: Leak tests. Br J Anaesth 54:572, 1982

41. Rendell-Baker L: Some gas machine hazards and their elimination. Anesth Analg 55:26, 1976

42. Rendell-Baker L, Meyer JA: Accidental disconnection and pulmonary barotrauma. Anesthesiology 58:186, 1983

43. Thompson PW: Prevention of the hazard of excessive airway pressure. Anaesthesia 35:593, 1979

44. Newton NI, Adams AP: Excessive airway pressure during anaesthesia: hazards, effects and prevention. Anaesthesia 3:689, 1978

45. Lahay WD: Defective pressure/flow alarm.

Can Anaesth Soc J 29:404, 1982

46. Shribman AJ: Failure of a ventilator alarm: not up to specification. Anaesthesia 37:1044, 1982

47. Mazza N, Wald A: Failure of battery-operated alarms. Anesthesiology 53:246, 1980

48. Chang JL, Larson CE, Bedger RC et al: An unusual malfunction of an anesthetic machine. Anesthesiology 52:446, 1980

49. Feeley TW, Bancroft ML: Problems with mechanical ventilators. Int Anesthesiol Clin 20:83, 1982

50. Steward DJ, Pelton DA, Brummitt WM: Audio vs visual oxygen alarm. Anesthesiology 52:192, 1980

51. Gissen D, Roaf ER: LED monitors and the color-blind. Anesthesiology 62:840, 1985

52. Rendell-Baker L: Problems with anesthetic gas machines and their solutions. Int Anesthesiol Clin 20:1, 1982

12

Risk Management and Quality Assurance for Anesthesia Machines

Publicity given to patient injuries caused by anesthesia machine failure is way out of proportion to the extremely small contribution machine failures actually make to anesthesia mortality. In the United States and Great Britain both the newspapers and government tend to emphasize equipment failures.[1, 2] Figure 12-1 is taken from the title page of a congressional hearing which investigated four deaths related to anesthesia machine failures. In one study 602 anesthesia accidents encompassing 16,000 man-years of anesthesia were analyzed and machine failure was not found to be a cause of any anesthesia-related accident.[3] A 10-year review of the maintenance records of 15 anesthesia machines that delivered a combined total of 7,000 anesthetics per year showed only minor malfunctions.[4] However, breathing circuit disconnections,[5-8] crossed internal pipelines for oxygen and nitrous oxide,[1] and other machine problems have contributed to anesthesia mortality and morbidity.[9] The few prospective studies examining factors which might contribute to error suggest the most common linking element to be human error.[7, 8, 10-12] Anesthesia equipment failures accounted for 115 of 1,089 critical incidents related to major errors in anesthesia management.[11] Only 16 of the 115 failures were specific anesthesia machine problems. Each year between 2,000 and 15,000 anesthetic deaths occur among the estimated 10 million anesthetized patients in the United States.[13]

Risk management and quality assurance in anesthesia are not easily separated in function. Risk management is a detection system designed to predict failures and ensure that precautions are taken to avoid patient harm.[14] Quality assurance deals with objective, systematic monitoring and the evaluation of the quality and appropriateness of patient care.[15]

RISK MANAGEMENT

Risk management has become an important subject in anesthesia as premiums for medical malpractice insurance skyrocket. Out-of-court and jury settlements are becoming higher each year. Hospitals, physicians, paraprofessionals, and health equipment manufacturers are prime targets for quick, easy money by so-

ANESTHESIA MACHINE FAILURES

HEARING
BEFORE THE

SUBCOMMITTEE ON
OVERSIGHT AND INVESTIGATIONS
OF THE

COMMITTEE ON
ENERGY AND COMMERCE
HOUSE OF REPRESENTATIVES

NINETY-EIGHTH CONGRESS

SECOND SESSION

SEPTEMBER 26, 1984

Serial No. 98-188

Printed for the use of the Committee on Energy and Commerce

Fig. 12-1 Hearing on anesthesia machine failures before members of Congress on 26 September 1984. (Taken from front page of Anesthesia Machine Failures. Hearing Subcommittee on Oversight and Investigations. U.S. Government Printing Office, Washington, DC, 1985.)

called "professional" lawyers and uninjured but cooperative patients.

Hospitals recognized the need for risk management from (1) the malpractice liability crisis of the 1970s and (2) their close association with the insurance industry, where risk managers have functioned successfully for a number of years. Hospital risk managers have emerged as a full-fledged member of the hospital administration staff. In small hospitals the administrator or assistant administrator accepts the responsibility. The risk manager identifies potential problems that can result in lawsuit. Patients are contacted early, a dialogue is established, and hopefully a lawsuit is avoided.

Anesthesiologists have recognized the problematic situation in which our specialty finds itself. Anesthesiologists make mistakes and patients can be injured as a consequence.

In this regard we are as Pogo, the great philosopher, once said: "We have identified the enemy, and they is us." Anesthesiologists recognize the limited patient–physician relationship and are encouraged to make pre- and post-anesthesia visits to each patient in order to improve the relationship.[16, 17] The Commission on Medical Professional Liability of the American Bar Association has found that patients treated indifferently by a physician seek redress through the courts for an incident.[18] A telephone survey in 1983 by the American Medical Society Group on Federation and Public Relations asked 1,000 randomly selected physicians their opinion on how to reduce risk in medicine. Better rapport between the physician and the patient was pinpointed as the best risk reduction strategy. Other less important strategies included peer review, continuing medical education, and seminars on risk management. Anesthesiologists must make time in their busy schedules to see patients. Patient perception and attitude are key elements in the formation of the public image of the anesthesiologist. The finest error-free anesthesia machines possible will not change high malpractice premiums unless efforts are made to modify the public image of the anesthesiologist at the grass roots level.

The American Society of Anesthesiologists (ASA) has recognized the importance of errors (human and mechanical) as contributing factors to the rise of malpractice premiums and patient injury. The ASA Risk Management and Patient Safety Committee was organized in 1983 to examine the factors leading to patient injury and devise means to assist anesthesiologists in decreasing the numbers of injuries to patients.[17] Six videotapes which address the issue of patient safety were produced by the committee (see Fig. 12-2).[19] Each videotape examines an area responsible for patient injury and suggests means to decrease or eliminate the problem. Every anesthesia department in the world could benefit from reviewing the videotapes. A concomitant examination of anesthesia standards of practice in each department with immediate imple-

An educational series covering a wide range of important topics.

Excellent for all hospital educational needs, including those of residency programs, the ASA series of six informative videotapes provides important information on current trends in patient safety techniques. Given the growing complexity of anesthesia practices and the increasing incidence of malpractice claims, these techniques are more important than ever.

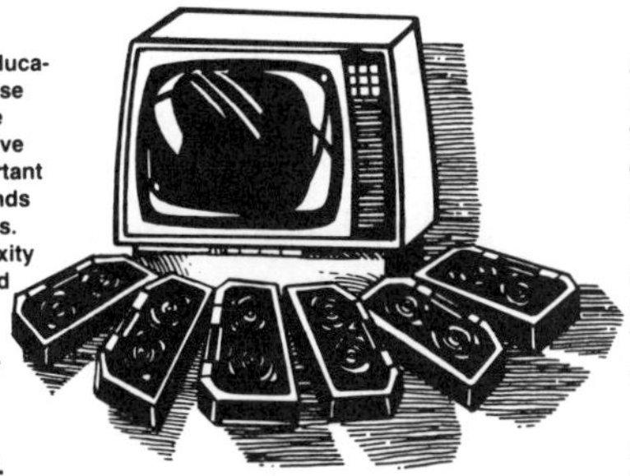

ASA Series Overview.
An introduction to the series, this tape provides a backdrop for examination of the variety of patient safety issues confronting the anesthesiologist. It provides examples of how the practice is being portrayed to the public, and then specifies the areas to be covered in the remaining tapes.

Preventing Disconnection in the Breathing Circuit.
An in-depth evaluation of the risks inherent with using this type of equipment, and the many reasons why mishaps of this variety occur. Includes current trends facilitating the detection of disconnections in the breathing circuit.

Anesthesia Machine Check-Out.
Important information about how to properly check this vital piece of equipment to help assure its most reliable operation. Invaluable advice for all resident as well as practicing anesthesiologists.

Adverse Events.
What to do in the event of an adverse patient reaction. This most difficult subject is analyzed both from the medical and legal perspectives.

Anesthesia Record-Keeping.
The importance of complete and legible anesthesia record-keeping. An imperative in today's environment because a significant quantity of today's losses is based on incomplete or illegible records.

Human Error.
Without doubt the most common cause of adverse events. This tape is vitally important to preventing the kinds of human error that can lead to disaster, and against which all anesthesiologists must remain ever vigilant.

Fig. 12-2 American Society of Anesthesiologists Patient Safety Program prepared by the Ad Hoc Committee on Patient Safety and Risk Management. The education series covers subjects that are major patient safety issues confronting the anesthesiologist. (Pamphlet, American Society of Anesthesiologists, Park Ridge, IL.)

mentation of many of the principles would decrease patient morbidity and mortality.

QUALITY ASSURANCE

Health care professionals have been encouraged for many years to "analyze, review and evaluate, and where necessary, improve the quality of clinical practice."[20] Since 1951 quality assurance under the joint Commission on Accreditation of Hospitals (JCAH) has been evolving from a subjective to an objective instrument in the evaluation of patient care.[21] In 1979 the JCAH began to focus on the identification and resolution of problems in patient care and clinical preformance.[22] The 1982 JCAH surveys made recommendations to 32

percent (372) of the hospitals for anesthesia improvement.[21] Fundamental principles of quality assurance are not being implemented in all anesthesia departments. Anesthesiologists must participate in the ongoing, objective, and systematic review of anesthesia care.

Presently the JCAH quality assurance program emphasizes an ongoing monitoring approach to identify and solve problems. Once a problem is identified by the anesthesia department, information is gathered in cooperation with the quality assurance director in order to evaluate the extent of the problem. Remedial actions are recommended by the chief of anesthesia upon advice of the members of the department of anesthesia. Periodic evaluations will ensure that the problem has been rectified and not recurred. Quality assurance in anesthesia is a planned and systematic process for monitoring and evaluating patient care.[21]

Increasing pressure will be applied to all medical service departments as members of the hospital governing boards recognize their responsibility for the quality of patient care.[15] The director of anesthesia has been designated by the JCAH to (1) recommend the type and amount of anesthesia equipment necessary for the administration of anesthesia, (2) develop regulations for anesthesia safety, and (3) ensure the monitoring of the quality and appropriateness of anesthesia care. Minimum standards related to the anesthesia machine include inspection and testing of anesthetic apparatus by the anesthetist prior to use, provision of a pin index safety system on every anesthesia machine, the recommendation of a gas-scavenging system and a oxygen pressure interlock system on every anesthesia machine, a planned and systematic process which will monitor and evaluate the standard of anesthesia care, and documentation of the effectiveness of the actions taken to improve and monitor the standard of anesthesia care.[15]

The chief of anesthesia will be able to improve the standard of patient care rendered by the anesthesia department by cooperating with the hospital risk manager and the quality assurance director. Documentation of morbidity and mortality in anesthesia has been insufficient in the United States. Lack of documentation makes it impossible to separate the extent of the contribution of human error from equipment failure in patient injury. Quality assurance review will help to remove the criticism that anesthesiologists are not doing everything possible to lower morbidity and mortality to the "irreducible minimum."[23] Active participation in risk management and quality assurance activities by the anesthesia department can be the "best evidence" that the department is aggressive in preventing foreseeable patient injury.[24]

The concepts of risk management and quality assurance are intertwined in function and purpose. When separate committees are established in hospitals for each subject, it is critical to have an interface between the committees to ensure nonduplication of work and proper cooperation. Risk management and quality assurance programs can identify problem areas in anesthesia related to the anesthesia machine, as well as delineate discrepancies in other aspects of anesthesia. We will examine areas which serve both risk management and quality assurance.

INCIDENT REPORTS

Any event which is inconsistent with the routine administration of anesthesia or care of the patient can be considered an incident.[25-27] Unfortunely every anesthesiologist in practice for more than 5 years can relate hair-raising tales of faults and hazards which were detected, corrected, and never reported. Each incident related to the anesthesia machine must be documented. Documentation can be used by the chief of anesthesia and the hospital risk manager to investigate the incident and make a written evaluation.[26, 27] Incident report evaluation and steps for follow-up are outlined in Figure 12-3. All incident reports must be discussed in the monthly meeting of the department of anesthesia. In-service programs related to incident reports should be documented. The monthly meeting is the place to instruct anesthesiologists on modifications on existing anesthesia machines and to conduct in-service education on new anesthesia machines.

Each machine should have an individual maintenance file.[28, 29] In addition to maintenance records, the file should contain (1) incident reports related to the machine, (2) any addition, alteration, or removal of equipment, (3) pollution control reports, and (4) the results of all vaporizer calibrations. Once a machine or a group of machines show a pattern of risk, the data should be accumulated, the risk manager consulted, and a document prepared to request the update of the machine(s) or the purchase of new ones.

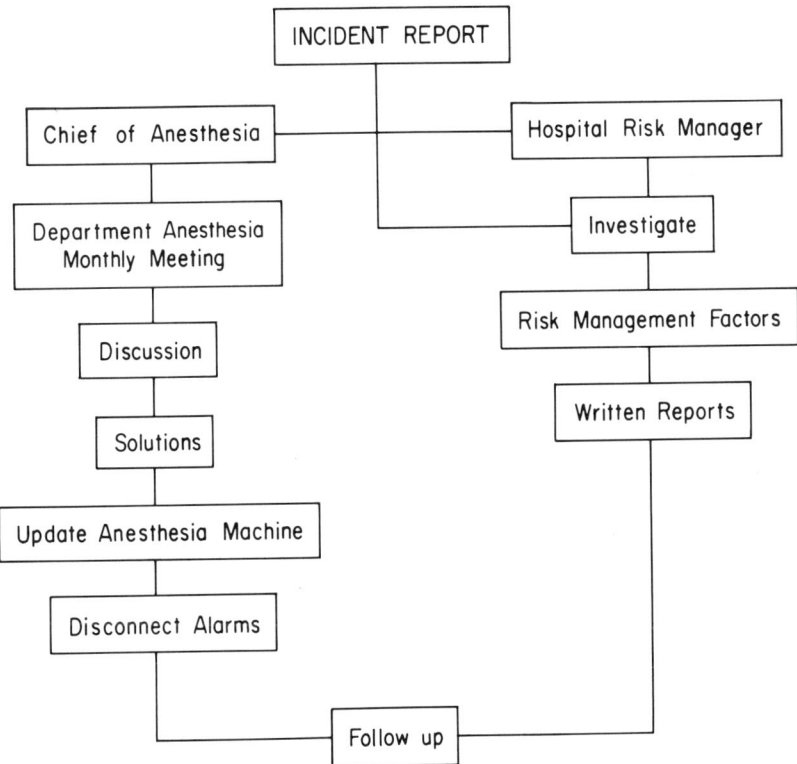

Fig. 12-3 Outline of how to approach an incident report generated by an anesthesia breathing circuit disconnect. Important features include investigation of the incident, discussion with the anesthesia department, recommended solutions, and follow-up.

Reluctance on the part of the anesthesiologist to initiate incident reports will only lead to further patient care problems and/or increase hospital liability. If an anesthesia machine malfunction causes or contributes to a serious injury or death, the anesthesiologist is responsbile for notifying the manufacturer, who in turn must notify the Food and Drug Administration.[30, 31] One quality assurance program designed to delineate clearly the types of occurrences to be looked for in anesthesia made a definite impact on the previous negative reactions of anesthesiologists.[25] The program was designed by the anesthesia department and the quality assurance directors. Specific incidents such as a recovery room time longer than 1 hour or malfunction of anesthesia equipment were identified as neces-sitating an incident report. Before the program was instituted 5,848 surgical cases resulted in 9 (0.1 percent) incident reports, as compared to 316 (4 percent) incident reports in the first 7,399 surgical cases under the new program. The program enhanced the quality of care in the hospital, strengthened the peer review process, and changed the clinical privileges of a few anesthesiologists.

PREANESTHESIA MACHINE CHECKOUT

Herr[8] summarily states that the majority of incidents involving anesthesia equipment failure are a result of failure of the anesthesiologist to check the equipment prior to use.

Cooper et al.[11] found 22 percent and Craig and Wilson[7] found 33 percent of "failures to inspect" to be an associated factor in anesthetic incidents. One of the standards for anesthesia services outlined by the JCAH Accreditation Manual is "prior to administering anesthesia, the anesthetist shall check the readiness . . . and working condition of all equipment used in the administration of anesthetic agents."[15] A number of investigators have supported the concept of an anesthesia machine checkout prior to the administration of anesthesia.[5, 7, 9, 11, 29, 32, 33] One question remaining to be answered for the anesthesia machine checkout is what is appropriate to check? There must be a balance between superficial observation of the machine and a three-page checkout list devised from the procedures recommended by certain anesthesia machine manufacturers. Perhaps a simple checkout list similar to the one in Figure 12-4 would be adequate. Some anesthesiologists keep a machine checkout list for each anesthetic along with the serial number of the anesthesia machine.

PRE-USE DAILY CHECK LIST

DATE _____

ANESTHESIA MACHINE SERIAL # _____

☐ CONTROLS OFF
☐ CYLINDER CONTENTS SUFFICIENT
☐ OXYGEN/N_2O RATIO ALARM
☐ PIPELINE SUPPLIES
☐ GAS FLOW CONTROLS
☐ VAPORIZERS FILLED
☐ MACHINE LEAK TEST
☐ OXYGEN ALARM TEST
☐ ABSORBER
☐ PATIENT CIRCUIT ASSEMBLY
☐ PATIENT CIRCUIT LEAK TEST
☐ PATIENT CIRCUIT FLOW
☐ VENTILATOR AND ALARM
☐ SCAVENGING SYSTEM

Fig. 12-4 A short daily anesthesia machine checklist to be completed prior to the first anesthetic. The anesthesia machine is identified by serial number, the date is noted, and the checklist either put in the patient's chart or filed in the department.

anesthesia machine. Others merely put an X in the anesthesia machine checkout box on the anesthesia record to document a completed preanesthesia checkout. Paulus et al.[33] found that some kind of written aid is necessary to make certain vital elements in the anesthesia machine checkout are remembered.

Anesthesiologists who fail to be enthusiastic about checking the anesthesia machine are exposed to high risk.[28] Anesthesia machines should be designed to facilitate easy checkout. The rushed anesthesiologist will skip the checkout if it is too time-consuming. Anesthesia machine checkouts on a nationwide basis cannot be achieved without major changes in the habits of many anesthesiologists. Arrival at the operating room 5 or 10 minutes prior to the start time of an anesthetic will never allow enough time for an adequate machine checkout. The user of the anesthesia machine has the same responsibility as the airline pilot (see Fig. 12-5) to check equipment prior to use. Neither competent anesthesia technicians nor biomedical technicians can accept the ultimate responsibility of checking the anesthesia machine prior to the administration of an anesthetic.[9, 34, 35] Anesthesiologists have to learn how to check an anesthesia machine as shown by a study conducted at an anesthesia meeting.[36] A total of 179 anesthesiologists were challenged to check out an anesthesia machine which had 5 intentionally created defects; the average number of faults discovered was 2.2, despite the knowledge that defects were present! Figure 12-6 indicates that the detection ability of the anesthesiologist was better in those who had 10 years or more of clinical experience.

Military anesthesiologists are now required to check all anesthesia equipment in detail before each administration of an anesthetic. The equipment check list, oxygen concentration, and flow rate must be included in each patient's medical record. The procedure was a directive of the secretary of defense after the recommendation of a task force report to the assistant secretary of defense for health affairs.[37]

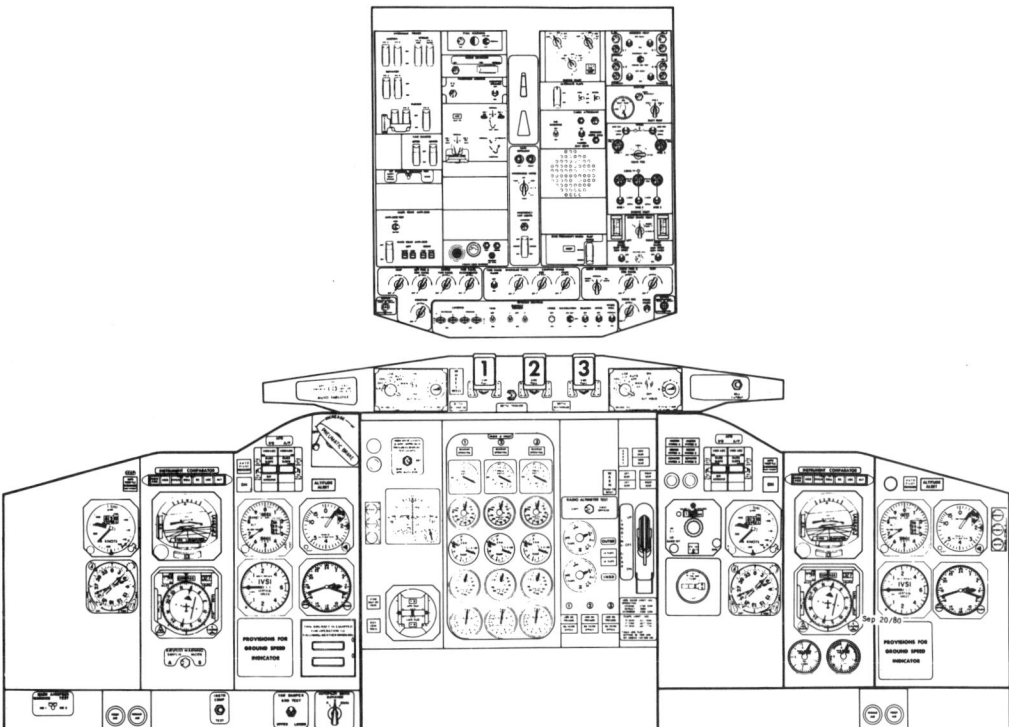

Fig. 12-5 The console of a small airplane. Checkout by the pilot must be done in detail prior to takeoff, during flight, prior to landing, and before leaving the aircraft. Anesthesiologists should develop similar habits when using the anesthesia machine.

STANDARDS FOR ANESTHESIA MACHINES

Extensive efforts have been made to develop a national standard for anesthesia machines. The American Society of Anesthesiologists was one of the founders of the American National Standards Institute (ANSI) Z79 committee formed to develop standards for anesthesia equipment. In 1983 the function of the ANSI Z79 committee was transferred to the F-29 Committee of the American Society for Testing and Materials because of possible liability to the ASA for standards-related activity.[16, 38, 39] Presently the ANSI has recommended standards for the anesthesia machine,[40] reservoir bags,[41] oxygen analyzers,[42] oro- and nasopharyngeal airways,[43] tracheal tube connectors and adapters,[44] breathing

tubes,[45] tracheal tubes,[46] and other related products used in anesthesia.[47] The voluntary standards have been written as a minimal requirement for the design and safety of anesthesia-related equipment. The standards cannot be enforced, and each booklet outlining a set of standards carries the following notation[40]:

> The existence of an American National Standard does not in any respect preclude anyone, whether he has approved the standard or not, from manufacturing, marketing, purchasing, or using products, processes, or procedures not conforming to the standard.

Each standard does represent a good general agreement among maker, seller, and user groups. Pressure is brought to bear on manufacturers of anesthesia equipment because in the development of the standards the ANSI

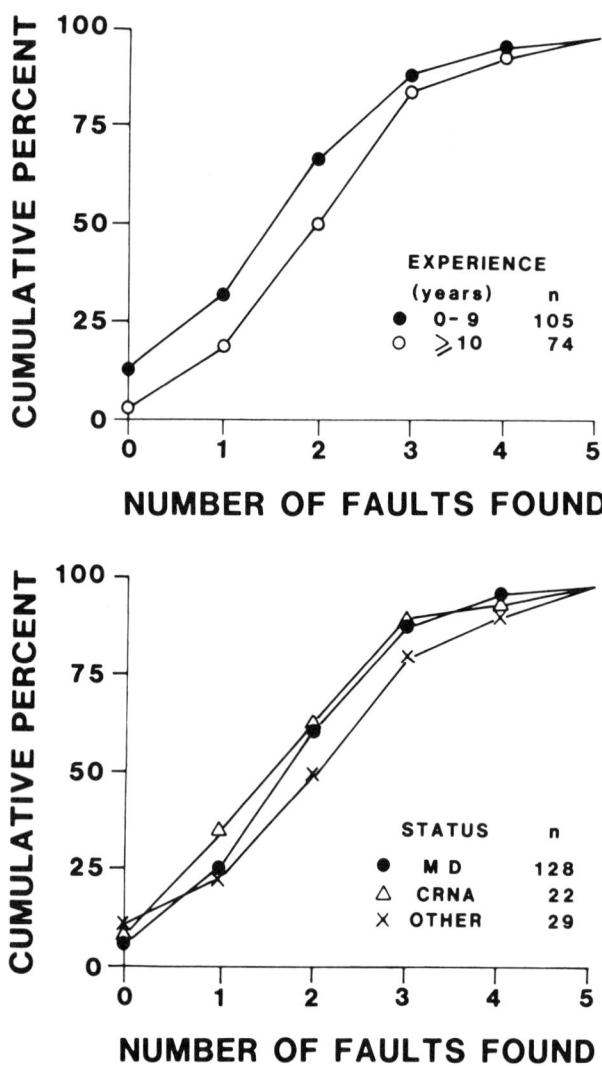

Fig. 12-6 Number of faults found in an anesthesia machine intentionally modified to create five faults. On the upper graph the number of faults detected is related to the years of experience of the 179 participants. The lower graph indicates that professional background did not influence the ability to find the faults. ("Other" includes dentists, anesthesia technicians, and persons involved in the design, manufacture, and service of anesthesia machines.) (Buffington CW, Ramanathan S, Turndorf H: Detection of anesthesia machine faults. Anesth Analg 63:79, 1984. Reprinted with permission, The International Anesthesia Research Society.)

attempted to reflect a national censensus of consumer, manufacturer, scientific, technical, and professional organizations, and government agencies.[40]

We are reminded to maintain simplicity in the practice of anesthesia.[48] Constant vigilance during anesthesia is the motto of the ASA. Complicated anesthesia machines tend to detract us from using our special senses as monitors. Additional patient care monitors remove us even further from the patient.[49] The Medical Device Amendments Act of 1976 provided a frame of reference for the development of two key concerns, safety and performance.[50] Anesthesiologists and manufacturers are encouraged to join in a unified approach to develop standards which could provide the highest standard of patient safety with the least degree of distraction for the anesthesiologist. Under the amendment the Food and Drug Administration has the authority to begin mandatory safety and performance standards for devices classified as class II. A device which does not comply to the standard cannot be sold 1 year after a standard has been developed, and devices sold prior to development of the standard do not have to be updated or removed from service.[39]

In 1978 Canada became the first country to have a published voluntary comprehensive standard for anesthesia machines.[51] One province, Manitoba, decided that a minimum standard was critical and by June 1980 had accommodated all anesthesia machines within the province to the standard.[52] Some anesthesia machines were updated and others discarded and replaced. As a result, every anesthesia machine achieved the goal of minimum design and safety features. The Canadian Bureau of Medical Devices and of Health and Welfare has plans to introduce nationwide mandatory standards for anesthesia machines.[53]

Hospitals in the United States should update anesthesia equipment to reduce risks to patients.[54] An argument has been made that a new standard alone is not reason enough to replace still-functional equipment.[55] A 1985 report resulting from the examination of the status of machines in one state stated the machines "appear to be obsolete and lacking in basic safety aspects."[56] Hospital risk managers and governing boards must be informed of the extremely high risk obsolete anesthesia machines carry for the hospital. Investments in new anesthesia machines are costly, bring no new revenue to the hospital when compared to a new magnetic resonance imager, and require long-term planning, since anesthesia machines are only adequate for 6 to 8 years. However, an investment in anesthesia machines can be cost effective and will mean improved safety for the anesthetized patient. The introduction of a new anesthesia machine must be made with caution during a carefully monitored period directly involving the anesthesia staff.[13]

Research and development in anesthesia machines is almost totally dependent on the manufacturers. Despite the risks related to the patient, the federal government has failed to recognize the need to support anesthesia machine research. Aviation, automobile, and boiler safety have all been improved by government support. Product liability problems have led some anesthesia manufacturers to withdraw from the market.[1, 39] Anesthesia machine sales are estimated to be about $40 million per year (0.4 percent of the annual amount spent for hospital equipment).[1] The relatively small market for anesthesia machines and the cost containment pressures inflicted by the prospective payment system will limit the funds manufacturers will be able to earmark for research and development.

Standards for anesthesia machines should be developed by those who manufacture anesthesia machines and those who use them. Greater emphasis must be given to anesthesia machines during the training of anesthesia personnel. Individuals must be taught how to check out an anesthesia machine, how to trace problems, what the limitations of the vital components of the anesthesia machine are, and when an anesthesia machine requires an update. Stress must be placed on preventive maintenance, cleanliness, and safety. Anesthesia residents could be markedly encouraged to learn about the anesthesia machine if questions pertaining to the subject were included in the written and oral examinations of the American Board of Anesthesiology. Cooperative seminars designed by the manufacturers and anesthesiologists which stress anesthesia machines through discussions and hands-on workshops would be another means to expose anesthesia personnel to technology-related training.

Perhaps voluntary standards should be made mandatory. A number of organizations have the power to develop, institute, and enforce the standards: (1) the ASA, (2) state societies of anesthesiology, (3) federal and state agencies, (4) the JCAH, and (5) malpractice insurance companies. An interesting restrictive endorsement clause in a malpractice insurance policy was recently suggested by the executive board of a medical liability insurance company.[57] The clause would invalidate the insurance policy unless the anesthesiologist had an oxygen analyzer in the breathing circuit and a low-pressure alarm on the anesthesia ventilator. The problem of how to stop the anesthesiologist with the Rube Goldberg anesthesia machine from moving it each day into more than one operating room, never doing a checkout, providing no maintenance until a malfunction occurs, and calling it the safest anesthesia machine (because "I know it from top to bottom") is a major threat to anesthesia malpractice liability and patient safety. Only cooperation on the part of the anesthesia community, regulatory agencies, manufacturers, and concerned citizens will improve anesthesia machine safety in the United States.

PREVENTIVE MAINTENANCE

Out of the industrial revolution came the concept of preventive maintenance: It is more efficient to inspect and service equipment periodically than to wait for a malfunction. Hospitals are usually held responsible for the maintenance of the anesthesia machines.[58] Anesthesia machines should be given preventive maintenance every 3 to 4 months by a qualified factory-trained serviceman.[9, 28, 29, 34, 36, 59] Each inspection should be documented on a form similar to the one in Figure 12-7 for each machine. Any modifications of the existing anesthesia machine should also be documented.[55] An individual file should be maintained for each anesthesia machine which can include final manufacturer inspection prior to use, all preventive maintenance checks, interim service calls, modifications, and any faults which are discovered during the use of the machine.[9, 28, 29] Only by maintaining individual anesthesia machine records can recurring problems be documented and risk management factors determined for each anesthesia machine.

Preventive maintenance checks should be done only by factory service representatives. Anesthesia or medicial electronic technicians hired by the hospital should not do periodic preventive maintenance checks. Outside servicemen are employed because of (1) access to parts, (2) off-hour services, (3) continuity of services with factory support, and (4) medicolegal liability.[9]

The preventive maintenance contract for the anesthesia machine should be considered an insurance policy. When an anesthesia machine malfunction causes damage to a patient, the anesthesiologist, hospital, and manufacturer are at risk.[14, 58] A higher number of medical malpractice cases are now including the manufacturer. Hospitals trying to save money by having in-house maintenance are allowing machine manufacturers to remove themselves from any product liability. A maintenance contract with the equipment manufacturer protects the hospital from charges of negligent maintenance.[58] The manufacturer can provide a diverse background of expertise when a lawsuit involves a possible malfunction of the anesthesia machine.

Today the Food and Drug Administration requires and approves the manufacturer's in-

Preventive Maintenance Check List

☐	1.0.	Sphygmanometer S/N _____	☐	13.0.	Alarm Circuit Delay Test
☐	2.0.	Vapor Exclusion System	☐	14.0.	Ventilation Monitor S/N _____
☐	3.0.	High Pressure Test	☐	14.10.	5.0 or 7.5 cm H_2O
☐	4.0.	Oxygen Supply Failure Protection	☐	14.13.	12.5 cm H_2O
☐	5.0.	NAD O_2 Monitor S/N _____	☐	14.15.	25 cm H_2O
☐	6.0.	Oxygen Concentration Test	☐	15.0.	Continuing Pressure Alarm
☐	7.0.	Flowmeter Test	☐	16.0.	High Pressure Alarm
☐	8.0.	Breathing System Leak Test	☐	17.0.	Sub-Atmospheric Pressure Alarm
☐	9.0.	Vapor Selector Valve	☐	18.0.	O_2 Ratio Monitor S/N _____
☐	10.0	APL Valve Test (Abs. S/N: _____)	☐	19.0.	O_2 Ratio Monitor Control S/N _____
☐	11.0.	Ventilator Test S/N _____	☐	20.0.	Scavenger Interface S/N _____
☐	11.1.	Pressure Test	☐	21.0.	Accessory Attachment
☐	11.2.	Inspiratory-Expiratory Ratio	☐	22.0.	Visual Inspection
☐	11.3.	Frequency	☐	23.0.	Oxygen Flush (100% Oxygen)
☐	11.4.	Frequency Divider	☐		_____
☐	12.0.	Flow Direction Test	☐		_____

Fig. 12-7 Preventive maintenance check list. A similar check list should be completed by the factory-authorized serviceman for each anesthesia machine during each quarterly inspection. (Courtesy of North American Drager, Telford, PA.)

structions and warnings for anesthesia machines. The anesthesiologist can be held responsible for the material in the operating manual, maintenance guide, and any warnings given by the manufacturer.[58]

Preventive maintenance of anesthesia machines used to be limited to simple mechanical devices, but in recent years a number of safety devices have incorporated electronic components. Traditional cleaning and inspection of moving parts is excellent for mechanical devices but may not be adequate for electronic devices.[60] Electronic devices may show subtle signs of impending failure, for example, a dimming diode light, which can only be detected by the user. It must be realized that preventive maintenance has certain limitations in finding faults.

Preventive maintenance can help prevent faults in the anesthesia machine related to the normal wear and deterioration of parts. In addition, anesthesia personnel must become aware of the function and limitations of the machine and how to detect a malfunction.

REFERENCES

1. Anesthesia Machine Failures. Hearing Subcommittee on Oversight and Investigations. Committee on Energy and Commerce. House of Rep. 98th Congress. Serial #98-188. U.S. Government Printing Office, Washington, DC, 1985
2. Heath ML: Accidents associated with equipment. Anaesthesia 39:57, 1984
3. Utting JE, Gray TC, Shelley FC: Human misadventures in anaesthesia. Can Anaesth Soc J 26:472, 1979
4. Mayer A: Malfunctions of anesthesia machines: a guide for maintenance. Anesth Analg 52:376, 1973
5. Cooper JB, Couvillon LA: Accidental breathing system disconnections. Interim report to Food and Drug Administration, Contract #223-82-5070, Boston, 1984
6. Cooper JB, Parker LA, Sears BE: Prevention of ventilator hazards. Anesthesiology 48:299, 1978
7. Craig J, Wilson ME: A survey of anaesthetic misadventures. Anaesthesia 36:933, 1981
8. Herr GP: Anesthesia mishaps: occurrence and prevention. Semin Anesth 2:213, 1983
9. Duberman S, Wald A: An integrated quality control program for anesthesia equipment. Qual Rev Bull 9:328, 1983
10. Cooper JB, Long CD, Newbower RS et al: Critical incidents associated with intraoperative exchanges of anesthesia personnel. Anesthesiology 56:456, 1982
11. Cooper JB, Newbower RS, Kitz RJ: An analysis of major errors and equipment failures in anesthesia management: considerations for pre-

vention and detection. Anesthesiology 60:34, 1984

12. Cooper JB, Newbower RS, Long CD et al: Preventable anesthesia mishaps: a study of human factors. Anesthesiology 49:399, 1978

13. Newbower RS, Cooper JB, Long CD: Learning from anesthesia mishaps. Qual Rev Bull 7:10, 1981

14. Petty C: Risk management in anesthesia. Curr Rev Clin Anesth 4:15, 1984

15. Joint Commission on Accreditation of Hospitals: Accreditation manual for hospitals. Joint Commission on Accreditation of Hospitals, Chicago, 1985

16. Capps RT: 1983 annual report of the president. ASA Newslett 47:1,4, 1983

17. Pierce EC: President's address. ASA Newslett 47:1, 1983

18. Parker S: Risk management: many solutions proposed and successes noted. Hospitals 52:157, 1978

19. Zauder HL: Medical liability crisis prompts action by patient safety committee. ASA Newslett 48:5, 1984

20. The Minimum Standard, American College of Surgeons, Chicago, 1917

21. Roberts JS, Walczak RM: Toward effective quality assurance: the evolution and current status of the JCAH QA standard. Qual Rev Bull 10:11, 1984

22. Joint Commission on Accreditation of Hospitals: Accreditation manual for hospitals. Joint Commission on Accreditation of Hospitals, Chicago, 1979

23. Adams AK: Quality assurance in anaesthesia. Anaesthesia 38:311, 1983

24. Gibbs RF: Ten commandments of anesthesia risk management. Leg Pers Anesth, Jan/Feb 1983

25. Beck B, Hardwick K: A concurrent surgical miniaudit procedure. Qual Rev Bull 7:60, 1981

26. Blake P: Incident investigation: a complete guide. Nurs Manage 15:36, 1984

27. Freilich H: Rapid incident identification, systematic follow-up key to preventive risk managing. Hospitals, p.53, August 1982

28. Cundy J, Baldock GJ: Safety check procedures to eliminate faults in anaesthetic machines. Anaesthesia 37:161, 1982

29. Paull JD: Anaesthetic machine hazards. Aust Family Phy 6:915, 1977

30. FDA issues medical device reporting requirement. Am Med News, 5 October 1984

31. Stringent reporting rules imposed on manufactures. Mod Healthcare, October 1984

32. Ditzler JW: Checking anesthesia machines. Anesthesiology 32:87, 1970

33. Paulus DA, Basta JW, Klie H et al: Preanesthetic checklist. Anesth Analg 64:264, 1985

34. Danner D: Attorney identifies potential legal hazards in routine anesthesia practice. Leg Pers Anesth, Sept/Oct 1983

35. Gibbs RF: Anesthesiology: a targeted specialty. Leg Pers Anesth, Jul/Aug 1983

36. Buffington CW, Ramanathan S, Turndorf H: Detection of anesthesia machine faults. Anesth Analg 63:79, 1984

37. Smith P: DOD requires closer checks by anesthetists. Army Times, 24 June 1985

38. American Society of Mechanical Engineers v. Hydrolevel Corp., 102s. Ct. 1935, U.S. Sup. Ct., 1982

39. Deaths during general anesthesia: technology-related, due to human error, or unavoidable? Emerg Care Res Inst, 5, 1985

40. American National Standard: Minimum Performance and Safety Requirements for Components and Systems of Continuous-Flow Anesthesia Machines for Human Use. Z79.8-1979. American National Standards Institute, New York, 1979

41. American National Standard for Anesthestic Equipment—Reservoir Bags. Z79.4-1983. American National Standards Institute, New York, 1983

42. American National Standard Requirements for Oxygen Analyzers for Monitoring Patient Breathing-Mixtures. Z79.10-1979. American National Standards Institute, New York, 1979

43. American National Standard for Anesthetic Equipment—Oropharyngeal and Nasopharyngeal Airways. Z79.3-1983. American National Standards Institute, New York, 1983

44. American National Standard for Tracheal Tube Connectors and Adapters. Z79.2-1976. American National Standards Institute, New York, 1976

45. American National Standard for Breathing Tubes. Z79.6-1975. American National Standards Institute, New York, 1975

46. American National Standard for Anesthetic

Equipment—Tracheal Tubes. Z79.14-1983. American National Standards Institute, New York, 1983

47. American National Standard for Breathing Machines for Medical Use. Z79.7-1976. American National Standards Institute, New York, 1976

48. Vandam LD: Simplicity and common sense in anesthesia. Med Instrum 14:157, 1980

49. Larcom GD: Who monitors the monitors? Surv Anesth 26:135, 1982

50. Miller MJ: Standards: a perspective. Med Instrum 14:157, 1980

51. Continuous flow inhalation anesthetic apparatus (anesthetic machines) for medical use. CSA Preliminary Standard 2168.3-M1978. Canadian Standards Association, Rexdale, Ontario, 1983

52. Craig DB, Longmuir J: Implementation of Canadian Standards Association Z168.3-M 1980 anaesthetic gas machine standard: the Manitoba experience. Can Anaesth Soc J 27:504, 1980

53. Craig DB: Personal communication, letter, 28 October 1983

54. Rendell-Baker L: Update anesthesia equipment to reduce risks. Hospitals, 16 November 1980

55. Is a new medical device standard valid reason to replace equipment? Emerg Care Res Inst, 3, September 1983

56. Hatchfield JH: Anesthesia mishaps. Letter (1985) to Keith Costell, in Office, State Senator Daniel J. Dalton, Box 100, RD #2, Turnersville, NJ 008012

57. Gibbs RF: Clamping down on the high cost of malpractice insurance. Leg Pers Anesth, Sept/Oct 1984

58. Peters JD, Fineberg KS, Kroll DA et al: Products Liability. Anesthesia and the Law. Health Administration Press, Ann Arbor, 1983

59. Risk management in anesthesia. Help News, September 1982

60. Wald A: Is preventive maintenance a Shibboleth? J Clin Eng 5:100, 1980

Index

Page numbers followed by *f* indicate figures; those followed by *t* indicate tables.